Imaging of the Athlete

Editors

ADAM C. ZOGA
JOHANNES B. ROEDL

RADIOLOGIC CLINICS OF NORTH AMERICA

www.radiologic.theclinics.com

Consulting Editor
FRANK H. MILLER

September 2016 • Volume 54 • Number 5

ELSEVIER

1600 John F. Kennedy Boulevard • Suite 1800 • Philadelphia, Pennsylvania, 19103-2899

http://www.theclinics.com

RADIOLOGIC CLINICS OF NORTH AMERICA Volume 54, Number 5
September 2016 ISSN 0033-8389, ISBN 13: 978-0-323-46266-2

Editor: John Vassallo (j.vassallo@elsevier.com)
Developmental Editor: Donald Mumford

Radiologic Clinics of North America (ISSN 0033-8389) is published bimonthly by Elsevier Inc., 360 Park Avenue South, New York, NY 10010-1710. Months of issue are January, March, May, July, September, and November. Periodicals postage paid at New York, NY and additional mailing offices. Subscription prices are USD 460 per year for US individuals, USD 784 per year for US institutions, USD 100 per year for US students and residents, USD 535 per year for Canadian individuals, USD 1002 per year for Canadian institutions, USD 660 per year for international individuals, USD 1002 per year for international institutions, and USD 315 per year for Canadian and international students/residents. To receive student and resident rate, orders must be accompanied by name of affiliated institution, date of term and the signature of program/residency coordinator on institution letterhead. Orders will be billed at individual rate until proof of status is received. Foreign air speed delivery is included in all *Clinics* subscription prices. All prices are subject to change without notice. **POSTMASTER:** Send address changes to *Radiologic Clinics of North America*, Elsevier Health Sciences Division, Subscription Customer Service, 3251 Riverport Lane, Maryland Heights, MO63043. **Customer Service: Telephone: 1-800-654-2452** (U.S. and Canada); **1-314-447-8871** (outside U.S. and Canada). **Fax: 1-314-447-8029. E-mail: journalscustomerservice-usa@ elsevier.com (for print support); journalsonlinesupport-usa@elsevier.com (for online support)**.

Reprints. For copies of 100 or more of articles in this publication, please contact the Commercial Reprints Department, Elsevier Inc., 360 Park Avenue South, New York, New York 10010-1710. Tel.: +1-212-633-3874; Fax: +1-212-633-3820; E-mail: reprints@elsevier.com.

Radiologic Clinics of North America also published in Greek Paschalidis Medical Publications, Athens, Greece.

Radiologic Clinics of North America is covered in *MEDLINE/PubMed (Index Medicus), EMBASE/Excerpta Medica, Current Contents/Life Sciences, Current Contents/Clinical Medicine, RSNA Index to Imaging Literature, BIOSIS, Science Citation Index,* and *ISI/BIOMED*.

Printed in the United States of America.

Contributors

CONSULTING EDITOR

FRANK H. MILLER, MD
Chief, Body Imaging Section and Fellowship Program; Medical Director of MRI; Professor, Department of Radiology, Northwestern University Feinberg School of Medicine, Chicago, Illinois

EDITORS

ADAM C. ZOGA, MD
Vice Chair for Clinical Practice; Director, Division of Musculoskeletal Imaging and Interventions, Associate Professor, Department of Radiology, Jefferson Medical College, Thomas Jefferson University Hospital, Thomas Jefferson University, Philadelphia, Pennsylvania

JOHANNES B. ROEDL, MD, PhD
Division of Musculoskeletal Imaging and Interventions, Assistant Professor, Department of Radiology, Jefferson Medical College, Thomas Jefferson University Hospital, Thomas Jefferson University, Philadelphia, Pennsylvania

AUTHORS

JEFFREY A. BELAIR, MD
Department of Radiology, Thomas Jefferson University Hospital, Philadelphia, Pennsylvania

KIERY A. BRAITHWAITE, MD
Assistant Professor of Radiology, Department of Radiology and Imaging Sciences, Emory University; Attending Physician, Department of Pediatric Radiology, Children's Healthcare of Atlanta at Egleston, Atlanta, Georgia

BETHANY U. CASAGRANDA, DO
Director, Division of Musculoskeletal Radiology, Department of Radiology; Program Director, Radiology Residency; Adjunct Associate Professor, Temple University; Allegheny General Hospital, Pittsburgh, Pennsylvania

I-YUAN JOSEPH CHANG, MD
Musculoskeletal Fellow, Imaging Institute, Cleveland Clinic, Cleveland, Ohio

ANNU CHOPRA, MRCS, FRCR
X-Ray Department, Musculoskeletal Centre, Leeds Teaching Hospitals, Chapel Allerton Hospital, Leeds, United Kingdom

JANA M. CRAIN, MD
Medical Director, National Orthopedic Imaging Associates, California Advanced Imaging at Atherton, Atherton, California

MOHAMMAD GHORBANHOSEINI, MD
Division of Foot and Ankle Surgery, Department of Orthopedic Surgery, Beth Israel Deaconess Medical Center, Harvard Medical School, Boston, Massachusetts

CRISTY N. GUSTAS, MD
Assistant Professor, Musculoskeletal Imaging, Department of Radiology, Penn State Milton S. Hershey Medical Center, Hershey, Pennsylvania

TAREK M. HEGAZI, MD, MBBS, FRCPC
Clinical Musculoskeletal Radiology Fellow,
Division of Musculoskeletal Imaging and
Interventions, Department of Radiology,
Jefferson Medical College, Thomas Jefferson
University Hospital, Thomas Jefferson
University, Philadelphia, Pennsylvania;
Department of Radiology, University of
Dammam, Dammam, Saudi Arabia

JOHN Y. KWON, MD
Assistant Professor; Chief of Division of Foot
and Ankle Surgery, Department of Orthopedic
Surgery, Beth Israel Deaconess Medical
Center, Harvard Medical School, Boston,
Massachusetts

KENNETH S. LEE, MD
Associate Professor, Musculoskeletal Imaging,
Department of Radiology, University of
Wisconsin School of Medicine and Public
Health, University of Wisconsin Hospital and
Clinics, Madison, Wisconsin

YU-CHING LIN, MD
Department of Medical Imaging and
Intervention, Chang Gung Memorial Hospital,
Keelung and Chang Gung University, Taoyuan,
Taiwan, China

KELLEY W. MARSHALL, MD
Assistant Professor of Radiology, Department
of Radiology and Imaging Sciences, Emory
University; Attending Physician, Department of
Pediatric Radiology, Children's Healthcare of
Atlanta at Egleston, Atlanta, Georgia

EOGHAN McCARTHY, MD
Division of Musculoskeletal Imaging and
Interventions, Department of Radiology,
Jefferson Medical College, Thomas Jefferson
University Hospital, Philadelphia, Pennsylvania

WILLIAM C. MEYERS, MD
General Surgery, Vincera Institute,
Philadelphia, Pennsylvania

WILLIAM B. MORRISON, MD
Professor, Division of Musculoskeletal Imaging
and Interventions, Department of Radiology,
Jefferson Medical College, Thomas Jefferson
University Hospital, Philadelphia,
Pennsylvania

MIKA T. NEVALAINEN, MD
Division of Musculoskeletal Imaging and
Interventions, Department of Radiology,
Jefferson Medical College, Thomas Jefferson
University Hospital, Philadelphia,
Pennsylvania

IMRAN M. OMAR, MD
Department of Radiology, Northwestern
Memorial Hospital, Chicago,
Illinois

JEAN-PIERRE PHANCAO, MD, MBA
Medical Director, National Orthopedic Imaging
Associates, California Pacific Advanced
Imaging, San Francisco,
California

JOSHUA M. POLSTER, MD
Associate Professor, Cleveland Clinic Lerner
College of Medicine; Staff Radiologist,
Musculoskeletal Section, Imaging Institute,
Cleveland Clinic, Cleveland, Ohio

ALEX E. POOR, MD
General Surgery, Vincera Institute,
Philadelphia, Pennsylvania

PAUL J. READ, MD
Clinical Assistant Professor, Division of
Musculoskeletal Radiology and Interventions,
Department of Radiology, Thomas Jefferson
University Hospital, Philadelphia,
Pennsylvania

PHILIP ROBINSON, MRCP, FRCR
X-Ray Department, Musculoskeletal Centre;
Leeds Musculoskeletal Biomedical Research
Unit, Leeds Teaching Hospitals, Chapel
Allerton Hospital, Leeds,
United Kingdom

JOHANNES B. ROEDL, MD, PhD
Division of Musculoskeletal Imaging and
Interventions, Assistant Professor, Department
of Radiology, Jefferson Medical College,
Thomas Jefferson University Hospital, Thomas
Jefferson University, Philadelphia,
Pennsylvania

PETER C. THURLOW, MD
Division of Musculoskeletal Radiology,
Department of Radiology, Allegheny
General Hospital, Pittsburgh,
Pennsylvania

DANIEL M. WALZ, MD
Chief, Division of Musculoskeletal Imaging,
Assistant Professor, Department of Radiology,
Hofstra Northwell School of Medicine,
Northwell Health, Great Neck,
New York

JIM S. WU, MD
Assistant Professor, Department of Radiology,
Beth Israel Deaconess Medical Center, Harvard
Medical School, Boston, Massachusetts

ADAM C. ZOGA, MD
Vice Chair for Clinical Practice; Director, Division
of Musculoskeletal Imaging and Interventions,
Associate Professor, Department of Radiology,
Jefferson Medical College, Thomas Jefferson
University Hospital, Thomas Jefferson
University, Philadelphia, Pennsylvania

Contents

Section I: The Throwing Athlete

Repetitive, high-velocity overhead throwing can lead to several adaptive changes in the throwing shoulder, which over time lead to structural microtrauma and eventually overt injury. MR imaging is a useful imaging modality to evaluate these changes and to characterize their acuity and severity. Understanding the throwing motion and the effects of this motion on the structures of the shoulder can help radiologists to recognize these findings and provide useful information to referring physicians, which may affect the treatment of these athletes. This article reviews shoulder pathomechanics and MR imaging findings in overhead throwing athletes.

Elbow pain in overhead sport athletes is not uncommon. Repetitive throwing can lead to chronic overuse and/or acute injury to tendons, ligaments, bones, or nerves about the elbow. A thorough history and physical examination of the thrower's elbow frequently establishes the diagnosis for pain. Imaging can provide additional information when the clinical picture is unclear or further information is necessary for risk stratification and treatment planning. This article focuses on current imaging concepts and image-guided treatments for injuries commonly affecting the adult throwing athlete's elbow.

Injuries to the shoulder and elbow in the pediatric and adolescent throwing athlete are common. Both knowledge of throwing mechanics and understanding of normal bone development in the immature skeleton are key to the diagnosis, treatment, and potential prevention of these common injuries. Pathologic changes from chronic repetitive trauma to the developing shoulder and elbow manifest as distinctly different injuries that can be predicted by the skeletal maturation of the patient. Sites of vulnerability and resulting patterns of injury change as the child evolves from the skeletally immature little league player to the skeletally mature high school/college athlete.

This review article describes injuries that occur in the upper extremities of athletes less commonly than those typically discussed with shoulders and elbows. A survey of osseous, musculotendinous, ligamentous, and neurovascular injuries is presented along with associated imaging findings and standard treatment options.

This article does not focus on the classic throwing injuries of the shoulder or elbow; the goal is to survey injuries in throwing sports that involve structures away from the glenohumeral, acromioclavicular, or elbow joints. The goal of this article is to introduce readers to these less common injuries, describe their clinical presentations, and characterize their typical imaging appearances.

Section II: The Musculoskeletal Core

radiography, MR imaging, MR arthrography, and even computed tomography to confirm diagnoses and support the need for potential intervention. Musculoskeletal radiologists should help referrers navigate available imaging options and protocols, while using both clinical information and imaging findings to arrive at a diagnosis that adds value to the treatment plan.

Section III: New Ideas for Imaging Sports Injuries in the Lower Extremity

PROGRAM OBJECTIVE
The objective of the *Radiologic Clinics of North America* is to keep practicing radiologists and radiology residents up to date with current clinical practice in radiology by providing timely articles reviewing the state of the art in patient care.

TARGET AUDIENCE
Practicing radiologists, radiology residents, and other health care professionals who provide patient care utilizing radiologic findings.

LEARNING OBJECTIVES
Upon completion of this activity, participants will be able to:
1. Review the role of imaging in diagnosing throwing injuries of the upper extremity.
2. Discuss the use of imaging in groin pain, pubic symphysis injuries, knee injuries, and other athletic injuries of the lower extremity.
3. Recognize the role of imaging in determining return to play following athletic injury.

ACCREDITATION
The Elsevier Office of Continuing Medical Education (EOCME) is accredited by the Accreditation Council for Continuing Medical Education (ACCME) to provide continuing medical education for physicians.

The EOCME designates this enduring material for a maximum of 15 *AMA PRA Category 1 Credit*(s)™. Physicians should claim only the credit commensurate with the extent of their participation in the activity.

All other health care professionals requesting continuing education credit for this enduring material will be issued a certificate of participation.

DISCLOSURE OF CONFLICTS OF INTEREST
The EOCME assesses conflict of interest with its instructors, faculty, planners, and other individuals who are in a position to control the content of CME activities. All relevant conflicts of interest that are identified are thoroughly vetted by EOCME for fair balance, scientific objectivity, and patient care recommendations. EOCME is committed to providing its learners with CME activities that promote improvements or quality in healthcare and not a specific proprietary business or a commercial interest.

The planning committee, staff, authors and editors listed below have identified no financial relationships or relationships to products or devices they or their spouse/life partner have with commercial interest related to the content of this CME activity:
Jeffrey A. Belair, MD; Kiery A. Braithwaite, MD; Bethany U. Casagranda, DO; I-Yuan Joseph Chang, MD; Annu Chopra, MRCS, FRCR; Jana M. Crain, MD; Anjali Fortna; Mohammad Ghorbanhoseini, MD; Cristy N. Gustas, MD; Tarek M. Hegazi, MD, MBBS, FRCPC; John Y. Kwon, MD; Yu-Ching Lin, MD; Kelley W. Marshall, MD; Eoghan McCarthy, MD; William C. Meyers, MD; William B. Morrison, MD; Mika T. Nevalainen, MD; Imran M. Omar, MD; Jean-Pierre Phancao, MD, MBA; Joshua M. Polster, MD; Alex E. Poor, MD; Paul J. Read, MD; Philip Robinson, MRCP, FRCR; Johannes B. Roedl, MD, PhD; Erin Scheckenbach; Karthik Subramaniam; Peter C. Thurlow, MD; John Vassallo; Daniel M. Walz, MD; Jim S. Wu, MD; Adam C. Zoga, MD.

The planning committee, staff, authors and editors listed below have identified financial relationships or relationships to products or devices they or their spouse/life partner have with commercial interest related to the content of this CME activity:
Kenneth S. Lee, MD has research support from Radiologic Society of North America; General Electric; National Basketball Association; and SuperSonic, receives royalties/patents from Elsevier, and is a consultant/advisor for Echometrix.

UNAPPROVED/OFF-LABEL USE DISCLOSURE
The EOCME requires CME faculty to disclose to the participants:
1. When products or procedures being discussed are off-label, unlabelled, experimental, and/or investigational (not US Food and Drug Administration [FDA] approved); and
2. Any limitations on the information presented, such as data that are preliminary or that represent ongoing research, interim analyses, and/or unsupported opinions. Faculty may discuss information about pharmaceutical agents that is outside of FDA-approved labelling. This information is intended solely for CME and is not intended to promote off-label use of these medications. If you have any questions, contact the medical affairs department of the manufacturer for the most recent prescribing information.

TO ENROLL
To enroll in the *Radiologic Clinics of North America* Continuing Medical Education program, call customer service at 1-800-654-2452 or sign up online at http://www.theclinics.com/home/cme. The CME program is available to subscribers for an additional annual fee of USD 315.

METHOD OF PARTICIPATION

In order to claim credit, participants must complete the following:

1. Complete enrolment as indicated above.
2. Read the activity.
3. Complete the CME Test and Evaluation. Participants must achieve a score of 70% on the test. All CME Tests and Evaluations must be completed online.

CME INQUIRIES/SPECIAL NEEDS

For all CME inquiries or special needs, please contact elsevierCME@elsevier.com.

RADIOLOGIC CLINICS OF NORTH AMERICA

ISSUE OF RELATED INTEREST

Magnetic Resonance Imaging Clinics, May 2016 (Vol. 24, Issue 2)
MR in the Emergency Room
Jorge A. Soto, *Editor*
Available at: http://www.mri.theclinics.com

THE CLINICS ARE AVAILABLE ONLINE!
Access your subscription at:
www.theclinics.com

Preface

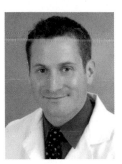 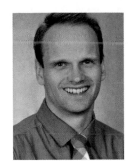

Adam C. Zoga, MD   Johannes B. Roedl, MD, PhD

Editors

Like it or not, the role of sports in our society seems to continuously increase. Professional and high-level amateur athletics reflect capitalism, with ever-increasing salaries, revenues, and media interest, and injuries are a variable central to all of these. There are daily media reports of professional athletes awaiting imaging results, which might determine the outcome of both the player's and the team's season or even a player's career. Recreational athletes or "weekend warriors" seem to find a new creative way to simultaneously express their competitiveness and achieve some level of physical fitness every few months. These folks have to get back to their lives and responsibilities after games, meets, or workouts, and there is often no place for nagging pains or physical limitations. For these two cultures, prompt diagnosis and treatment planning are crucial, and imaging plays a huge part in both. We designed this issue of *Radiologic Clinics of North America* with the hope that it will help radiologists generate imaging algorithms and provide and interpret value-based imaging for health care professionals treating athletes, parents of athletes, and the athletes themselves.

The musculoskeletal radiologist has become an important part of the medical team for many athletic franchises, playing a key role in not only the care of acute injuries but also the evaluation of chronic and remote lesions in free agents, trade prospects, and potential new signings. Not surprisingly, athletes are generally not very forthcoming about symptoms when they are in line to sign a lucrative, new contract. The evolution of joint-specific MRI protocols and the now widely established field of musculoskeletal ultrasound with its dynamic capabilities have resulted in the niche subspecialty of "sports imaging." And not surprisingly, given the prevalence of imaging among high-level players, recreational athletes expect or request medical care on par with the pros they watch on multimedia.

We have assembled a group of gifted academic and clinical sports imagers as authors for this issue of *Radiologic Clinics of North America*. Four articles are dedicated to the throwing athlete: both skeletally mature and immature, both intra-articular and extra-articular lesions, and both static and dynamic imaging techniques. The next four articles center on the musculoskeletal core, including diagnostic as well as potentially therapeutic imaging tools. This section includes forward-thinking imaging algorithms for musculoskeletal lesions spanning the pubic symphysis to the hips and iliac crests. The final four articles each tackle an old problem for sports imagers but with state-of-the-art imaging and fresh biophysical concepts. The final submission is a guidebook on how to best answer the question perhaps

Radiol Clin N Am 54 (2016) xiii–xiv
http://dx.doi.org/10.1016/j.rcl.2016.07.001
0033-8389/16/© 2016 Published by Elsevier Inc.

most frequently asked to sports imagers, "When can I/he/she return to play?" We sincerely hope you find the issue as valuable as we found it fun during production.

Adam C. Zoga, MD
Musculoskeletal MRI
Thomas Jefferson University
132 South 10th Street, Suite 1096
Philadelphia, PA 19107, USA

Johannes B. Roedl, MD, PhD
Musculoskeletal Division
Thomas Jefferson University
132 South 10th Street
10 Main Radiology
Philadelphia, PA 19107, USA

E-mail addresses:
adam.zoga@jefferson.edu (A.C. Zoga)
Johannes.roedl@jefferson.edu (J.B. Roedl)

Section I - The Throwing Athlete

Pathomechanics and Magnetic Resonance Imaging of the Thrower's Shoulder

I-Yuan Joseph Chang, MD[a], Joshua M. Polster, MD[b,c],*

KEYWORDS

- MR imaging • Throwing • Baseball • Shoulder • Rotator cuff • SLAP tear • Internal impingement
- GIRD

KEY POINTS

- Overhead throwing generates supraphysiologic forces that lead to bone and soft tissue adaptations, chronic microtrauma, and eventually overt injury.
- Understanding the throwing motion can help radiologists understand the patterns of shoulder injury in overhead throwing athletes.
- MR imaging is useful for characterizing soft tissue and osseous changes that occur in overhead throwing athletes and can provide useful information for treatment.

INTRODUCTION

Overhead throwing by a baseball pitcher is perhaps the fastest human athletic movement. In this movement, humeral internal rotation has been documented to reach an angular velocity in excess of 7500°/s in professional athletes.[1] Such extreme velocity is achieved by the human body functioning as a kinetic chain, whereby the large muscles of the legs and trunk generate great force and transfer that energy through the shoulder and upper extremity to the ball at release.[2] Because of the complex anatomy, extremes of shoulder motion, and great force, a wide variety of injuries to the osseous and soft tissue structures of the shoulder and elbow may occur. This article focuses on the pathomechanics and MR imaging findings of overuse shoulder injuries encountered in throwing athletes.

NORMAL ANATOMY

The glenohumeral joint is a ball-and-socket joint with the greatest range of motion of all joints in the human body.[3] This range is achieved by the spherical humeral head being fitted into a cuplike depression of the bony glenoid, akin to a golf ball steadied atop a tee. To overcome the lack of osseous stability that comes with such freedom of motion, the shoulder has an elaborate system of static and dynamic soft tissue stabilizers.[4]

The static soft tissue stabilizers of the shoulder include the glenoid labrum, the glenohumeral ligaments, and the joint capsule (**Fig. 1**).[4] The glenoid labrum is a fibrocartilaginous structure that deepens the glenoid rim and provides a functional seal around the humeral articular surface, generating a weak vacuum effect that helps to keep the humeral head in place.[3] The anterior, middle, and

Conflict of Interest: The authors declare no competing financial interests.
[a] Imaging Institute, Cleveland Clinic, 9500 Euclid Avenue, A21, Cleveland, OH 44195, USA; [b] Cleveland Clinic Lerner College of Medicine, 9500 Euclid Avenue, A21, Cleveland, OH 44195, USA; [c] Musculoskeletal Section, Imaging Institute, Cleveland Clinic, 9500 Euclid Avenue, A21, Cleveland, OH 44195, USA
* Corresponding author.
E-mail address: Polstej@ccf.org

Radiol Clin N Am 54 (2016) 801–815
http://dx.doi.org/10.1016/j.rcl.2016.04.004

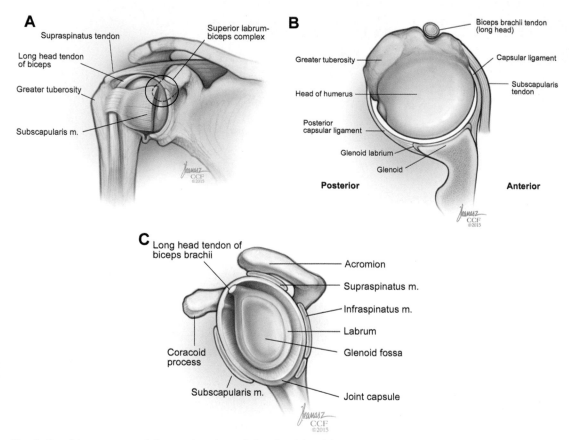

Fig. 1. Shoulder anatomy. (*A*) Anterior view of the shoulder. (*B*) Superior view. (*C*) Lateral view with humerus removed. Copyright © The Cleveland Clinic Foundation 2015.

inferior glenohumeral ligaments are focal thickenings of the joint capsule that help to resist excess motion and prevent shoulder dislocation.[4]

The dynamic stabilizers of the glenohumeral joint include the rotator cuff and the long head of the biceps tendon. The rotator cuff muscles and tendons encase the anterior, superior, and posterior aspects of the joint capsule, contracting and relaxing to resist humeral head decentering on the glenoid during shoulder motion.[4] The rotator cuff consists of 4 muscle-tendon units: the supraspinatus, infraspinatus, teres minor, and subscapularis.[3] The rotator cuff is the primary dynamic stabilizer of the glenohumeral joint.[4]

The long head of the biceps tendon and muscle reinforces the anterior-superior aspect of the glenohumeral joint.[4] It originates from the supraglenoid tubercle and passes anterolaterally over the humeral head, through the rotator interval between the supraspinatus and subscapularis tendons, and into the intertubercular groove inside a tendon sheath that is contiguous with the joint capsule.[3] The coracohumeral and superior glenohumeral ligaments, which abut the superficial side and undersurface of

the long head of the biceps tendon in the rotator interval, form the biceps sling that stabilizes the biceps tendon and anterosuperior glenohumeral joint.[4]

MR IMAGING TECHNIQUE

MR imaging of the shoulder is optimally performed on either a 1.5-T or 3-T scanner (**Table 1**). Fat-suppressed fluid-sensitive sequences are useful for detecting subtle areas of injury-related edema in soft tissue structures and bone marrow. However, fat suppression results in a lower signal/noise ratio compared with non–fat-suppressed sequences. The use of intermediate-weighted sequences improves the signal/noise ratio compared with longer echo time (TE) T2-weighted sequences; however, these sequences are more prone to magic angle artifact than longer TE sequences. The authors typically rely primarily on intermediate-weighted sequences to evaluate the glenoid labrum and glenohumeral articular cartilage and confirm cuff disorders on longer TE T2-weighted sequences. The use of T1-weighted sequences or non–fat-suppressed proton-density or T2-weighted images

Table 1
MR imaging protocols at our institution

Equipment	1.5-T or 3-T scanner Dedicated multichannel shoulder coil or a body phased array coil wrapped around the shoulder
Position	Patient supine and the arm in neutral position to slight external rotation (arm by the side, palm supinated)
Spatial parameters	Field of view: 12–14 cm Section thickness: 2.5–3 mm, with an intersecting gap of 0.4–0.5 mm In-plane resolution, 0.4 × 0.4–0.5 mm
Standard shoulder MR imaging sequences	Fat-saturated T2 coronal oblique and sagittal oblique Fat-saturated intermediate-weighted (echo time, 40–45 ms) coronal oblique and axial Non–fat-saturated T1 sagittal oblique
Direct shoulder MR arthrography sequences	Following intra-articular injection of dilute gadolinium-based contrast (1:200 gadoterate meglumine): Fat-saturated T1 coronal oblique and axial Fat-saturated T2 coronal oblique and sagittal oblique Fat-saturated intermediate-weighted axial Non–fat-saturated T1 sagittal oblique

Fig. 4. Two axia
(B, arrow) in a

increased exte
anism: the sho
shift of the gle
and superiorly,
greater tuberos
meral externa
throwing arc
impingement c
curs (**Fig. 5**).[13]
glenohumeral c
of the humera
humeral ligam
external rotatic
curs.[15] This inc
the throwing a
at a higher vel

Osseous Char

Osseous ada
torsion and g

A

Fig. 5. Effect of
ing, there is phy:
margin (arrow),
posterosuperior
(straight arrow)
© The Clevelanc

allows clear definition of anatomy by providing tissue contrast between fat and low-signal structures, which can be particularly useful in the context of chronic injuries. T1-weighted images can also be used to evaluate evidence of fractures, cortical thickening, heterotopic ossification, and joint bodies. Direct MR arthrography offers greater sensitivity for detecting labral tears and articular-sided partial-thickness rotator cuff tears because of high MR tissue contrast and joint distension.[5–7] However, direct arthrography is invasive, and patients occasionally experience a painful contrast-induced synovitis in the days following the procedure.[8] Given the already high accuracy of high-quality images available with 3-T MR imaging and multichannel shoulder coils, the authors do not typically perform MR arthrography except in the case of prior labral repair. However, practice varies from institution to institution. Use of the shoulder abduction external rotation (ABER) position has been shown to increase detection of nondisplaced anteroinferior labral tears, superior labral tears through the peel-back mechanism, and articular-sided partial-thickness rotator cuff tears,[9–12] but this position is not routinely used at our institution because of added scan time and the risk of iatrogenic shoulder dislocation in patients with known instability.

BIOMECHANICS OF THE THROWING MOTION

To understand the forces encountered by the shoulder that may result in injury, it is helpful to divide the overhead throwing motion into phases: wind-up, stride, arm cocking, arm acceleration, arm deceleration, and follow-through (**Fig. 2**).[13,14]

Most of the relevant forces occur between late cocking and follow-through. The arm cocking phase begins when the lead foot makes contact; the pitcher rotates the torso forward to face the target while the humerus moves into a position of 90° of abduction (in line with the axis of the shoulders) and the humerus externally rotates. The late cocking phase ends when the pitcher has achieved the maximum humeral external rotation, in which the forearm can be nearly perpendicular to the vertical axis of the torso.

Achieving high angular velocity during humeral internal rotation in the arm acceleration phase is the most crucial component of attaining high pitching velocity.[15] The maximum humeral internal rotation velocity depends on the length of the throwing arc: a longer arc provides a longer acceleration time and produces a higher peak velocity.[15] This arc length is determined by the maximal external rotation position. Approximately 90 N·m of internal rotation torque is generated about the shoulder at the end of the late cocking phase,[16] which equals half of the maximal torque available in the 2-L engine of a 2016 Honda Civic. At the whiplike transition between late cocking and early acceleration, this force can result in supraphysiologic posterior shoulder impingement and anterior capsule stretching.[1,15,17]

From the cocked position, the pitcher initiates arm acceleration by extending the elbow and internally rotating the shoulder toward the target. The arm acceleration phase ends with ball release. At the time of ball release, the pitcher transfers momentum energy from the hip through the upper torso to the ball.[2] During the arm cocking and arm acceleration phases, the biceps muscle than in the nondominant arm.[27,28] The external rotation torque produced by adolescent pitchers in the late cocking phase has been shown to exert significant stress on the proximal humeral physis,[29] which may cause the asymmetric humeral remodeling that is frequently seen in baseball pitchers.[30,31]

Humeral retrotorsion provides theoretic advantages for pitching. Higher degrees of retrotorsion may enable pitchers to achieve higher maximum external rotation of the arm, a longer pitching arc of motion, and thus higher ball velocity.[32]

Glenoid retroversion

Glenoid version describes the angular relationship between the axis of the glenoid articular surface and the scapular axis; these axes are usually approximately perpendicular to each other.[33] Any posterior angulation of the glenoid surface from this perpendicular plane is termed glenoid retroversion (**Fig. 6**).[33] On average, glenoid retroversion in healthy individuals measures 1° ± 3°.[34] That number jumps to 8.6° ± 6° in the throwing shoulders of major league pitchers versus 4.9° ± 4.8° in their nonthrowing shoulders.[35] Such side-to-side differences in glenoid retroversion have long been observed in pitchers, leading to the belief that these changes are morphologic adaptations to pitching stress.[27,35]

Secondary ossification centers for the inferior two-thirds of the glenoid develop at approximately age 14 to 15 years as small islands of ossifications around the glenoid rim.[36] Complete fusion of the epiphysis with the glenoid surface does not occur until age 17 or 18 years,[37] providing a window for bony remodeling before physeal closure. There

may also be adaptive bone remodeling after physeal closure. Pitchers have increased glenoid subchondral bone density compared with healthy nonathletes, reflecting increased mechanical pitching stress in the anteroinferior and posterosuperior glenoid (**Fig. 7**),[38] which correlates with a large anterior shearing force of 310 N and posterior glenoid compressive force of 480 N during the late cocking phase.[1] The authors believe that during skeletal maturation, the posterior glenoid physis is repeatedly injured by the compressive force of pitching, leading to its stunted growth.

Mechanically, glenoid retroversion affords increased clearance between the humeral head and posterior glenoid (**Fig. 8**), which allows greater external rotation of the humeral head before the greater tuberosity contacts the glenoid, lengthening the throwing arc and leading to higher pitching speed. Greater clearance between the greater tuberosity and glenoid also lessens the likelihood of impingement and injury. This hypothesis was supported by a recent study showing an increased incidence of superior labral anteroposterior (SLAP) tears in professional pitchers without glenoid retroversion in their throwing shoulders relative to pitchers with glenoid retroversion.[39]

INJURIES RELATED TO THE LATE COCKING PHASE OF PITCHING
Internal Impingement

Posterosuperior impingement of the glenohumeral joint is the most common cause of shoulder pain in throwing athletes,[40] usually occurring in the late cocking and early acceleration phases.[41,42] There is physiologic contact of the undersurface of the

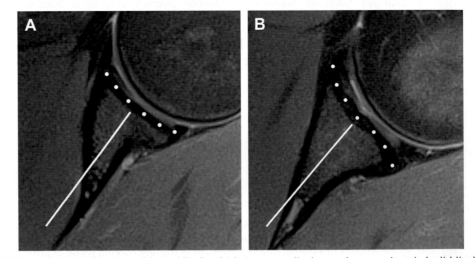

Fig. 6. (A) Normal glenoid contour (*dotted line*), which is perpendicular to the scapula axis (*solid line*). (B) Glenoid retroversion. Note the loss of perpendicular relationship between the posterior glenoid surface and scapula axis, and the convex contour of the posterior glenoid articular surface.

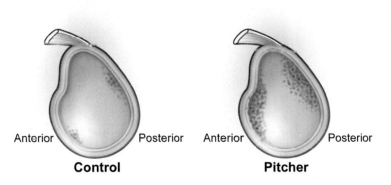

Fig. 7. Controls (*left*). Professional baseball pitcher (*right*). Pitchers show increased subchondral bone density (*shaded areas*), representing bone stress localizing to the posterosuperior and anteroinferior glenoid. (*Data from* Shimizu T, Iwasaki N, Nishida K, et al. Glenoid stress distribution in baseball players using computed tomography osteoabsorptiometry: a pilot study. Clin Orthop Relat Res 2012;470:1534–9.)

rotator cuff between the greater tuberosity and the posterosuperior glenoid and labrum when the shoulder is in ABER.[22] This contact has been observed in healthy nonathletes and pitchers.[43,44] However, pitching results in repeated contact and supraphysiologic compressive force generated in arm cocking, subjecting the rotator cuff and posterosuperior labrum to pathologic posterosuperior impingement and resulting in rotator cuff and labrum tears.[41,45]

Typical imaging findings of posterosuperior impingement include articular-sided partial-thickness tears of the posterior supraspinatus and

anterior infraspinatus tendons and superior labral tears.[46] Articular-sided partial-thickness rotator cuff tears are seen as focal high signal extending to the humeral articular surface on proton-density or T2 fat-saturated sequences.[46] Most cuff injuries associated with posterosuperior impingement are seen at the posterior supraspinatus and anterior infraspinatus tendons (**Fig. 9**).[22] It is important to assess the depth of partial-thickness cuff tears as well as their location in the cuff tendon relative to tendon insertion. Because of the high risk of progression to full-thickness tears, partial cuff tears involving greater

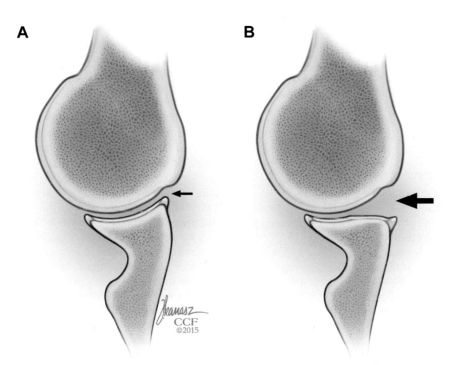

Fig. 8. Posterior glenoid remodeling from pitching. (*A*) Normal glenoid contour. In the ABER position, the greater tuberosity comes close to the glenoid margin (*arrow*). (*B*) Posterior glenoid remodeling in a pitcher increases clearance between the greater tuberosity and posterior glenoid (*arrow*), therefore increasing maximal external rotation and reducing the risk of impingement injury. Copyright © The Cleveland Clinic Foundation 2015.

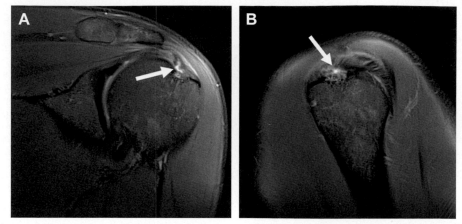

Fig. 9. (*A*) Coronal T2-weighted MR image of the left shoulder shows a small articular-side partial-thickness tear at the junction of posterior supraspinatus and anterior infraspinatus tendons (*arrow*). The tear involves the medial aspect of the insertion on the greater tuberosity. (*B*) Sagittal T2-weighted MR image of the left shoulder shows the small articular-side partial-thickness tear at the junction of posterior supraspinatus and anterior infraspinatus tendons (*arrow*).

than 50% of the tendon thickness at the site of tendon insertion are often treated with surgery, whereas more superficial tears and those occurring medial to the insertion are often treated conservatively.[5,6]

Superior Labral Tear

SLAP tears are superior labrum injuries seen in 3.9% to 6% of patients undergoing shoulder arthroscopy.[47–49] SLAP lesions are divided into 4 main types (**Table 2**); type II lesions are the most common and are thought to be associated with repetitive overhead activity.[47–49] A total of 62% of type II SLAP lesions extend to the posterosuperior labrum, which is thought to contribute to posterior-superior instability and undersurface rotator cuff tear.[50]

Table 2 Types of SLAP lesions	
Type I	Fraying of the superior labrum without discrete tear
Type II	Discrete tear with detachment of the superior labrum and adjoining biceps-labral anchor from the underlying glenoid cartilage
Type III	Bucket-handle tear of the superior labrum without extension into the biceps tendon
Type IV	Bucket-handle tear of the superior labrum with extension into the biceps tendon

Data from Snyder SJ, Karzel RP, Del Pizzo W, et al. SLAP lesions of the shoulder. Arthroscopy 1990;6:274–9.

There are 2 main theories on the pathogenesis of type II SLAP lesions in athletes. Cadaveric and arthroscopic demonstrations of impingement of the posterosuperior labrum between the greater tuberosity and glenoid with the shoulder in ABER led to the hypothesis that posterosuperior impingement causes SLAP and cuff tears (**Fig. 10**).[20,22] Other investigators favor a peel-back mechanism, wherein humeral hyperexternal rotation in the late cocking phase generates a posteriorly directed torsional force on the biceps tendon, leading to twisting and peel-back and detachment of the biceps root and posterosuperior labrum from the underlying glenoid cartilage.[15,50] Given how often posterosuperior impingement, SLAP lesions, and rotator cuff undersurface tears occur concurrently, both of these proposed mechanisms likely contribute to the pathogenesis of SLAP lesions.

Because hyperexternal rotation in abduction results in significant twisting and shearing stress on the rotator cuff, long head of the biceps tendon, and superior labrum,[51] humeral retrotorsion also may confer an advantage of decreased injury risk by requiring less external rotation of the proximal humerus (humeral head and tuberosities) to achieve maximum external rotation (**Fig. 11**). This protective effect of humeral retrotorsion against injury is supported by studies showing a higher incidence and severity of shoulder injuries in professional baseball players with lower degrees of humeral torsion in the throwing arm.[27,28]

MR imaging is useful for diagnosing SLAP lesions, although a broad range of accuracy numbers have been reported with a sensitivity of 38% to 98%, specificity of 75% to 100%, and

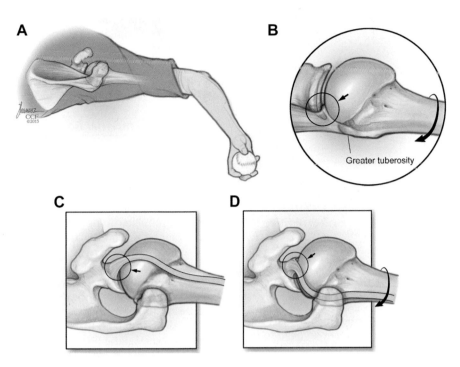

Fig. 10. Pathomechanics of a SLAP tear. (*A*) Overhead large field of view of the shoulder in ABER position in late cocking phase of pitching. (*B*) Posterosuperior impingement causes impingement of the rotator cuff and labrum between the greater tuberosity and posterior glenoid margin (*small arrow*). (*C*) There is no tension on the biceps-labral complex (*arrow*) when the shoulder is in neutral position. (*D*) Shoulder external rotation (*rotating arrow*) induces tension and peel-back of the biceps tendon from the superior labrum (*small arrow*). Copyright © The Cleveland Clinic Foundation 2015.

accuracy of 63% to 96%.[7,52–56] Higher sensitivity and specificity numbers were reported in studies performed on 3-T scanners and read by musculoskeletal fellowship–trained radiologists.[7,52–56] Although the glenoid labrum is routinely imaged in 3 planes, imaging of the coronal plane is most sensitive for the detection of SLAP lesions.[57] MR imaging findings in patients with SLAP lesions can include abnormal signal and fraying of the superior labrum (type I lesions), fluid signal within the labrum substance or at the labral cartilage junction (type II lesions), displaced bucket-handle tear of the superior labrum (type III lesions), and large displaced tear with extension into the biceps tendon (type IV lesions).[7] Subclassification of SLAP tears can be difficult. The most useful imaging distinction is between labral detachment requiring surgery (types II–IV) and normal or nondetached labral abnormalities (type I).[58] Anecdotally, a concurrent finding of perilabral edema seems to be associated with acute injury (**Figs. 12** and **13**), which can be a useful sign when evaluating high-level pitchers who often have chronic labral disorders when they present with acute symptoms. Studies have shown MR arthrogram to be more

sensitive (84%–98%) but less specific (58%–99%) than noncontrast MR imaging in the detection of SLAP lesions.[7,56,59,60]

It is often difficult to distinguish between a normal variant sublabral recess and a superior labral tear. The recess or sulcus is a normal separation of the superior labrum from the glenoid cartilage located at the 11-o'clock to 1-o'clock position and thus appears similar to a detached labral tear on MR imaging (ie, as a cleft of high signal between the labrum and the adjacent articular cartilage).[61] There are several MR imaging features that may be useful in distinguishing a tear from a normal recess, although none is definitive. The features favoring a tear rather than a recess include extension of the cleft laterally away from the glenoid margin and into the substance of the labrum, a cleft with a depth of 2 mm or greater in a patient less than 40 years of age, wider separation of the labrum from the underlying cartilage, irregular or globular margins of the cleft, and greater posterior extension beyond the level of the biceps tendon attachment.[62]

SLAP lesions in overhead athletes usually must be repaired to allow a return to preinjury level of

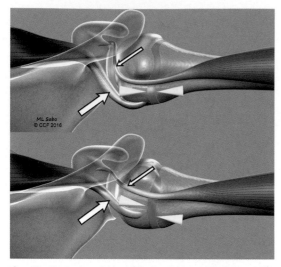

Fig. 11. Posterior views of 2 shoulders with the arms in 90° of abduction and in the same degree of external rotation. (*Top*) Shoulder with low degree of humeral retrotorsion. (*Bottom*) Shoulder with high degree of humeral retrotorsion. The thin white arrows point to the long head of the biceps tendon, the thick *white arrows* point to the supraspinatus tendon, and the orange bands represent the proximal humeral physes. Despite the same degree of external rotation of the arm in both cases, the shoulder in *B* is able to achieve this position with less external rotation of the humeral head and tuberosities. As a result, the long head of the biceps and supraspinatus tendons experience less twisting and traction. Copyright © The Cleveland Clinic Foundation 2015.

play.[63] Reattachment of the labrobicipital complex with suture anchors has a higher success rate than reattachment with bioabsorbable tacks.[63,64] Performing concomitant rotator cuff repair and biceps

tenodesis at the time of SLAP repair has been associated with a higher rate of return to function than performing SLAP repair alone.[65]

INJURIES RELATED TO THE DECELERATION AND FOLLOW-THROUGH PHASES OF PITCHING
Glenohumeral Internal Rotation Deficit

Glenohumeral internal rotation deficit (GIRD) describes a loss of internal humeral rotation in excess of the degree of the adaptive gain of external rotation and loss of the degree of attainable humeral internal rotation in the throwing shoulder relative to the contralateral nonthrowing shoulder.[15,66] Glenohumeral rotation is measured with the patient supine, the humerus in 90° abduction in the plane of the body, the elbow flexed 90°, and the scapula stabilized against the examination table; the degree of anterior and posterior forearm rotation from the vertical position determines the amount of internal and external rotation of the humerus at the shoulder (**Fig. 14**).[15] A biomechanical model by Burkhart and colleagues[15] attributes GIRD to pathologic contracture of the posterior capsule and postulates that GIRD is the most important cause of decreased horizontal adduction and performance loss. A review of MR arthrograms from 6 professional baseball players with GIRD showed a thickened posterior joint capsule (**Fig. 15**) along with findings of posterosuperior impingement.[67]

Although GIRD greater than 25° has previously been associated with shoulder injury,[15] newer data suggest that external rotation insufficiency (external rotation in the throwing arm that is <5° greater than external rotation in the nonthrowing

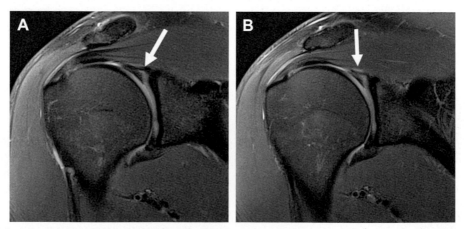

Fig. 12. (*A*) Coronal intermediate-weighted MR image of the right shoulder. Cleft of high signal through the posterosuperior labrum at its attachment (*arrow*), consistent with a SLAP tear. The cleft is wide, deep, and extends laterally into the labrum. (*B*) Slightly more anteriorly, there is continuation of the labral tear, with mild perilabral edema (*arrow*). This finding suggests an acute injury.

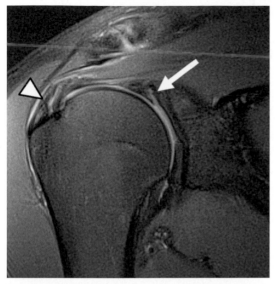

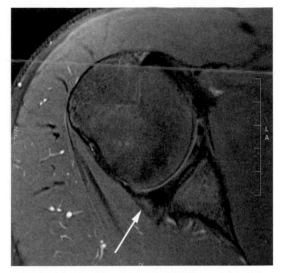

Fig. 15. Very thick posterior capsule (*arrow*) in pitcher with GIRD.

Fig. 13. Coronal intermediate-weighted MR image in a different patient showing superior labral tear (*arrow*) and tendinosis of the supraspinatus tendon (*arrowhead*). There is no adjacent perilabral edema, suggesting chronic injury.

arm) rather than GIRD is the measurement of glenohumeral rotation that is most closely linked to injury.[16] Clinical experience suggests that 90% of symptomatic GIRD cases improve with a posterior capsule stretching program; the remaining 10% require surgery (eg, posterior capsulotomy and SLAP tear repair).[15]

Bennett Lesion

A Bennett lesion is a bony protuberance of the posteroinferior glenoid cortex adjacent to the posterior band of the inferior glenohumeral ligament complex (**Fig. 16**).[68,69] This lesion is thought to

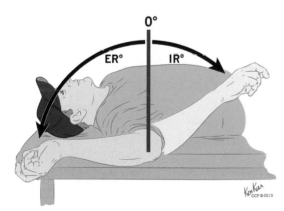

Fig. 14. Measurement of internal rotation (IR) and external rotation (ER) of the shoulder by physical examination. Copyright © The Cleveland Clinic Foundation 2015.

represent reactive new bone formation in response to repetitive traction injury to the posterior capsule during follow-through and impaction of the humeral head on the posterior glenoid during late cocking.[70–72] A Bennett lesion is not thought to be an osteophyte and is usually not associated with cartilage loss. It is therefore different from the osteophytes seen in the posteromedial elbow (ulnotrochlear joint) in throwers, which in most cases are associated with cartilage defects and posteromedial elbow impingement.[73] Bennett lesions are seen in 22% to 47% of baseball pitchers and are usually asymptomatic.[70,74,75] However, Bennett lesions may irritate the adjacent axillary nerve or cause impingement of the joint capsule and labrum, resulting in posterior shoulder pain with throwing (painful Bennett lesion).[71,72,74,76] Painful Bennett lesions are more likely to be large (>20% of the width of the glenoid fossa), to show fibrosis and synovial proliferation of the posteroinferior glenohumeral ligament, and to have an avulsed bone fragment if there is acute-onset throwing pain.[75] Although studies have suggested an association between Bennett lesions and rotator cuff/labrum injuries, which often occur concurrently,[22] there are no statistically significant data to prove a causal relationship.[75]

On MR imaging, a Bennett lesion manifests as low-signal ossification along the posteroinferior glenoid cortex with adjacent capsular thickening and fibrosis; edemalike high signal in the ossification or capsule may be seen if there is synovial proliferation or an acute-on-chronic component (**Fig. 17**).

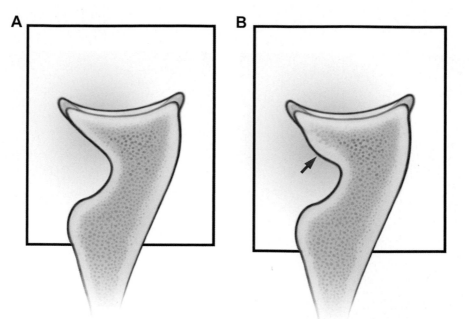

Fig. 16. Comparison of normal shoulder (*A*) to Bennett lesion (*B*). Note the bony protuberance of the posterior glenoid cortex (*arrow*) in the Bennett lesion.

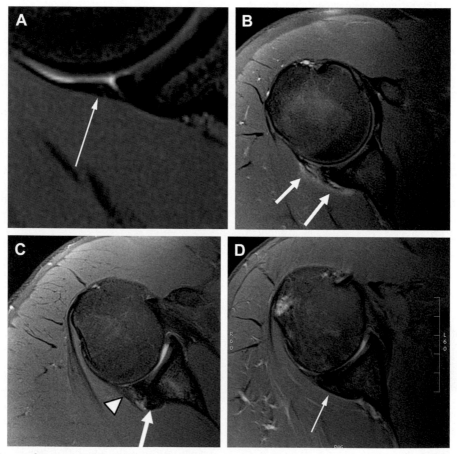

Fig. 17. Phases of Bennett lesion development. (*A*) Normal posterior capsule (*arrow*). (*B*) Axial MR image with acute/subacute lesion with edema in the thickened posterior capsule (*arrows*) and periosteal edema about the posterior glenoid; there is no bony hypertrophy yet. (*C*) Thickened posterior capsule without edema (*arrowhead*) and periosteal new bone along the posterior glenoid (*arrow*) consistent with subacute-chronic change. (*D*) Mature hypertrophic bone and marrow formation along the posterior glenoid margin consistent with a chronic Bennett lesion (*arrow*).

Treatment of Bennett lesions is controversial, because some investigators have questioned whether these lesions are the cause of posterior shoulder pain or whether they occur concurrently alongside the true cause.[74] Other bony changes in overhead athletes, especially in skeletally immature patients, include overuse injuries at the proximal humerus (proximal humeral epiphysiolysis) and at the acromioclavicular joint,[77,78] such as the recently described stress response at the acromial synchondrosis (acromial apophysiolysis).[77] These injuries are described elsewhere in this issue.

SUMMARY

Repetitive, high-velocity overhead throwing can lead to several adaptive changes in the throwing shoulder, which over time lead to structural microtrauma and eventually overt injury. MR imaging is useful for evaluating these changes and characterizing their acuity and severity. Understanding the throwing motion and the effects of this motion on the structures of the shoulder can help radiologists to recognize these findings and provide useful information to referring physicians.

ACKNOWLEDGMENTS

We would like to thank Joe Kanasz and Mark Sabo for figures 1,2,3,5,7,10, and 16.

REFERENCES

1. Fleisig GS. Biomechanics of baseball pitching: implications for injury and performance. Proceedings of the 28th Conference of the International Society of Biomechanics in Sports. Michigan, July 19–23, 2010.
2. Calabrese GJ. Pitching mechanics, revisited. Int J Sports Phys Ther 2013;8:652–60.
3. Drake R, Vogl AW, Mitchell AW. Gray's anatomy for students. 2nd edition. Philadelphia: Churchill Livingstone/Elsevier; 2010.
4. Hsu HC, Boardman ND 3rd, Luo ZP, et al. Tendon-defect and muscle-unloaded models for relating a rotator cuff tear to glenohumeral stability. J Orthop Res 2000;18:952–8.
5. Matava MJ, Purcell DB, Rudzki JR. Partial-thickness rotator cuff tears. Am J Sports Med 2005;33:1405–17.
6. Schreinemachers SA, van der Hulst VP, Willems WJ, et al. Detection of partial-thickness supraspinatus tendon tears: is a single direct MR arthrography series in ABER position as accurate as conventional MR arthrography? Skeletal Radiol 2009;38:967–75.
7. Dinauer PA, Flemming DJ, Murphy KP, et al. Diagnosis of superior labral lesions: comparison of non-contrast MRI with indirect MR arthrography in unexercised shoulders. Skeletal Radiol 2007;36:195–202.
8. Saupe N, Zanetti M, Pfirrmann CW, et al. Pain and other side effects after MR arthrography: prospective evaluation in 1085 patients. Radiology 2009;250:830–8.
9. Herold T, Bachthaler M, Hamer OW, et al. Indirect MR arthrography of the shoulder: use of abduction and external rotation to detect full- and partial-thickness tears of the supraspinatus tendon. Radiology 2006;240:152–60.
10. Tirman PF, Bost FW, Steinbach LS, et al. MR arthrographic depiction of tears of the rotator cuff: benefit of abduction and external rotation of the arm. Radiology 1994;192:851–6.
11. Lee SY, Lee JK. Horizontal component of partial-thickness tears of rotator cuff: imaging characteristics and comparison of ABER view with oblique coronal view at MR arthrography initial results. Radiology 2002;224:470–6.
12. Borrero CG, Casagranda BU, Towers JD, et al. Magnetic resonance appearance of posterosuperior labral peel back during humeral abduction and external rotation. Skeletal Radiol 2010;39:19–26.
13. Fleisig GS, Barrentine SW, Escamilla RF, et al. Biomechanics of overhead throwing with implications for injuries. Sports Med 1996;21:421–37.
14. Werner SL, Gill TJ, Murray TA, et al. Relationships between throwing mechanics and shoulder distraction in professional baseball pitchers. Am J Sports Med 2001;29:354–8.
15. Burkhart SS, Morgan CD, Kibler WB. The disabled throwing shoulder: spectrum of pathology. Part I: pathoanatomy and biomechanics. Arthroscopy 2003;19:404–20.
16. Wilk KE, Macrina LC, Fleisig GS, et al. Deficits in glenohumeral passive range of motion increase risk of shoulder injury in professional baseball pitchers: a prospective study. Am J Sports Med 2015;43:2379–85.
17. Heyworth BE, Williams RJ 3rd. Internal impingement of the shoulder. Am J Sports Med 2009;37:1024–37.
18. Gowan ID, Jobe FW, Tibone JE, et al. A comparative electromyographic analysis of the shoulder during pitching. Professional versus amateur pitchers. Am J Sports Med 1987;15:586–90.
19. Jobe FW, Moynes DR, Tibone JE, et al. An EMG analysis of the shoulder in pitching. A second report. Am J Sports Med 1984;12:218–20.
20. Jobe CM. Posterior superior glenoid impingement: expanded spectrum. Arthroscopy 1995;11:530–6.
21. Jobe FW, Giangarra CE, Kvitne RS, et al. Anterior capsulolabral reconstruction of the shoulder in athletes in overhead sports. Am J Sports Med 1991;19:428–34.
22. Walch G, Boileau P, Noel E, et al. Impingement of the deep surface of the supraspinatus tendon on the posterosuperior glenoid rim: an arthroscopic study. J Shoulder Elbow Surg 1992;1:238–45.
23. Halbrecht JL, Tirman P, Atkin D. Internal impingement of the shoulder: comparison of findings

Multimodality Imaging of the Painful Elbow

Current Imaging Concepts and Image-Guided Treatments for the Injured Thrower's Elbow

Cristy N. Gustas, MD[a],*, Kenneth S. Lee, MD[b]

KEYWORDS

- Elbow injuries • Ultrasound • Throwing athlete • UCL • Epicondylosis
- Valgus extension overload syndrome • PRP

KEY POINTS

- Overhead sport athletes are at risk for several causes of elbow pain, including epicondylosis, ulnar collateral ligament injury, and bony and nerve injury.
- During the throwing motion, large valgus and extension forces lead to tensile stress on the medial structures, compressive forces laterally, and shear forces on the posterior structures resulting in characteristic injuries.
- Throwing athletes are subject to chronic repetitive overuse injuries of the elbow.
- Imaging can serve as an adjunct tool to establish a diagnosis or to guide treatment.
- Ultrasound-guided percutaneous injection therapies are emerging as an alternative treatment for some ligament and chronic tendon injuries about the elbow.

INTRODUCTION

Recent decades have seen a sharp increase in overhead throwing athletes competing in sports such as baseball, softball, football, tennis, volleyball, and various track and field events. Not surprisingly, this growth in participation has led to an increase in the incidence of elbow injuries. More than 50% of high school, college, and professional baseball players experience elbow pain.[1] Sports that require repetitive gripping and throwing impart high valgus and extension loads to the athlete's elbow. These forces lead to tensile stress on the medial structures, compressive

forces laterally, and shear forces on the posterior structures. A characteristic pattern of acute and chronic injuries or progressive structural changes is often the result.

A thorough history and physical examination of the thrower's elbow frequently establishes the diagnosis for elbow pain. Imaging can afford additional information when the clinical picture is unclear or further information is necessary for risk stratification and treatment planning. Radiographs and computed tomography (CT) play a role in the evaluation of osseous lesions (bony avulsions, calcifications, intraarticular bodies). The large field of view in MR imaging is particularly useful in cases

[a] Musculoskeletal Imaging, Department of Radiology, Penn State Milton S. Hershey Medical Center, 500 University Drive-H066, Hershey, PA 17033, USA; [b] Musculoskeletal Imaging, Department of Radiology, University of Wisconsin School of Medicine & Public Health, University of Wisconsin Hospital and Clinics, E3/366, 600 Highland Avenue, Madison, WI 53792, USA
* Corresponding author.
E-mail address: cgustas@hmc.psu.edu

Radiol Clin N Am 54 (2016) 817–839
http://dx.doi.org/10.1016/j.rcl.2016.04.005
0033-8389/16/$ – see front matter © 2016 Elsevier Inc. All rights reserved.

of vague or diffuse elbow pain. Superior contrast resolution enables quick recognition of bone and soft tissue pathology and provides a planning tool for rehabilitation or surgery. Ultrasound (US) imaging is rapidly growing in popularity and offers focused high-resolution imaging of tendons, ligaments, and nerves about the elbow. Unique advantages of US include accessibility as well as the capability for dynamic assessment and quick comparison with the contralateral side. US imaging is also useful for guided therapeutic procedures. This article focuses on current imaging concepts and image-guided treatments for injuries commonly affecting the adult throwing athlete's elbow. Topics discussed include lateral and medial epicondylosis, ulnar collateral ligament (UCL) injury, bony injuries, and nerve impingement. Conditions typically seen in the skeletally immature thrower's elbow, such as medial epicondyle apophysitis (little league elbow), medial epicondyle avulsion fracture in adolescent pitchers, and osteochondritis dissecans are addressed in other dedicated articles in this issue.

TENDINOSIS

Tendon injuries about the elbow may result from an acute traumatic event, repetitive microtrauma, or a combination of these processes. In overhead throwing athletes, tendinopathies are often related to overuse resulting in microtearing and progressive tendon degeneration owing to an incomplete reparative response.[2,3] Histologic analysis of the pathologic tendon reveals angiofibroblastic hyperplasia, mucoid degeneration, chondroid metaplasia, and fibrillary degeneration of collagen.[4] Over time, scar tissue forms that is vulnerable to chronic repetitive trauma. This vicious cycle of microtear and disorganized repair can lead to larger tears with worsening symptoms and eventual biomechanical failure of the tendon.[3] Inflammation is noted only in the earliest stages of the healing process and declines by postinjury day 10 as the proliferative healing phase begins.[5,6] Indeed, 1 study found no histopathologic evidence of either acute or chronic inflammation to correspond with areas of tendon signal abnormality on MR imaging.[7] For this reason "tendinosis," rather than "tendinitis," is considered the preferred name for the clinical entity of chronic tendon degeneration.

Lateral Epicondylosis

Lateral epicondylosis, or "tennis elbow," is the most common cause of lateral elbow pain in skeletally mature athletes, occurring in more than 50% of racquet sport players.[2,8] Repetitive activities involving wrist extension and supination (eg, the backhand swing in racquet sports) can result in degeneration of the common extensor tendon (CET) origin at the lateral epicondyle. Several studies have identified the extensor carpi radialis brevis component of the CET as almost universally affected in lateral epicondylosis.[3,7,9] The anterior edge of the extensor digitorum communis is involved 50% of the time.[2] Typical symptoms include focal tenderness at the lateral epicondyle and lateral elbow pain, particularly with wrist extension. Patients occasionally report weakened grip strength.[3]

Lateral epicondylosis is diagnosed by history and physical examination in most cases, but imaging may be helpful to confirm the diagnosis or evaluate the extent of tissue injury in recalcitrant cases of lateral elbow pain. Elbow radiographs are often negative, but may show enthesophytes or heterotopic ossification along the lateral epicondyle.[3] On MR imaging, tendon morphology is assessed most easily on the coronal and axial images. The normal CET should be uniformly low in signal on all sequences. Tendinosis presents as intermediate intratendinous signal on both T1-weighted and fluid-sensitive sequences with or without tendon thickening (**Fig. 1**A, B).[3,10] Partial or complete tears can result from acute traumatic events or as a sequelae of chronic advanced tendinosis. Partial thickness tears are seen as hyperintense fluid signal interrupting a portion of the tendon fibers with associated tendon thinning (**Fig. 2**A–C). A full-thickness tear appears as a fluid signal intensity gap completely interrupting the tendon fibers or a fluid signal gap between the proximal tendon and lateral epicondyle in the setting of avulsion injury.

On US imaging, the extensor carpi radialis brevis makes up a major portion of the CET attachment and is the most anteriorly located of the tendons at the lateral epicondyle. On long axis imaging, the normal CET demonstrates a compact fibrillar pattern of uniform echogenicity.[8,11] Tendinosis commonly presents as tendon thickening with hypoechogenicity and loss of the typical compact fibrillar pattern.[12] Hyperemia representative of neovascularity may be seen on Doppler investigation (**Fig. 1**C).[8] Other US findings occasionally seen in lateral epicondylosis include intratendinous calcification and bone irregularity in the adjacent lateral epicondyle.[13] Tears appear as a focal anechoic or fluid-filled gap in the tendon with accompanying tendon discontinuity (**Fig. 2**D). Previous studies have shown that US is accurate for the diagnosis of lateral epicondylosis with a similar specificity (67%–100%) but slightly diminished sensitivity (64%–82%) compared with

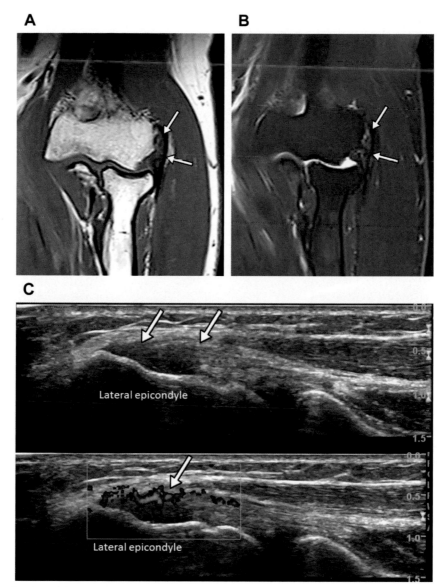

Fig. 1. Lateral epicondylosis in a 34-year-old professional fisherman complaining of lateral elbow pain during casting. (*A*) Coronal T1 and (*B*) coronal proton density (PD) with fat suppression sequences show marked thickening and intermediate signal in the common extensor tendon (CET; *arrows*). (*C*) Long axis gray-scale and power Doppler ultrasound (US) images of the same patient demonstrates thickening and hypoechogenicity (*arrows*) of the CET with hyperemia. (*D*) Long axis US images during guided therapeutic needle fenestration (*arrows*) and platelet-rich plasma (PRP) injection (*arrowheads*). (*E*) A 48-year-old woman with lateral epicondylosis (*arrow in top image*) and improved US appearance of the CET 12 weeks after PRP injection (*bottom image*).

MR imaging (90%–100% sensitivity).[13–15] Hypoechogenicity of the CET origin has the best combination of diagnostic sensitivity and specificity for the diagnosis of common extensor tendinosis.[16] Neovascularity, calcifications, and cortical irregularities have strong specificity for chronic lateral epicondylalgia.[16] Sonoelastography is an emerging US technique to detect increased compressibility or tendon softening in areas of tendinosis. It demonstrated not only excellent

sensitivity, but also excellent correlation with US findings in early studies of lateral epicondylosis.[17] In addition to these diagnostic capabilities, US provides target localization during image-guided percutaneous therapy.

Treatment
Several percutaneous injection therapies for chronic tendinosis have emerged and been subjected to randomized, controlled trials. Although

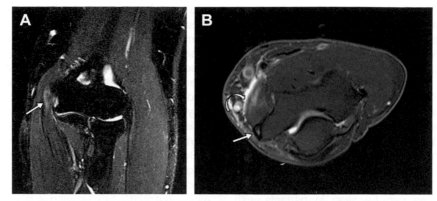

Fig. 3. Flexor–pronator strain in a 45-year-old tennis player with medial elbow pain after an overhand tennis serve. (A) Coronal T2 fat suppression (FS) and (B) axial T2 FS sequence shows high signal in the common flexor tendon origin (arrow) and feathery edema in the pronator teres muscle (curved arrow).

confirm these anecdotal findings. Operative therapy for recalcitrant cases includes variations of tendinosis debridement, open release of the flexor muscle origin, and medial epicondylectomy, but excessive debridement can damage the adjacent UCL or ulnar nerve.[54,61] For professional athletes, early surgery to repair areas of high-grade tendon tearing or reattachment of an avulsed flexor–pronator origin may be indicated.[62]

ULNAR COLLATERAL LIGAMENT

The UCL or medial collateral ligament is the primary soft tissue stabilizer against valgus stress in the medial elbow. Athletes participating in overhead sports, such as javelin, tennis, football, wrestling, softball, gymnastics, and baseball—

particularly high velocity pitchers—are especially susceptible to UCL injury.[63] Clinical assessment of UCL integrity can prove challenging. Therefore, imaging serves an important adjunct role in the diagnosis of UCL injury or reinjury after operative intervention.

Anatomy

The UCL complex is composed of 3 separate bundles: anterior, posterior, and transverse. The anterior bundle originates from the anteroinferior aspect of the medial epicondyle, both distal and lateral to the origin of the adjacent common flexor tendon. The ligament is round at the origin and tapers distally.[64] The anterior bundle inserts on the sublime tubercle of the coronoid process,

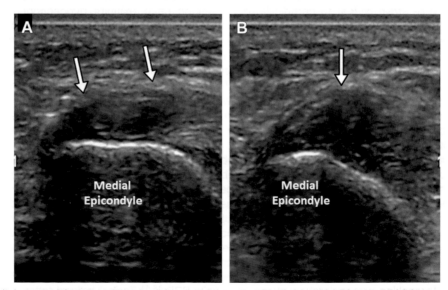

Fig. 4. Medial epicondylosis in a 52-year-old archer. (A) Long-axis ultrasound (US) view and (B) short-axis US view of the medial elbow demonstrates a thickened and hypoechoic common flexor tendon origin (arrows).

approximately 5 mm beyond the ulnar cartilage, with a long tapered attachment running down an osseous ridge along the medial ulna.[65–67]

The UCL provides the primary restraint against valgus stress in the arc of the overhead throwing motion (30°–120° of flexion).[68,69] The anterior bundle itself is composed of an anterior and posterior band that work in a reciprocal fashion to resist valgus stress through the range of motion.[56,64,66] However, these functional bands of the anterior bundle are not detected as separate structures on imaging.

The overhead throwing motion generates extreme valgus and extension forces on the elbow, particularly during the late cocking and early acceleration phases.[1,56] During this motion, loads approach the maximal tensile strength of the UCL. Repetitive near-failure loads can cause microtrauma to the anterior band of the UCL and may eventually lead to ligament attenuation or tear.[1]

Diagnosis

Athletes with acute UCL tears owing to spontaneous failure of the ligamentous complex may experience a "pop" sensation accompanied by immediate pain and possibly soft tissue edema or ecchymosis. Another subset of athletes with chronic injury may experience vague onset of medial elbow pain, usually during the late cocking/early acceleration phase of throwing, associated with a decrease in performance.[1,63] Patients with UCL tears typically have medial elbow tenderness 2 cm distal to the medial epicondyle. Associated injuries to the flexor–pronator muscles can present as medical epicondyle pain worsened by resisted wrist flexion. Several physical examination tests have been described for assessing UCL injury and thus valgus stability of the elbow.[68] The clinical diagnosis of acute, complete tears is often straightforward, but partial tears and chronic ligament laxity often present a considerable diagnostic challenge.[70]

Radiographs should be evaluated for arthritic changes, osseous UCL avulsions from the medial epicondyle or sublime tubercle, traction enthesophytes, calcifications in the ligament, and posteromedial olecranon osteophytes. Olecranon osteophytes and heterotopic calcification within the UCL substance were the most common radiographic findings in 1 large series of patients with a UCL tear.[63]

MR Imaging

Advanced imaging can be helpful to document the presence and severity of UCL injury to distinguish this entity from other causes of medial elbow pain and to direct appropriate treatment. In an early study of 25 baseball players with confirmed UCL tear, Timmerman and colleagues[71] found that MR imaging and CT arthrography were equally accurate for detection of complete tears. For partial tears the sensitivity of MR imaging decreased to 57% with specificity of 100%, whereas the sensitivity and specificity of CT arthrogram was 86% and 91%, respectively. Today, MR arthrography is the study of choice for most orthopedic surgeons and sports medicine physicians. It has a high sensitivity and specificity of 92% and 100% and has the best interobserver reliability.[64,72–74] Future developments in 3-dimensional sequence imaging offer potential advantages, such as thinner slice acquisition and the ability to evaluate ligaments in any orientation through multiplanar reformats.

It is important to understand the normal MR imaging appearance of the UCL to avoid diagnostic error. The anterior bundle is best seen in the coronal and axial planes over 2 to 3 consecutive slices. The normal UCL is low signal on both T1-weighted and fluid-sensitive sequences (**Fig. 5**A, B). At the proximal humeral attachment, the UCL may have a slightly striated appearance, particularly on short TE sequences, owing to interspersed fat (see **Fig. 5**A).[75] The overlying common flexor tendon attachment lies in close proximity to the UCL, but should always occur cephalad and medial with respect to the proximal attachment of the anterior bundle. The UCL takes a slightly anterior to posterior course and tapers at the far distal attachment on the medial aspect of the coronoid process of the ulna, otherwise known as the sublime tubercle. Munshi and colleagues[75] observed variability in this distal attachment of the anterior bundle. In cadaveric specimens they found the normal anterior bundle inserted 3 to 4 mm beyond the articular margin of the sublime tubercle, thus resulting in slight separation between the distal ligament and bone.[67,75] This finding becomes important in the diagnosis of partial thickness tears, described below.

The MR appearance of the pathologic UCL in the overhead athlete depends on the timing and severity of injury. Acute complete tears of the anterior bundle typically present as discontinuity of the ligament, often accompanied by laxity, irregularity, and poor definition of the ligament. They are often accompanied by increased T2 signal intensity edema within and around the ligament.[76] Extracapsular leakage of injected contrast on MR arthrogram is another sign of complete tear.[76] Early literature reported a large majority of tears to be midsubstance.[73,77] But MR imaging often

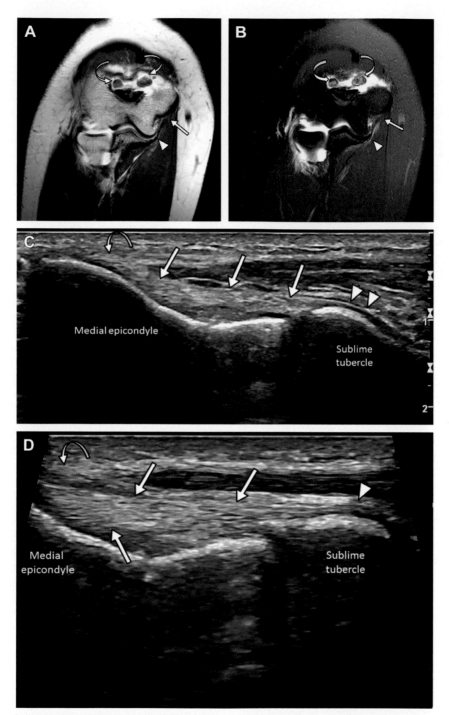

Fig. 5. Normal ulnar collateral ligament (UCL) in a 20-year-old baseball player with elbow pain and locking but no instability. (*A*) Coronal T1 arthrogram and (*B*) T2 fat suppression arthrogram sequences show a normal UCL (*arrow*) with striated signal in the proximal portion owing to interspersed fat. The distal insertion is intact at the sublime tubercle (*arrowhead*). Intraarticular bodies (*curved arrows*) were the cause for elbow pain. (*C, D*) Long axis ultrasound image shows the common flexor tendon (*curved arrow*) superficial to the normal hyperechoic compact fibrillar appearance of the UCL (*arrow*) with intact insertion on the sublime tubercle (*arrowhead*).

demonstrates both proximal and distal avulsions, often in greater frequency than midsubstance tears.[73]

Sprains are characterized by alterations in ligament morphology (thickening) and signal intensity (intermediate T1 and T2) without discontinuity.[73] Most partial thickness tears involve injury to the deep capsular layer of the anterior bundle. They present on MR imaging as focal areas of hyperintense ligamentous interruption on fluid sensitive sequences with varying degrees of residual intact fibers (**Fig. 6**A). Timmerman and colleagues[71,78] identified an undersurface tear or partial detachment of the distal UCL from the insertion on the sublime tubercle. The authors described an arthrographic "T-sign" in which contrast extending distally beyond the articular surface margin of the ulna represented a partial tear of the deep UCL fibers (**Fig. 7**). Subsequent studies with cadaveric correlation revealed normal variation in the distal insertion of the anterior bundle up to 3 or 4 mm distal to the articular margin of the sublime tubercle and normal separation between the 2 structures on MR imaging.[67,75] Thus, caution is required when describing an arthrographic "T-sign." To increase accuracy, the reader should assess for other supporting signs of injury (alternations in ligament morphology or signal and adjacent soft tissue edema) when diagnosing a partial thickness distal undersurface tear or detachment. Distal UCL injuries can also present as an avulsion fracture or stress reaction of the sublime tubercle. These injuries are typically seen as bone marrow edema, with or without discrete linear fracture, in the setting of an intact or chronically thickened UCL (**Fig. 8**).[79]

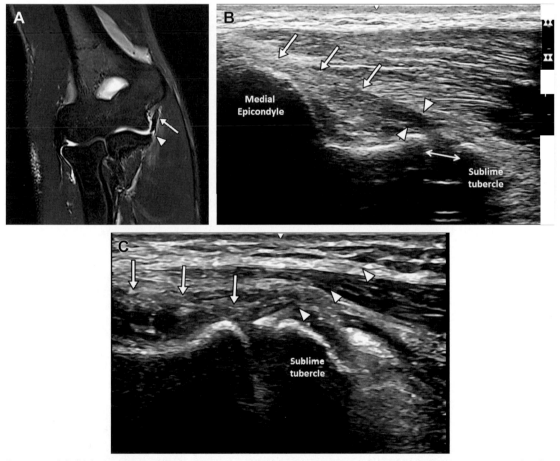

Fig. 6. Partial-thickness ulnar collateral ligament (UCL) tear superimposed on chronic ligament attenuation in a 22-year-old javelin athlete. (*A*) Coronal T2 fat suppression arthrogram image shows thickening and chronic degenerative changes of the UCL (*arrow*) with an acute high-grade partial-thickness tear of the distal insertion (*arrowhead*). (*B*) Long axis ultrasound (US) image shows the hypoechoic partial-thickness tear (*arrowheads*) in the distal UCL (*arrows*) and gapping of the medial joint space (*double headed arrow*). (*C*) US-guided needle placement (*arrowheads*) in the distal UCL (*arrows*) for platelet-rich plasma injection.

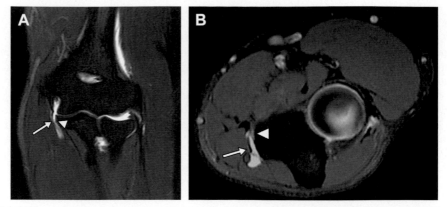

Fig. 7. Partial-thickness distal ulnar collateral ligament (UCL) tear in a 21-year-old football quarterback. (*A*) Coronal T2 fat suppression (FS) arthrogram and (*B*) axial T1 FS arthrogram images of the "T-sign" in the form of arthrogram solution separating the distal UCL (*arrow*) and sublime tubercle (*arrowhead*). PRP, platelet-rich plasma.

MR imaging "abnormalities" in the UCL may represent an adaptive change related to chronic repetitive forces of throwing or overhead sports.[80] For example, Kooima and colleagues[81] found that UCL changes, such as thickening, signal heterogeneity, or even discontinuity, were present on MR imaging in the dominant elbow of 87% (14/16) of asymptomatic professional baseball pitchers (**Fig. 9**C). Throwing athletes may also develop asymptomatic degenerative calcification or heterotopic ossification within the UCL from chronic repetitive stress.

Ultrasound imaging

Musculoskeletal US may be an effective complementary tool for diagnosing UCL tears. Advantages of US are its high resolution, dynamic capability, and the ability to compare findings with the asymptomatic side.[59]

To image the anterior band of the UCL, the elbow should be placed in 30° of flexion with the proximal portion of the probe over the medial epicondyle. The somewhat broader and multi-fibrillar proximal attachment as well as the distal attachment on the sublime tubercle are better appreciated on US owing to the increased spatial resolution (**Fig. 5**C, D).[82] Anisotropy can be used to the operator's benefit to better differentiate the ligament from adjacent structures.[59]

Both De Smet and colleagues[83] and Wood and colleagues[84] showed that the added dynamic capability of US to demonstrate medial joint instability during valgus stress imaging could reliably identify UCL tears as accurately as MR imaging

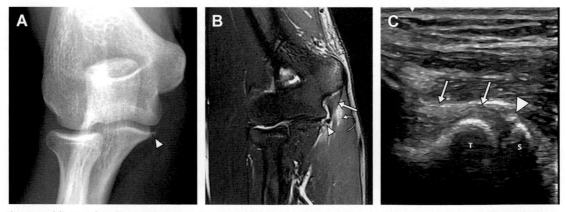

Fig. 8. Sublime tubercle avulsion in a 17-year-old javelin athlete. (*A*) Anteroposterior elbow radiograph shows acute avulsion fracture of the sublime tubercle (*arrowhead*). (*B*) Coronal T2 fat suppression MR image and (*C*) long axis ultrasound image shows an intact proximal ulnar collateral ligament (*arrows*) and distal sublime tubercle avulsion (*arrowhead*). Feathery edema from strain is seen in the flexor pronator mass on the MR image (*curved arrow*). S, sublime tubercle; T, trochlea.

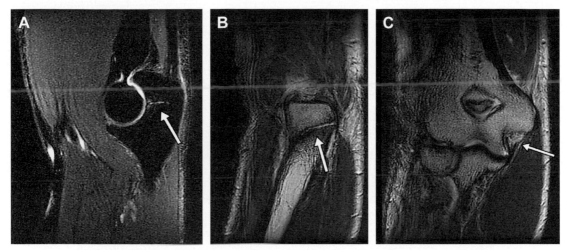

Fig. 9. Olecranon stress fracture nonunion in a 33-year-old professional baseball pitcher. (*A*) Sagittal T2 fat suppression and (*B*) coronal T2 sequences demonstrate a linear olecranon fracture with surrounding marrow edema. (*C*) Coronal T2 image of the same player shows a thickened ulnar collateral ligament (*arrow*) with intermediate signal compatible with chronic attenuation, probably predisposing this player to olecranon stress injury. (*Courtesy of* Tim Sanders, MD, Medical Director NationalRad.)

in collegiate-level baseball pitchers (**Fig. 10**). Miller and colleagues[85] later showed that US can detect UCL tears accurately, even without dynamic stress. Complete UCL rupture manifests on US imaging as an anechoic fluid gap in the normally hyperechoic fibrillary ligament or as heterogeneous hypoechoic tissue in the expected location of the ligament. Medial epicondyle avulsions may show a detached echogenic bony fragment. Sprain manifests as thickening and decreased echogenicity of the injured ligament often with surrounding hypoechoic edema. Partial thickness tears of the distal ligament often present as anechoic fluid between the deep surface of the ligament and ulnar attachment (**Fig. 6B**).[85] Asymmetrical widening of the ulnohumeral joint compared with the normal contralateral side during valgus stress imaging correlates with tear of the deep UCL layer described by Timmerman and Andrews[78] (**Fig. 11**).

Similar to MR imaging, US can detect chronic changes in UCL morphology in overhead throwing athletes. Multiple studies have looked at the UCL in asymptomatic collegiate and professional baseball players. These studies show consistently that the UCL in the dominant elbow is thicker, more likely to have hypoechoic foci and/or calcifications, and more lax, with valgus stress than the nondominant elbow. Importantly, dynamic US indicated that these athletes may demonstrate increased joint space gapping with stress over time.[86–88] In contrast with conventional US and MR imaging, which depend on the direct visualization of tears, stress US can diagnose an

insufficient UCL indirectly by measuring UCL laxity and compare it with the contralateral side.[86] UCL tears may not be directly visible on US or MR imaging when they are too small, filled with granulation tissue, or obscured by artifacts like ligament calcifications. In these situations, increased UCL laxity can help in making the diagnosis by measuring the widening of the ulnotrochlear joint and by comparing it with the contralateral uninjured elbow. The feasibility of stress US has initially been described by the group at Thomas Jefferson University by Nazarian and colleagues.[86] Subsequently, a prospective study from the same group on asymptomatic professional baseball pitchers by Ciccotti and colleagues[87] showed that the UCL in the dominant elbow has increased laxity with stress US over time compared with the contralateral elbow. However, baseball players evaluated in that study did not have UCL tears at the time of the US examination. The most recent study (in press) from the Thomas Jefferson group by Roedl and colleagues[88] shows that relative gapping (relative to the contralateral elbow) of more than 1.5 mm yields a sensitivity of 81% and a specificity of 91%. Full-thickness tears resulted in a mean increase of joint gapping by 3.3 mm.

Recent studies have tried to elucidate the natural history of chronic UCL changes in adolescent athletes. Marshall and colleagues[89] showed that preseason US examination of high school pitchers lacked the chronic adaptive changes seen in professional pitchers. But stresses from only one season of pitching can create these changes in multiple structures about the elbow, including

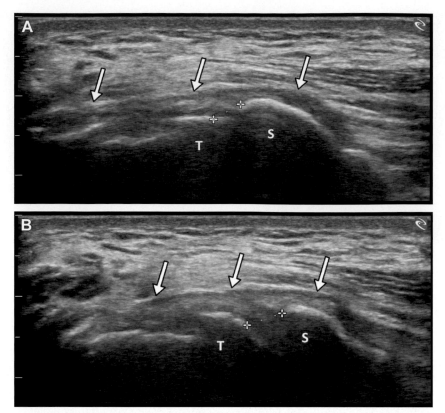

Fig. 10. Recurrent partial thickness tear of the reconstructed ulnar collateral ligament (UCL) graft in a baseball pitcher. Dynamic ultrasound assessment demonstrates ulnotrochlear joint space widening (calipers) between the (*A*) nonstressed and (*B*) stressed images of the anterior band UCL (*arrows*). S, sublime tubercle; T, trochlea. (*Courtesy of* Adam Zoga, MD, Thomas Jefferson University, Philadelphia.)

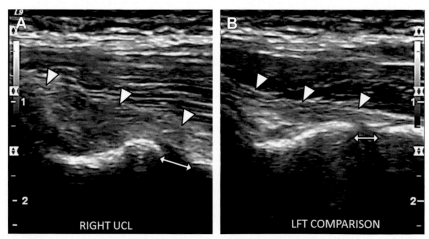

Fig. 11. Partial thickness anterior bundle ulnar collateral ligament (UCL) tear in a 17-year-old pitcher. Long axis ultrasound of the injured right elbow (*A*) shows a thickened, hypoechoic UCL (*arrowheads*) and greater than 2 mm of gapping of the medial joint space (*double-head arrow*) compared with the normal left (*B*) UCL. (*From* Lee KS, Tuite MJ, Rosas HG. Elbow injuries in sports: essentials for radiologists and clinicians. In: Robinson P, editors. Essential radiology for sports medicine. New York; Dordrecht (Netherlands); Heidelberg (Germany); London: Springer; 2010. p. 132; with permission of Springer Science + Business Media.)

UCL heterogeneity and thickening, increased ulnohumeral joint space laxity, and enlargement of the ulnar nerve.[90] Atanda and colleagues[91] showed that UCL thickening may be one of the first changes to develop in young professional baseball pitchers.

Treatment

Nonoperative treatment for UCL injuries can have acceptable results in low demand patient populations.[66] Conservative management has even proven effective for low-grade partial tears in some baseball players.[92] However, Rettig and colleagues[93] found only 42% of throwing athletes with a UCL tear were able to return to play after 3 months of rest and rehabilitation. As outlined, PRP is theorized to improve the tissue healing environment and decrease healing time in various tendons and ligaments throughout the body

(**Fig. 6C**). Podesta and colleagues[94] noted encouraging results in patients with partial thickness UCL tears that were treated with PRP injection under US guidance (**Fig. 12**). Of 34 athletes, 30 (88%) returned to the same level of asymptomatic play in an average of 12 weeks. Objectively, medial elbow joint space opening with valgus stress also decreased.[94] This substantially shorter return to play period and alternative to season-ending surgery may seem appealing, but more studies are required to determine the long-term outcome before definitive recommendations can be made.

Operative UCL treatment is indicated for the overhead athlete with a complete tear or partial thickness tear that has failed a comprehensive rehabilitation program. Primary repair of the torn UCL is considered in young athletes and in the case of acute avulsion injury,[95,96] but ligament reconstruction is now the standard of care for most acute and chronic UCL injuries in adult

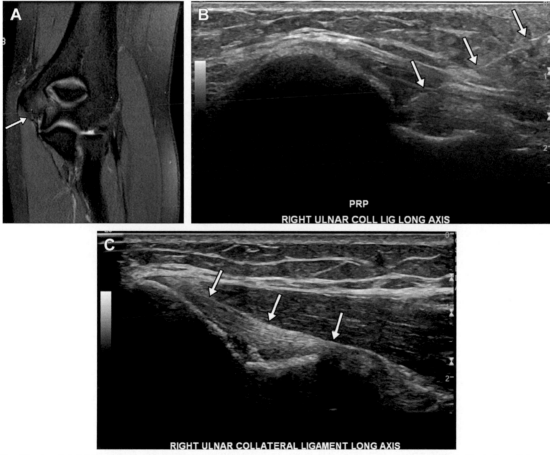

Fig. 12. Partial thickness proximal ulnar collateral ligament (UCL) tear in an 18-year-old baseball pitcher. (*A*) Coronal T2 fat suppression image of a partial thickness proximal UCL tear (*arrow*). (*B*) Long axis ultrasound (US) image of platelet-rich plasma (PRP) injection (*arrows*) in the proximal UCL. (*C*) Long axis routine follow-up US of the UCL (*arrows*) 16 weeks after PRP therapy.

overhead athletes.[66,68] The surgical procedure centers on restoration of the anterior band with the use of an autologous free tendon graft. Since the original report by Jobe and colleagues,[97] numerous technical refinements for UCL reconstruction have been proposed, and the popularity of the procedure has grown steadily. The main differences between techniques involve variation in ulnar nerve transposition, graft configuration, and how the graft is attached to the ulna and medial epicondyle.[1,66,98] The overall rate of return to play is approximately 79% to 83% and transient ulnar neuropraxia is the most commonly reported complication.[63,99]

Postoperative Imaging

Although excellent results have been reported in UCL reconstruction,[100] retears of the reconstruction graft do occur. Most surgeons prefer MR arthrogram for postoperative graft evaluation over routine MR imaging. The intraarticular contrast distends the joint and can insinuate between torn fibers thus, facilitating distinction between a heterogeneous graft with granulation tissue and a true tear. In addition to assessing the graft, intraarticular contrast can be helpful to characterize other causes of elbow pain including intraarticular bodies and osteochondral injury.

In general, most surgical permutations in UCL reconstruction have a similar appearance on MR imaging. The reconstructed ligament is considerably larger than the native UCL because it typically constitutes a looped length (double bundle) of graft that is subsequently sewn together. In addition, the native UCL is usually not excised but left in place and sutured for extra stability. The proximal attachment of the graft is much broader than the native UCL and thus should not be confused with common flexor pathology. Although the graft may be thickened on postoperative imaging, it should be taut. If the graft seems to be wavy, it may be lax and functionally insufficient, particularly in flexion.[101] With regard to postoperative graft signal, Wear and colleagues[101] found that approximately 70% (29/41) of normal intact UCL grafts demonstrated homogeneously low signal on both T1- and T2-weighted images (**Fig. 13A–E**). Intermediate T1 or intermediate to high T2 signal was noted within the remaining intact grafts and was most commonly seen proximally.

Diagnosis of large grafts tears is typically straightforward with visualization of a discrete disruption of the graft fibers and high T2 fluid signal or intraarticular contrast in the graft on T1 arthrogram sequences. Contrast leakage outside the joint capsule is suggestive of a full-thickness graft tear. Smaller tears may not show discrete disruption of the fibers, but rather a striated intraligamentous signal on T1 sequences owing to subtle imbibition of contrast into the torn fibers.[101] One important distinction in assessing the native UCL versus the reconstructed graft is interpretation of the "T-sign" or contrast extension between the distal graft and sublime tubercle. Although this finding may indicate partial distal tear of the native UCL, it does not necessarily apply in the postoperative patient, because the ulnar tunnels for the reconstruction graft are typically placed 3 to 4 mm distal to the articular surface.[101]

POSTEROMEDIAL OSSEOUS IMPINGEMENT

Posteromedial elbow pain in overhead sport athletes is a common phenomenon.[1] Repetitive stress of overhead throwing and the often accompanying progressive medial elbow laxity can lead to excessive shear forces in the posterior elbow.[81,102] This stress often results in impingement of the posteromedial tip of the olecranon process on the medial wall of the olecranon fossa. Over time, this impingement leads to osteophyte formation on the posteromedial tip of the olecranon and associated synovitis.[103] Throwers typically complain of posterior elbow pain, particularly at release, rather than at the onset of arm acceleration as is seen with UCL pathology.[102] On physical examination they present with posteromedial olecranon tenderness and reproducible pain, particularly in terminal extension while applying a valgus stress to the elbow. This motion correlates with the deceleration or follow-through phase of throwing.[103] Valgus extension overload syndrome is the name for the clinical condition corresponding with the aforementioned radiologic findings.[102]

Radiographs may be negative in early disease but usually reveal a posteromedial olecranon osteophyte or loose body.[102] On MR imaging, a pathology pattern includes osteochondral changes to the posterior trochlea and anteromedial olecranon along with posteromedial gutter synovitis.[104] On T2-weighted sequences, the findings range from an abnormal edemalike signal in the hyaline cartilage (grade 1 chondrosis) to partial thickness cartilage defects with subchondral marrow edema (grade 2 or 3 chondrosis).[104] Posteromedial olecranon fossa and olecranon tip osteophytes are often seen on T1-weighted imaging and CT scan (**Fig. 14**). These osteophytes may subsequently fracture leading to intraarticular bodies, best seen on MR arthrogram or in the setting of joint effusion. MR arthrogram may also reveal posteromedial recess synovitis and

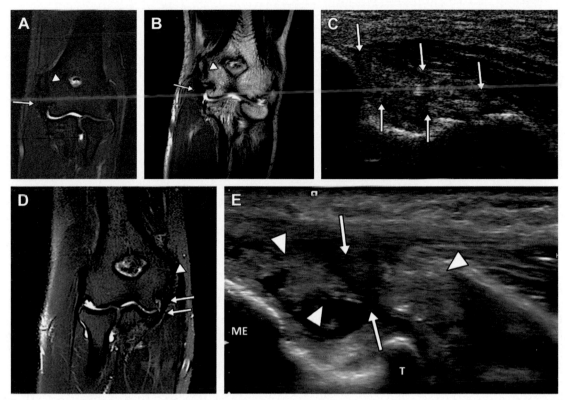

Fig. 13. Professional baseball pitchers with a history of Tommy John surgery. (*A*) Coronal T2 fat suppression (FS) arthrogram and (*B*) coronal T1 arthrogram sequences show changes of ulnar collateral ligament (UCL) reconstruction with a thick but hypointense graft (*arrow*) and fixation tunnel in the medial epicondyle (*arrowhead*). (*C*) Ultrasound (US) image of an intact UCL graft (*arrows*) in a different patient. The graft seems to be thicker and more hyperechoic compared with a native UCL. (*D*) Coronal T2 FS arthrogram image in a different patient shows changes of UCL reconstruction with an intact graft (*arrows* and *arrowhead*). (*E*) US of the same patient after acute injury shows an anechoic fluid cleft (*arrows*) within the UCL graft (*arrowheads*) consistent with a full-thickness graft tear. (*Courtesy of* [*E*] Patricia Delzell, MD, Cleveland Clinic, Cleveland, OH.)

adjacent soft tissue edema.[104] In a recent study by Roedl and colleagues[88] from the group at Thomas Jefferson University, 48 of 144 baseball players undergoing surgery or arthroscopy for medial elbow pain were found to have posteromedial elbow impingement. MR arthrography had a sensitivity, specificity, and accuracy of 94% (45/48), 98% (94/96), and 97% (139/144), respectively, for diagnosing posteromedial impingement. In addition to the typical findings of Valgus extension overload syndrome, it is important to look for associated conditions, such as chronic UCL pathology or findings of ulnar neuritis.[81] As mentioned, most repetitive throwing athletes have chronic UCL

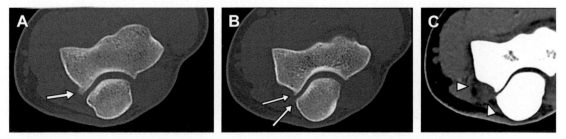

Fig. 14. Posteromedial impingement in a 22-year-old college football quarterback. Axial noncontrast computed tomography images show (*A, B*) early posteromedial olecranon and trochlear osteophyte formation (*arrows*) and (*C*) associated synovitis (*arrowheads*).

changes on MR imaging, often with accompanying laxity. In these instances, the clinical history and physical examination are critical to the proper diagnosis and treatment. The presence of these conditions may alter surgical planning to return the athlete to competitive play successfully.[102] Treatment typically includes minimally invasive or arthroscopic surgery for osteophyte resection and chondral debridement.

OLECRANON STRESS FRACTURE

Osseous stress response at the shoulder and elbow[105,106] and olecranon stress fractures (OSF)[107] are especially seen in younger athletes and in overhead sports, such as baseball, tennis, weightlifting, and gymnastics.[107] Forced extension can result in excessive tensile stress from the triceps tendon and posterior impingement of the olecranon against the olecranon fossa.[102] Repetitive injury can lead to olecranon stress reaction or fracture. OSF presents clinically as insidious posterior olecranon pain that may occur during or after throwing. Localized tenderness is typically more distal and lateral on the olecranon versus the posteromedial pain in valgus extension overload syndrome.[102] Because the frequency of OSF is low (only about 5% of baseball-related elbow disorders), it can be missed during clinical examination.[107] There is a high prevalence (71%–95%) of concomitant medial UCL injuries, suggesting it may be a major risk factor for OSF development.[107]

In adolescent throwers, olecranon injuries present as delayed closure and nonunion of the epiphyseal plate.[107] The most common adult-type OSFs present as on oblique fracture arising from the middle third of the olecranon articular surface coursing proximally or distally toward the dorsal cortex.[107] On CT scan, the typical fracture pattern is a linear lucency, often with surrounding sclerotic reparative bone, perpendicular to the long axis of the olecranon. MR imaging can assist in the diagnosis of stress reaction, demonstrating high signal in the olecranon marrow on fluid-sensitive sequences. When stress reaction progresses to fracture, an irregular hypointense line with surrounding marrow edema is noted (**Fig. 9**A, B).[55]

ULNAR NEURITIS

Ulnar neuritis can be an isolated or concurrent cause of medial sided elbow pain. Many athletes with valgus instability and symptoms of medial epicondylosis also tend to have ulnar nerve symptoms.[76] Forty percent of patients with UCL instability also develop ulnar nerve traction injury.[8] Other causes include posteromedial osteophytes, flexor–pronator muscle hypertrophy, an accessory anconeus epitrochlearis, and congenital subluxation of the nerve.[55,108]

MR imaging and US are useful for evaluation of ulnar neuritis. On MR imaging, nerves are normally low to intermediate signal intensity on all pulse sequences.[108] Nerve inflammation results in enlargement and hyperintense signal on fluid sensitive sequences (**Fig. 15**A).[108] Caution is required; a recent study demonstrated isolated high signal in the ulnar nerve in 60% of asymptomatic individuals.[109] In a recent study[88] (online, ahead of print) by Roedl and colleagues, 31 of 144 baseball players presenting with medial elbow pain had ulnar neuritis. The most accurate size threshold to predict ulnar neuritis with MR imaging was 10 mm². Defining ulnar neuritis as increased signal intensity and size greater than 10 mm², MR arthrography had a sensitivity, specificity, and accuracy of 74% (23/31), 92% (104/113), and 88% (127/144), respectively. For conventional US,

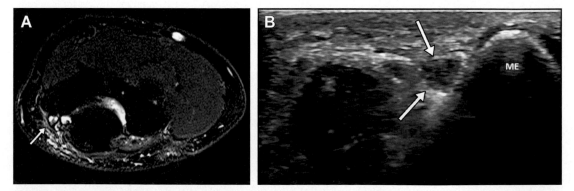

Fig. 15. Ulnar neuritis in a 19-year-old baseball pitcher related to neuropraxia and medial elbow instability. (*A*) Axial T2 fat suppression image shows increased caliber and signal hyperintensity in the ulnar nerve (*arrow*) within the cubital tunnel. (*B*) Transverse ultrasound image of the ulnar nerve shows a similar enlargement and hypoechogenicity of the nerve (*arrows*). ME, medial epicondyle.

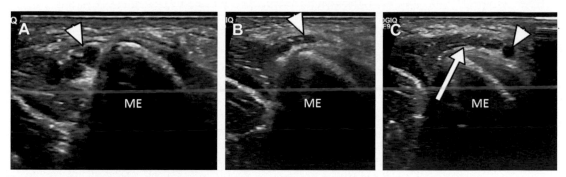

Fig. 16. Ultrasound (US) images of ulnar nerve subluxation. (*A–C*) Transverse US images of the cubital tunnel show progressive subluxation of the ulnar nerve (*arrowhead*) and medial head of the triceps muscle (*arrow*) over the medial epicondyle as the elbow moves dynamically from (*A*) extension to (*C*) flexion.

greater than 9 mm² was the most accurate threshold to predict ulnar neuritis with a sensitivity, specificity, and accuracy of 94% (29/31), 74% (84/113), and 79% (113/144), respectively. A logistic regression analysis with ulnar neuritis as the dependent variable and with MR signal intensity, nerve size on MR imaging, nerve size on conventional US, and ulnar nerve subluxation as independent variables showed that the combination of nerve size on US, subluxation, and MR imaging signal was the best predictor of ulnar neuritis. Based on this combined model, ulnar neuritis was defined as increased nerve size on US (>9 mm²) and either subluxation on US or increased signal intensity on MR imaging. This combined approach had a sensitivity, specificity and accuracy of 90% (28/31), 100% (113/113), and 98% (141/144), respectively. Compared with MR arthrography alone, the combined approach did not increase sensitivity significantly (*P* = .07; McNemar), but did increase specificity (*P*<.001) and accuracy 98% (*P*<.001). Compared with conventional US alone, the combined approach did not increase sensitivity (*P*>.999; McNemar), but did increase specificity (*P*<.001) and accuracy (*P*<.001). Ultimately, ulnar nerve transposition was performed in 12 of the 31 patients with ulnar neuritis.

In cases of denervation injury, MR imaging may show feathery T2 hyperintense edema or T1 hyperintense fatty atrophy in the flexor digitorum profundus, flexor carpi ulnaris muscles, or intrinsic musculature of the hand.[55]

High-resolution US is also a useful focused imaging tool for ulnar neuritis.[108] The normal US appearance of the nerve is that of hypoechoic nerve fascicles separated by echogenic perineurium septae resulting in a "honeycomb" appearance. A normal nerve is hyperechoic compared with muscle but hypoechoic compared with tendon. In cases of entrapment, the nerve may become enlarged, edematous, and hypoechoic proximal to the site of entrapment.[110] Long axis extended field-of-view technique can be helpful to discern the area of nerve caliber change.[8] Neuropraxic injury presents as a swollen hypoechoic nerve (**Fig. 15B**). US is capable of continuous visualization of the ulnar nerve during dynamic maneuvers. Elbow flexion may provoke subluxation or dislocation of the nerve from the cubital tunnel and over the medial epicondyle.[8] It can be accompanied by pain and an audible "snap" and is often accompanied by dislocation of the medial head of the triceps muscle, also known as snapping triceps syndrome (**Fig. 16A–C**).[111]

SUMMARY

Forces acting on the elbow in the overhead throwing motion can lead to chronic overuse and acute injuries to tendons, ligaments, bones or nerves. Various imaging methods can supplement history and physical examination to establish a diagnosis or guide treatment. US-guided injection therapies are an emerging treatment option, but more studies are needed to determine their long-term efficacy.

REFERENCES

1. Cain EL Jr, Dugas JR, Wolf RS, et al. Elbow injuries in throwing athletes: a current concepts review. Am J Sports Med 2003;31(4):621–35.
2. Frick MA, Murthy NS. Imaging of the elbow: muscle and tendon injuries. Semin Musculoskelet Radiol 2010;14(4):430–7.
3. Walz DM, Newman JS, Konin GP, et al. Epicondylitis: pathogenesis, imaging, and treatment. Radiographics 2010;30(1):167–84.
4. Nirschl RP, Pettrone FA. Tennis elbow. The surgical treatment of lateral epicondylitis. J Bone Joint Surg Am 1979;61(6A):832–9.

5. Chiavaras MM, Jacobson JA. Ultrasound-guided tendon fenestration. Semin Musculoskelet Radiol 2013;17(1):85–90.

6. Pitzer ME, Seidenberg PH, Bader DA. Elbow tendinopathy. Med Clin North Am 2014;98(4):833–49, xiii.

7. Potter HG, Hannafin JA, Morwessel RM, et al. Lateral epicondylitis: correlation of MR imaging, surgical, and histopathologic findings. Radiology 1995;196(1):43–6.

8. Lee KS, Rosas HG, Craig JG. Musculoskeletal ultrasound: elbow imaging and procedures. Semin Musculoskelet Radiol 2010;14(4):449–60.

9. Jobe FW, Ciccotti MG. Lateral and medial epicondylitis of the elbow. J Am Acad Orthop Surg 1994;2(1):1–8.

10. Martin CE, Schweitzer ME. MR imaging of epicondylitis. Skeletal Radiol 1998;27(3):133–8.

11. Lee KS. Musculoskeletal sonography of the tendon. J Ultrasound Med 2012;31(12):1879–84.

12. Lee MH, Cha JG, Jin W, et al. Utility of sonographic measurement of the common tensor tendon in patients with lateral epicondylitis. AJR Am J Roentgenol 2011;196(6):1363–7.

13. Levin D, Nazarian LN, Miller TT, et al. Lateral epicondylitis of the elbow: US findings. Radiology 2005;237(1):230–4.

14. Miller TT, Shapiro MA, Schultz E, et al. Comparison of sonography and MRI for diagnosing epicondylitis. J Clin Ultrasound 2002;30(4):193–202.

15. Chourasia AO, Buhr KA, Rabago DP, et al. Relationships between biomechanics, tendon pathology, and function in individuals with lateral epicondylosis. J Orthop Sports Phys Ther 2013; 43(6):368–78.

16. Dones VC 3rd, Grimmer K, Thoirs K, et al. The diagnostic validity of musculoskeletal ultrasound in lateral epicondylalgia: a systematic review. BMC Med Imaging 2014;14:10.

17. De Zordo T, Lill SR, Fink C, et al. Real-time sonoelastography of lateral epicondylitis: comparison of findings between patients and healthy volunteers. AJR Am J Roentgenol 2009;193(1):180–5.

18. Ljung BO, Alfredson H, Forsgren S. Neurokinin 1-receptors and sensory neuropeptides in tendon insertions at the medial and lateral epicondyles of the humerus. Studies on tennis elbow and medial epicondylalgia. J Orthop Res 2004;22(2):321–7.

19. Coombes BK, Bisset L, Vicenzino B. Efficacy and safety of corticosteroid injections and other injections for management of tendinopathy: a systematic review of randomised controlled trials. Lancet 2010;376(9754):1751–67.

20. Smidt N, van der Windt DA, Assendelft WJ, et al. Corticosteroid injections, physiotherapy, or a wait-and-see policy for lateral epicondylitis: a randomised controlled trial. Lancet 2002;359(9307):657–62.

21. Krogh TP, Bartels EM, Ellingsen T, et al. Comparative effectiveness of injection therapies in lateral epicondylitis: a systematic review and network meta-analysis of randomized controlled trials. Am J Sports Med 2013;41(6):1435–46.

22. Coombes BK, Bisset L, Brooks P, et al. Effect of corticosteroid injection, physiotherapy, or both on clinical outcomes in patients with unilateral lateral epicondylalgia: a randomized controlled trial. JAMA 2013;309(5):461–9.

23. Mishra AK, Skrepnik NV, Edwards SG, et al. Efficacy of platelet-rich plasma for chronic tennis elbow: a double-blind, prospective, multicenter, randomized controlled trial of 230 patients. Am J Sports Med 2014;42(2):463–71.

24. Sims SE, Miller K, Elfar JC, et al. Non-surgical treatment of lateral epicondylitis: a systematic review of randomized controlled trials. Hand (N Y) 2014;9(4): 419–46.

25. Lee KS, Wilson JJ, Rabago DP, et al. Musculoskeletal applications of platelet-rich plasma: fad or future? AJR Am J Roentgenol 2011;196(3):628–36.

26. Foster TE, Puskas BL, Mandelbaum BR, et al. Platelet-rich plasma: from basic science to clinical applications. Am J Sports Med 2009;37(11): 2259–72.

27. Davidson J, Jayaraman S. Guided interventions in musculoskeletal ultrasound: what's the evidence? Clin Radiol 2011;66(2):140–52.

28. Housner JA, Jacobson JA, Misko R. Sonographically guided percutaneous needle tenotomy for the treatment of chronic tendinosis. J Ultrasound Med 2009;28(9):1187–92.

29. McShane JM, Nazarian LN, Harwood MI. Sonographically guided percutaneous needle tenotomy for treatment of common extensor tendinosis in the elbow. J Ultrasound Med 2006;25(10):1281–9.

30. McShane JM, Shah VN, Nazarian LN. Sonographically guided percutaneous needle tenotomy for treatment of common extensor tendinosis in the elbow: is a corticosteroid necessary? J Ultrasound Med 2008;27(8):1137–44.

31. Rabago D, Best TM, Beamsley M, et al. A systematic review of prolotherapy for chronic musculoskeletal pain. Clin J Sport Med 2005; 15(5):376–80.

32. Scarpone M, Rabago DP, Zgierska A, et al. The efficacy of prolotherapy for lateral epicondylosis: a pilot study. Clin J Sport Med 2008;18(3):248–54.

33. Dong W, Goost H, Lin XB, et al. Injection therapies for lateral epicondylalgia: a systematic review and Bayesian network meta-analysis. Br J Sports Med 2015;1–10.

34. Rabago D, Lee KS, Ryan M, et al. Hypertonic dextrose and morrhuate sodium injections (prolotherapy) for lateral epicondylosis (tennis elbow): results of a single-blind, pilot-level, randomized

controlled trial. Am J Phys Med Rehabil 2013;92(7): 587–96.

35. Rabago D, Best TM, Zgierska AE, et al. A systematic review of four injection therapies for lateral epicondylosis: prolotherapy, polidocanol, whole blood and platelet-rich plasma. Br J Sports Med 2009;43(7):471–81.

36. Paoloni J, De Vos RJ, Hamilton B, et al. Platelet-rich plasma treatment for ligament and tendon injuries. Clin J Sport Med 2011;21(1):37–45.

37. Hsu WK, Mishra A, Rodeo SR, et al. Platelet-rich plasma in orthopaedic applications: evidence-based recommendations for treatment. J Am Acad Orthop Surg 2013;21(12):739–48.

38. Mishra A, Harmon K, Woodall J, et al. Sports medicine applications of platelet rich plasma. Curr Pharm Biotechnol 2012;13(7):1185–95.

39. DeLong JM, Russell RP, Mazzocca AD. Platelet-rich plasma: the PAW classification system. Arthroscopy 2012;28(7):998–1009.

40. Moraes VY, Lenza M, Tamaoki MJ, et al. Platelet-rich therapies for musculoskeletal soft tissue injuries. Cochrane Database Syst Rev 2014;(4):CD010071.

41. Mishra A, Pavelko T. Treatment of chronic elbow tendinosis with buffered platelet-rich plasma. Am J Sports Med 2006;34(11):1774–8.

42. Peerbooms JC, Sluimer J, Bruijn DJ, et al. Positive effect of an autologous platelet concentrate in lateral epicondylitis in a double-blind randomized controlled trial: platelet-rich plasma versus corticosteroid injection with a 1-year follow-up. Am J Sports Med 2010;38(2):255–62.

43. Gosens T, Peerbooms JC, van Laar W, et al. Ongoing positive effect of platelet-rich plasma versus corticosteroid injection in lateral epicondylitis: a double-blind randomized controlled trial with 2-year follow-up. Am J Sports Med 2011;39(6): 1200–8.

44. Wolf JM, Ozer K, Scott F, et al. Comparison of autologous blood, corticosteroid, and saline injection in the treatment of lateral epicondylitis: a prospective, randomized, controlled multicenter study. J Hand Surg Am 2011;36(8):1269–72.

45. de Vos RJ, Windt J, Weir A. Strong evidence against platelet-rich plasma injections for chronic lateral epicondylar tendinopathy: a systematic review. Br J Sports Med 2014;48(12):952–6.

46. Thanasas C, Papadimitriou G, Charalambidis C, et al. Platelet-rich plasma versus autologous whole blood for the treatment of chronic lateral elbow epicondylitis: a randomized controlled clinical trial. Am J Sports Med 2011;39(10):2130–4.

47. Creaney L, Wallace A, Curtis M, et al. Growth factor-based therapies provide additional benefit beyond physical therapy in resistant elbow tendinopathy: a prospective, single-blind, randomised trial of autologous blood injections versus platelet-rich plasma injections. Br J Sports Med 2011;45(12):966–71.

48. Glanzmann MC, Audige L. Platelet-rich plasma for chronic lateral epicondylitis: is one injection sufficient? Arch Orthop Trauma Surg 2015;135(12). 1637–45.

49. Chiavaras MM, Jacobson JA, Carlos R, et al. IMpact of Platelet Rich plasma OVer alternative therapies in patients with lateral Epicondylitis (IMPROVE): protocol for a multicenter randomized controlled study: a multicenter, randomized trial comparing autologous platelet-rich plasma, autologous whole blood, dry needle tendon fenestration, and physical therapy exercises alone on pain and quality of life in patients with lateral epicondylitis. Acad Radiol 2014;21(9):1144–55.

50. Chaudhury S, de La Lama M, Adler RS, et al. Platelet-rich plasma for the treatment of lateral epicondylitis: sonographic assessment of tendon morphology and vascularity (pilot study). Skeletal Radiol 2013;42(1):91–7.

51. Finnoff JT, Fowler SP, Lai JK, et al. Treatment of chronic tendinopathy with ultrasound-guided needle tenotomy and platelet-rich plasma injection. PM R 2011;3(10):900–11.

52. Bredella MA, Tirman PF, Fritz RC, et al. MR imaging findings of lateral ulnar collateral ligament abnormalities in patients with lateral epicondylitis. AJR Am J Roentgenol 1999;173(5):1379–82.

53. Ford RD, Schmitt WP, Lineberry K, et al. A retrospective comparison of the management of recalcitrant lateral elbow tendinosis: platelet-rich plasma injections versus surgery. Hand (N Y) 2015;10(2):285–91.

54. Mishra A, Pirolo JM, Gosens T. Treatment of medial epicondylar tendinopathy in athletes. Sports Med Arthrosc 2014;22(3):164–8.

55. Wenzke DR. MR imaging of the elbow in the injured athlete. Radiol Clin North Am 2013;51(2): 195–213.

56. Kancherla VK, Caggiano NM, Matullo KS. Elbow injuries in the throwing athlete. Orthop Clin North Am 2014;45(4):571–85.

57. Kijowski R, De Smet AA. Magnetic resonance imaging findings in patients with medial epicondylitis. Skeletal Radiol 2005;34(4):196–202.

58. Park GY, Lee SM, Lee MY. Diagnostic value of ultrasonography for clinical medial epicondylitis. Arch Phys Med Rehabil 2008;89(4):738–42.

59. De Maeseneer M, Brigido MK, Antic M, et al. Ultrasound of the elbow with emphasis on detailed assessment of ligaments, tendons, and nerves. Eur J Radiol 2015;84(4):671–81.

60. Konin GP, Nazarian LN, Walz DM. US of the elbow: indications, technique, normal anatomy, and pathologic conditions. Radiographics 2013;33(4): E125–47.

61. Shahid M, Wu F, Deshmukh SC. Operative treatment improves patient function in recalcitrant medial epicondylitis. Ann R Coll Surg Engl 2013; 95(7):486–8.

62. Ciccotti MC, Schwartz MA, Ciccotti MG. Diagnosis and treatment of medial epicondylitis of the elbow. Clin Sports Med 2004;23(4):693–705, xi.

63. Cain EL Jr, Andrews JR, Dugas JR, et al. Outcome of ulnar collateral ligament reconstruction of the elbow in 1281 athletes: results in 743 athletes with minimum 2-year follow-up. Am J Sports Med 2010;38(12):2426–34.

64. Erickson BJ, Harris JD, Chalmers PN, et al. Ulnar collateral ligament reconstruction: anatomy, indications, techniques, and outcomes. Sports Health 2015;7(6):511–7.

65. Farrow LD, Mahoney AJ, Stefancin JJ, et al. Quantitative analysis of the medial ulnar collateral ligament ulnar footprint and its relationship to the ulnar sublime tubercle. Am J Sports Med 2011; 39(9):1936–41.

66. Dugas J, Chronister J, Cain EL Jr, et al. Ulnar collateral ligament in the overhead athlete: a current review. Sports Med Arthrosc 2014;22(3):169–82.

67. Dugas JR, Ostrander RV, Cain EL, et al. Anatomy of the anterior bundle of the ulnar collateral ligament. J Shoulder Elbow Surg 2007;16(5):657–60.

68. Bruce JR, Andrews JR. Ulnar collateral ligament injuries in the throwing athlete. J Am Acad Orthop Surg 2014;22(5):315–25.

69. Regan WD, Korinek SL, Morrey BF, et al. Biomechanical study of ligaments around the elbow joint. Clin Orthop Relat Res 1991;271:170–9.

70. O'Driscoll SW, Lawton RL, Smith AM. The "moving valgus stress test" for medial collateral ligament tears of the elbow. Am J Sports Med 2005;33(2): 231–9.

71. Timmerman LA, Schwartz ML, Andrews JR. Preoperative evaluation of the ulnar collateral ligament by magnetic resonance imaging and computed tomography arthrography. Evaluation in 25 baseball players with surgical confirmation. Am J Sports Med 1994;22(1):26–31 [discussion: 32].

72. Schwartz ML, al-Zahrani S, Morwessel RM, et al. Ulnar collateral ligament injury in the throwing athlete: evaluation with saline-enhanced MR arthrography. Radiology 1995;197(1):297–9.

73. Carrino JA, Morrison WB, Zou KH, et al. Noncontrast MR imaging and MR arthrography of the ulnar collateral ligament of the elbow: prospective evaluation of two-dimensional pulse sequences for detection of complete tears. Skeletal Radiol 2001; 30(11):625–32.

74. Magee T. Accuracy of 3-T MR arthrography versus conventional 3-T MRI of elbow tendons and ligaments compared with surgery. AJR Am J Roentgenol 2015;204(1):W70–5.

75. Munshi M, Pretterklieber ML, Chung CB, et al. Anterior bundle of ulnar collateral ligament: evaluation of anatomic relationships by using MR imaging, MR arthrography, and gross anatomic and histologic analysis. Radiology 2004;231(3): 797–803.

76. Ouellette H, Bredella M, Labis J, et al. MR imaging of the elbow in baseball pitchers. Skeletal Radiol 2008;37(2):115–21.

77. Conway JE, Jobe FW, Glousman RE, et al. Medial instability of the elbow in throwing athletes. Treatment by repair or reconstruction of the ulnar collateral ligament. J Bone Joint Surg Am 1992;74(1): 67–83.

78. Timmerman LA, Andrews JR. Undersurface tear of the ulnar collateral ligament in baseball players. A newly recognized lesion. Am J Sports Med 1994; 22(1):33–6.

79. Salvo JP, Rizio L 3rd, Zvijac JE, et al. Avulsion fracture of the ulnar sublime tubercle in overhead throwing athletes. Am J Sports Med 2002;30(3): 426–31.

80. Del Grande F, Aro M, Farahani SJ, et al. Three-Tesla MR imaging of the elbow in non-symptomatic professional baseball pitchers. Skeletal Radiol 2015; 44(1):115–23.

81. Kooima CL, Anderson K, Craig JV, et al. Evidence of subclinical medial collateral ligament injury and posteromedial impingement in professional baseball players. Am J Sports Med 2004;32(7):1602–6.

82. Farrow LD, Mahoney AP, Sheppard JE, et al. Sonographic assessment of the medial ulnar collateral ligament distal ulnar attachment. J Ultrasound Med 2014;33(8):1485–90.

83. De Smet AA, Winter TC, Best TM, et al. Dynamic sonography with valgus stress to assess elbow ulnar collateral ligament injury in baseball pitchers. Skeletal Radiol 2002;31(11):671–6.

84. Wood N, Konin JG, Nofsinger C. Diagnosis of an ulnar collateral ligament tear using musculoskeletal ultrasound in a collegiate baseball pitcher: a case report. N Am J Sports Phys Ther 2010;5(4):227–33.

85. Miller TT, Adler RS, Friedman L. Sonography of injury of the ulnar collateral ligament of the elbow-initial experience. Skeletal Radiol 2004; 33(7):386–91.

86. Nazarian LN, McShane JM, Ciccotti MG, et al. Dynamic US of the anterior band of the ulnar collateral ligament of the elbow in asymptomatic major league baseball pitchers. Radiology 2003;227(1): 149–54.

87. Ciccotti MG, Atanda A Jr, Nazarian LN, et al. Stress sonography of the ulnar collateral ligament of the elbow in professional baseball pitchers: a 10-year study. Am J Sports Med 2014;42(3):544–51.

88. Roedl JB, Gonzalez FM, Zoga AC, et al. Potential utility of a combined approach with US and MR

arthrography to image medial elbow pain in baseball players. Radiology 2016;279(3):827–37.

89. Marshall NE, Keller RA, Van Holsbeeck M, et al. Ulnar collateral ligament and elbow adaptations in high school baseball pitchers. Sports Health 2015;7(6):484–8.

90. Keller RA, Marshall NE, Bey MJ, et al. Pre- and postseason dynamic ultrasound evaluation of the pitching elbow. Arthroscopy 2015;31(9):1708–15.

91. Atanda A Jr, Buckley PS, Hammoud S, et al. Early anatomic changes of the ulnar collateral ligament identified by stress ultrasound of the elbow in young professional baseball pitchers. Am J Sports Med 2015;43(12):2943–9.

92. Kim NR, Moon SG, Ko SM, et al. MR imaging of ulnar collateral ligament injury in baseball players: value for predicting rehabilitation outcome. Eur J Radiol 2011;80(3):e422–6.

93. Rettig AC, Sherrill C, Snead DS, et al. Nonoperative treatment of ulnar collateral ligament injuries in throwing athletes. Am J Sports Med 2001;29(1):15–7.

94. Podesta L, Crow SA, Volkmer D, et al. Treatment of partial ulnar collateral ligament tears in the elbow with platelet-rich plasma. Am J Sports Med 2013;41(7):1689–94.

95. Savoie FH 3rd, Trenhaile SW, Roberts J, et al. Primary repair of ulnar collateral ligament injuries of the elbow in young athletes: a case series of injuries to the proximal and distal ends of the ligament. Am J Sports Med 2008;36(6):1066–72.

96. Richard MJ, Aldridge JM 3rd, Wiesler ER, et al. Traumatic valgus instability of the elbow: pathoanatomy and results of direct repair. J Bone Joint Surg Am 2008;90(11):2416–22.

97. Jobe FW, Stark H, Lombardo SJ. Reconstruction of the ulnar collateral ligament in athletes. J Bone Joint Surg Am 1986;68(8):1158–63.

98. Osbahr DC, Cain EL Jr, Raines BT, et al. Long-term outcomes after ulnar collateral ligament reconstruction in competitive baseball players: minimum 10-year follow-up. Am J Sports Med 2014;42(6):1333–42.

99. Watson JN, McQueen P, Hutchinson MR. A systematic review of ulnar collateral ligament reconstruction techniques. Am J Sports Med 2014;42(10):2510–6.

100. Vitale MA, Ahmad CS. The outcome of elbow ulnar collateral ligament reconstruction in overhead athletes: a systematic review. Am J Sports Med 2008;36(6):1193–205.

101. Wear SA, Thornton DD, Schwartz ML, et al. MRI of the reconstructed ulnar collateral ligament. AJR Am J Roentgenol 2011;197(5):1198–204.

102. Dugas JR. Valgus extension overload: diagnosis and treatment. Clin Sports Med 2010;29(4):645–54.

103. Osbahr DC, Dines JS, Breazeale NM, et al. Ulnohumeral chondral and ligamentous overload: biomechanical correlation for posteromedial chondromalacia of the elbow in throwing athletes. Am J Sports Med 2010;38(12):2535–41.

104. Cohen SB, Valko C, Zoga A, et al. Posteromedial elbow impingement: magnetic resonance imaging findings in overhead throwing athletes and results of arthroscopic treatment. Arthroscopy 2011; 27(10):1364–70.

105. Roedl JB, Morrison WB, Ciccotti MG, et al. Acromial apophysiolysis: superior shoulder pain and acromial nonfusion in the young throwing athlete. Radiology 2015;274(1):201–9.

106. Roedl JB, Nevalainen M, Gonzalez FM, et al. Frequency, imaging findings, risk factors, and long-term sequelae of distal clavicular osteolysis in young patients. Skeletal Radiol 2015;44(5):659–66.

107. Furushima K, Itoh Y, Iwabu S, et al. Classification of Olecranon stress fractures in baseball players. Am J Sports Med 2014;42(6):1343–51.

108. Andreisek G, Crook DW, Burg D, et al. Peripheral neuropathies of the median, radial, and ulnar nerves: MR imaging features. Radiographics 2006;26(5):1267–87.

109. Husarik DB, Saupe N, Pfirrmann CW, et al. Elbow nerves: MR findings in 60 asymptomatic subjects–normal anatomy, variants, and pitfalls. Radiology 2009;252(1):148–56.

110. Beekman R, Visser LH, Verhagen WI. Ultrasonography in ulnar neuropathy at the elbow: a critical review. Muscle Nerve 2011;43(5):627–35.

111. Jacobson JA, Jebson PJ, Jeffers AW, et al. Ulnar nerve dislocation and snapping triceps syndrome: diagnosis with dynamic sonography–report of three cases. Radiology 2001;220(3):601–5.

The Skeletally Immature and Newly Mature Throwing Athlete

Kiery A. Braithwaite, MD[a,b,*], Kelley W. Marshall, MD[a,b]

KEYWORDS

- Physeal injury • Pediatric • Throwing athlete • Skeletally immature • Overuse • Shoulder • Elbow
- Little league

KEY POINTS

- Knowledge of normal endochondral bone growth is key to understanding overuse injuries in the skeletally immature patient.
- Vulnerability of the maturing physis and newly formed metaphyseal bone, susceptible to both acute and chronic injuries, makes pediatric injuries unique.
- Injury patterns evolve in a relatively predictable fashion as the pediatric skeleton matures.
- Pathophysiologic changes of repetitive microtrauma seen within the physis (such as little league shoulder) also occur in the epiphyses and apophyses: chronic physeal injuries, medial epicondylitis, and juvenile osteochondritis dissecans are different manifestations of the same underlying pathophysiology.
- "Little League Elbow" refers to a spectrum of injuries, related to the patient's skeletal maturity: radiologists should strive to be more specific in their descriptions of injury.

INTRODUCTION

Familiarity with normal skeletal growth is essential for the accurate interpretation of pediatric musculoskeletal imaging studies. Disruption of normal endochondral ossification is the unifying pathophysiology seen in most chronic overuse injuries involving the pediatric skeleton. The chondroosseous junction located at the physeal-metaphyseal junction of any growing bone is the most vulnerable structure to overuse injuries observed in the young pediatric athlete.[1,2] For example, in the rapidly growing peripubescent pitcher, vulnerability of the proximal humeral physis results in the classic throwing injury "little league shoulder" (LLS), named for the sport in which the term was first coined.[3]

As the adolescent matures, proximal humeral integrity strengthens with physeal fusion and areas of vulnerability shift to remaining open physes and apophyses. In the throwing late pubescent athlete, this may manifest as acromial or clavicular stress injuries. At the elbow, a spectrum of overuse injuries can develop in response to the complex forces occurring across the growing skeleton during throwing. These injuries, although quite specific and predictable, are often vaguely lumped under the broad diagnostic category of "little league elbow" (LLE).

The authors have nothing to disclose.
a Department of Radiology & Imaging Sciences, Emory University, 1364 Clifton Road, NE Suite D112, Atlanta, GA 30322, USA; b Department of Pediatric Radiology, Children's Healthcare of Atlanta at Egleston, 1405 Clifton Road Northeast, Atlanta, GA 30322, USA
* Corresponding author. Department of Pediatric Radiology, Children's Healthcare of Atlanta at Egleston, 1405 Clifton Road Northeast, Atlanta, GA 30322.
E-mail address: kiery.braithwaite@choa.org

Radiol Clin N Am 54 (2016) 841–855
http://dx.doi.org/10.1016/j.rcl.2016.04.006
0033-8389/16/$ – see front matter © 2016 Elsevier Inc. All rights reserved.

NORMAL ANATOMY: NORMAL SKELETAL GROWTH

Development of the pediatric skeleton begins prenatally and continues throughout childhood and adolescence. Two types of bone growth contribute[4–6]:

- Intramembranous ossification occurs along the diaphyseal surface of long bones and within the flat bones of the axial skeleton, including the skull and pelvis.
- Endochondral (enchondral) ossification occurs primarily within the long bones of the appendicular skeleton, contributing to most skeletal growth and elongation.

Endochondral ossification, which is the focus of the following discussion, occurs at the level of the growth plates, or physes, throughout the skeleton.

Growth Plate Anatomy

Growth plates can be divided morphologically into 2 types: (1) the discoid primary physis, and (2) the spherical secondary physis.[5]

The physis (or primary physis) refers to the typical discoid-shaped growth plate residing between the metaphysis and epiphysis at the end of long bones. A morphologically similar growth plate is also situated between the apophyses and their adjacent bony shafts.[5]

The secondary physes denote the smaller spherical growth plates located at the periphery of epiphyseal and epiphyseal-equivalent bones (apophyses, carpal/tarsal bones, and sesamoid bones). Other terms used to describe this cohort of secondary physes include acrophysis and the growth plate for the secondary ossification center[5,7] (**Fig. 1**).

It is important to understand that endochondral ossification, the process of converting physeal cartilage to metaphyseal bone, occurs wherever a cartilaginous growth plate exists in the growing skeleton.[5]

Endochondral Ossification Within the Primary Physis

The primary physis is responsible for the elongation of bone achieved throughout childhood, most rapidly during infancy and puberty. New metaphyseal bone is created on a framework of maturing chondrocytes within the physis, which are subsequently replaced by bone[6] (**Fig. 2**).

Histologically, the sequential process of endochondral ossification is characterized by an orderly architecture with horizontal bands of developing

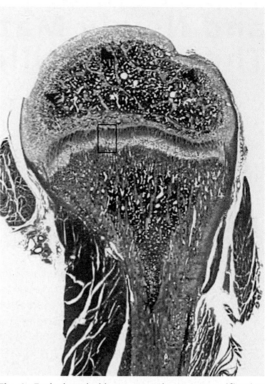

Fig. 1. Endochondral bone growth. Low-magnification light micrograph of a developing humerus. A portion of the primary physis with its columnar structure highlighted in the black rectangle is demonstrated in **Fig. 2**. Arrowheads denote the smaller peripheral secondary physis. (*From* Vaughan DW. A learning system in histology: CD ROM and guide. Oxford: Oxford University Press, 2002; with permission.)

chondrocytes categorized into resting, proliferating, and hypertrophied zones.[7]

Resting quiescent chondrocytes populate the superficial layer of the physis, derived from aggregated mesenchymal cells. Maturation of these progenitor chondrocytes into long columns of rapidly proliferating chondrocytes serves as the cartilaginous framework for bone elongation at the physeal-metaphyseal junction. In the final zone, the deep hypertrophied chondrocytes located closest to the metaphysis release growth factors, thereby recruiting adjacent metaphyseal vessels to form and deposit minerals and osteoblasts. This orchestrated interaction between hypertrophied chondrocytes and metaphyseal vessels in the deepest layer of the physis promotes chondrocyte mineralization, apoptosis of hypertrophic chondrocytes, and subsequent osteogenesis. Osteoblasts deposit bony matrix on the degrading calcified cartilage framework in the final steps of endochondral ossification.[1,6–9] Recent studies have suggested that not all hypertrophied chondrocytes undergo terminal

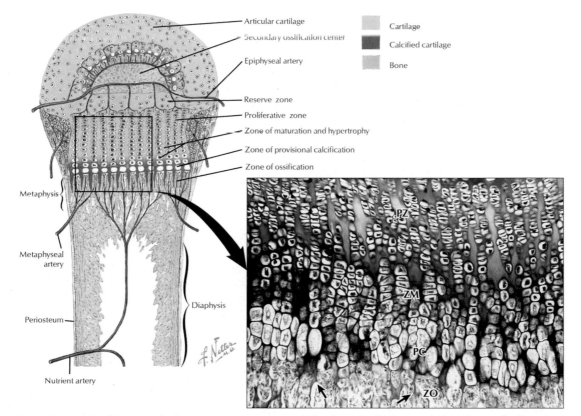

Articular cartilage
Secondary ossification center
Epiphyseal artery

Reserve zone
Proliferative zone
Zone of maturation and hypertrophy
Zone of provisional calcification
Zone of ossification

Cartilage
Calcified cartilage
Bone

Metaphysis

Metaphyseal
artery

Diaphysis

Periosteum

Nutrient artery

PZ
ZM
PC
ZO

Fig. 2. Schematic of the growth plate showing structure and blood supply. The 2 growth plates in a typical long bone are peripheral extensions of the primary ossification center. The primary center grows and expands centrifugally in all directions until it becomes confined to the bone ends. A growth plate consists mostly of a cartilaginous portion with various histologic zones and a bony component known as the metaphysis. (*Insert*) Low-magnification of the growth plate in longitudinal section. The proliferative zone (PZ) shows closely packed stacks of flattened chondrocytes. Zones of maturation and hypertrophy (ZM) contain enlarged cells, which create small open cavities in the provisional calcification (PC) zone. The cartilage matrix becomes more basophilic as it calcifies and gives rise to slender spicules (*arrows*) of the zone of ossification (ZO) that project into the marrow cavity (Wright stain, original magnification ×150).

apoptosis, but some may directly transform into osteoblasts and osteoclasts, further contributing to the development of mature bone.[10]

The zone of provisional calcification is the deepest portion of the growth plate, demarcating the final transition from cartilage to bone. This chondro-osseus junction is also the weakest part of the growth plate.[2,4,5]

Endochondral Ossification Within the Secondary Physes

The secondary physis contributes to transverse and spherical growth within the epiphyses and apophyses at the end of long bones.

In the fetus and newborn, the epiphysis is composed of 3 types of hyaline cartilage: epiphyseal, physeal, and articular.[1] During skeletal growth, 1 or more secondary ossification centers (SOC) develops from precursor epiphyseal hyaline

chondrocytes. The SOC is surrounded circumferentially by the secondary physis, which is then surrounded by germinal hyaline cartilage and finally the articular cartilage along the outer periphery.[1,5] The SOC is initially spherical but later becomes hemispherical as the ossified portion of the epiphysis grows, eventually abutting the primary physis.[1,7]

The process of endochondral ossification here mirrors that in the primary physis discussed previously. Minor differences include that the secondary physis is thinner than the primary physis, and zonal architecture has been shown histologically to be less orderly.[6,11] Vascular supply to the SOC is by epiphyseal vascular cartilage channels.[4,7,12]

Areas of vulnerability in the maturing epiphysis and apophyses mirror that within the primary physeal-metaphyseal junction. The newly formed peripheral bone created by the secondary physis has been coined "metaphyseal equivalent" bone, even though it is within the epiphysis or epiphyseal-equivalent bone.[1,13]

MR Imaging of Normal Physeal Anatomy

The normal physeal-metaphyseal junction has a trilaminar appearance on T2-weighted MR images (**Fig. 3**). The physis is high signal intensity on water-sensitive sequences. The deepest layer of the physis, the zone of provisional calcification, is uniquely low signal on all sequences, outlining the chondro-osseous junction.[1,2,14] On MR, the normal healthy physis is uniform in thickness and signal intensity, with a continuous zone of provisional calcification. Physeal undulation is normal and increases with age.[14] High signal intensity within the primary spongiosa distinguishes the superficial metaphysis, the third and final layer of the trilaminar physeal-metaphyseal junction.[1,2,14]

Within the epiphysis, the thinner circumferential secondary physis mirrors the MR signal intensity of the primary physis. The ossified portion of the epiphysis (SOC) follows signal characteristics of normal epiphyseal marrow, which changes from hematopoietic to fatty within 6 months of ossification.[14]

VULNERABILITY OF THE PHYSIS: PATHOPHYSIOLOGY OF PHYSEAL INJURIES

An experimental study in skeletally immature rabbits provides insight into the pathophysiology of

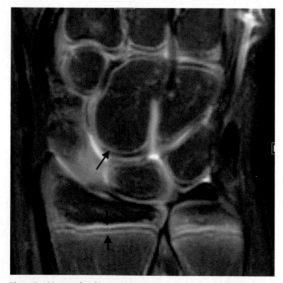

Fig. 3. Normal physes. Proton density weighted fat saturated coronal image of a 5-year-old child demonstrates the normal trilaminar appearance of the growing distal radial primary physis (*red arrows*) and the peripheral secondary physes seen deep to the articular cartilage in the ossifying carpal bones (*black arrow*).

primary physeal injuries observed in pediatric athletes.[15]

In this study, induced metaphyseal injury in skeletally immature bone resulted in disruption of normal endochondral ossification at the level of the physis. Histologically, this was evidenced by thickening of the hypertrophic physeal zone of developing chondrocytes. Corresponding MR findings included abnormal widening of the growth plate with abnormal extension of nonmineralized foci of cartilage signal into the metaphysis.[15]

Subsequent retrospective MR studies revealed similar findings of abnormal physeal widening in pediatric patients following an assortment of prior metaphyseal insults,[16] including chronic overuse in pediatric athletes.[17] These studies laid the groundwork for understanding that disruption of endochondral ossification was the unifying pathophysiology occurring in chronic physeal injuries in the skeletally immature. Disruption of vascular supply to the metaphysis interrupts the final steps of endochondral ossification including mineralization and apoptosis of the hypertrophied chondrocytes in the deepest layer of the physis. By imaging, this injury results in widening of the physis diffusely or even focally with foci of high signal physeal tissue extending into the metaphysis, as seen in "little league shoulder".[15,17]

IMAGING PROTOCOLS

Conventional radiographs are the recommended initial imaging modality for patients presenting with acute or chronic upper extremity pain. In the skeletally immature patient, comparison images with the nondominant throwing arm can be used in distinguishing ossification variants in the developing skeleton from pathology. When additional imaging is indicated, either because of failure of conservative management, continued pain, and/or indeterminate radiographic findings, MR is the imaging study of choice. For sports-related injuries, MR is routinely performed without intravenous contrast. Similar to the adult throwing athlete population, the addition of arthrographic contrast can be particularly beneficial in the maturing pediatric athlete presenting with shoulder or elbow pain. These recommendations are in accordance with the American College of Radiology appropriateness criteria.

IMAGING FINDINGS/PATHOLOGY: SHOULDER
Little League Shoulder: Proximal Humeral Physeal Stress Injury

The proximal humeral physis contributes to 80% of overall humeral longitudinal growth,[4] contributing to its increased susceptibility of chronic physeal injury. The typical age of presentation of LLS occurs between 11 and 16 years.[18] This correlates expectedly with the time of accelerated growth and therefore increased physeal vulnerability. Physiologic closure of the proximal humeral physis occurs typically between 14 and 17 years of age.[19,20] Most common in pitchers, LLS results from repetitive rotational torque across the proximal humeral physis generated during the acceleration phase of throwing.[4,18,20,21]

By plain radiography, LLS is characterized by abnormal widening of the proximal humeral physis, leading early investigators to erroneously suspect a chronic Salter Harris type 1 fracture as the underlying etiology.[22–24] As detailed previously, it is now recognized that chronic microtrauma causing disruption of endochondral ossification predisposes to the classic overuse physeal injuries seen in pediatric athletes. The growth spurt occurring in conjunction with the onset of puberty increases the vulnerability of the developing skeleton.[2]

LLS is often diagnosed clinically: typically insidious proximal humeral pain during throwing with associated point tenderness over the proximal humeral physis, particularly laterally. Standard anteroposterior (AP) shoulder radiographs can often confirm the clinical diagnosis with characteristic abnormal widening of the proximal humeral physis. Additional radiographic findings may include lateral metaphyseal fragmentation, demineralization, and sclerosis of the proximal humeral metaphysis[18,20,21,25] (Fig. 4). Comparison to the contralateral asymptomatic humerus may be useful. Advanced imaging is rarely necessary, but may be performed in cases that do not respond to conservative treatment[18,20,26] (Fig. 5).

Treatment is conservative with rest from throwing. In a case series of 23 patients diagnosed with LLS based on symptomology and supportive radiographs, 21 (91%) of 23 patients had resolution of symptoms with return to baseball following an average of 3 months of rest.[27]

Acromial Apophyseal Stress Injury (Acromial Apophysitis or Acromial Apophysiolysis)

Following closure of the proximal humeral physis, continued shoulder stress in the older high school or collegiate pitcher may shift to remaining open physes about the shoulder, such as the acromion. Greatest stress to the acromion during pitching occurs during the deceleration phase of throwing.[28]

The scapular acromion consists of up to 3 ossification centers that ossify and often coalesce

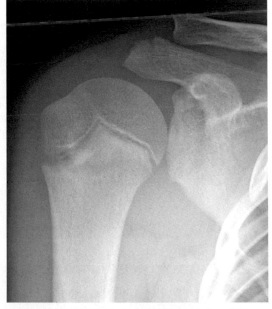

Fig. 4. Proximal humeral physeal stress injury, LLS. Anteroposterior external rotation radiograph demonstrates proximal humeral physeal widening and irregularity evident laterally.

during adolescence. Proximal to distal, these centers include the meta-acromion, mesa-acromion, and pre-acromion respectively. Fusion of these centers is variable, but can normally be as late as the early 20s, long after the proximal humeral physis has closed.[19,29] Failure to fuse by 25 years of age, coined "os acromiale," is an uncommon entity occurring in approximately 1% to 8% of patients, typically along the 2 largest ossification centers (meta-acromion and meso-acromion).[13,29–31] Although often asymptomatic, os acromiale also may be a source of chronic shoulder pain in the adult population.[19,28]

Sporadic case reports in pediatric patients have described clinically symptomatic changes of "acromial apophysitis" supported by abnormal imaging.[31–33] Typically patients complain of shoulder pain during sports with resolution at rest, typical of other physeal injuries elsewhere. Radiographic findings of this traction apophyseal stress injury include irregularity, sclerosis, and fragmentation of the acromion apophysis but this can be difficult to differentiate from normal ossification variation in the skeletally immature child.[32,33] In these cases, the diagnosis is often made clinically as the patient is point tender over the open acromial physis or by MR imaging where edema at the junction of the apophysis and body of the acromion is often seen in addition to physeal widening and irregularity similar to MR findings observed in the proximal humeral physis in patients with LLS[31] (Fig. 6).

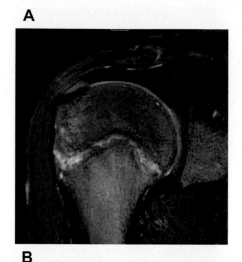

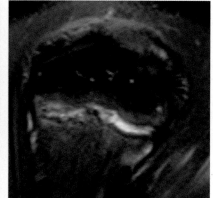

Fig. 5. LLS MR imaging findings. (*A*) Coronal oblique fat-saturated T2-weighted image in a 12-year-old pitcher demonstrates diffuse proximal humeral primary physeal widening and undulation with bone marrow edema within the metaphysis and lateral epiphysis. (*B*) Two sagittal oblique fat-saturated T2-weighted images obtained in a 13-year-old pitcher demonstrate preservation of the normal anterior medial humeral physis (*red arrows*) in contrast to the widened irregular physis posteriorly and laterally.

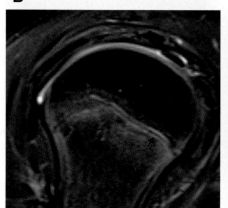

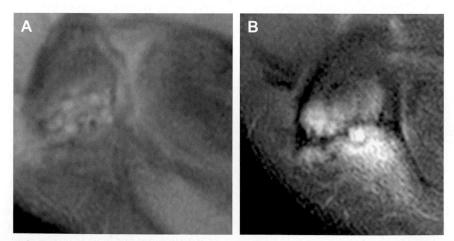

Fig. 6. Acromial physeal stress injury. Axial T1-weighted fat-saturated (*A*) and axial T2-weighted fat-saturated images (*B*) demonstrate classic physeal widening, irregularity, and disorganization with surrounding bone marrow edema of overuse injury demonstrated in this competitive 14-year-old female pole vaulter.

A large retrospective study by Roedl and colleagues[30] identified 61 patients (ages 15–25 years old) with shoulder MR performed for shoulder pain, where the only abnormal finding identified was acromion apophyseal edema. "Acromial apophysiolysis" was defined by MR as incomplete fusion and edema (relative to the distal clavicle) along the acromion apophysis, typically along the 2 largest ossification centers (meta-acromion and meso-acromion). Risk factor for development included pitching (both baseball and softball): 40% of patients were noted to have pitch counts that exceeded 100 per week.[30]

Further, follow-up imaging in patients with MR diagnosis of acromial apophyseal stress injury revealed that the vast majority (86% of patients) subsequently failed to fuse consistent with an os acromiale (vs only 4% in the control group). This carries long-term morbidity implications manifesting as increased risk of rotator cuff tears in the adult population secondary to subacromial impingement related to the hypermobile os acromiale.[13,29,30,34]

Clavicular Osteolysis: Distal Clavicular Stress Injury

In children, injury to the acromioclavicular joint is more likely to result in a distal clavicular physeal injury rather than a true acromioclavicular separation. The strength of the capsule and ligaments supporting the acromioclavicular joint far exceeds that of the immature physis as seen elsewhere in the pediatric patient.[21,35,36]

Chronic stress injury to the distal clavicle termed "distal clavicular osteolysis" has recently been reported in adolescent athletes, previously predominantly seen in adult weight lifters.[37,38] Implicated in a variety of overhead sports, only the combination of weightlifting and overhead activity resulted in increased risk of this injury in a study involving pediatric patients. MR findings include distal clavicular marrow edema, subchondral fracture, and subchondral cystic change[38] (**Fig. 7**).

Rare sporadic case reports of medial physeal stress fractures have been reported in pediatric competitive gymnasts.[27] Similar to the acromial physis, the medial clavicular physis is one of the last to close, remaining unfused into the patient's early 20s.[21]

IMAGING FINDINGS/PATHOLOGY: ELBOW
Little League Elbow Injury Spectrum

The term "little league elbow" is traditionally used to describe medial elbow pain in skeletally immature throwers, consistent with the first description in 2 little league players with symptomatic medial elbow injuries.[39] However, one should avoid using this nonspecific term to describe elbow pathology in the young throwing athlete. Elbow pain in the pediatric throwing athlete rather encompasses a predictable spectrum of specific injuries that can involve different aspects of the elbow.[2]

Manifestations of overuse injury are related to both throwing mechanics as well as evolving areas of vulnerability related to the skeletal maturation of the elbow's multiple ossification centers, which include both epiphyseal and apophyseal centers. Understanding the directionality of the force vectors across the elbow, the position of the elbow throughout the throwing motion, and most importantly the skeletal maturation of the throwing athlete, the radiologist can predict the injury pattern.

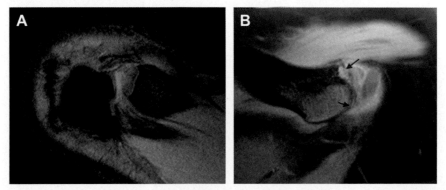

Fig. 7. Distal clavicular stress injury. (*A*) Note the normal thin open distal clavicular physis demonstrated on an axial T2*-weighted image in this 15-year-old boy (*red arrow*). (*B*) An 18-year-old young man presenting with a 6-month history of acromioclavicular joint pain with bench-pressing. Axial fat-saturated T1-weighted image demonstrates changes of distal clavicular physeal stress injury in the ventral half of the clavicle with widening and irregularity of the physis evident (*black arrow*). A remnant of the normal posterior physis is noted dorsally (*red arrow*).

The stress across the different compartments of the elbow during pitching has been coined "valgus extension overload (VEO) syndrome."[40,41] In brief, distraction forces are applied medially as the elbow is placed in maximum valgus. In turn, compressive forces are delivered to the 90° flexed lateral compartment during this valgus posture. As the medial stabilizers over time become lax or fail, excessive translational freedom of the humeral-ulnar articulation occurs allowing more posterior compartmental reactive changes and/or injury.

Little League Elbow: Medial Injuries

During pitching, valgus positioning of the elbow creates tensile force between the medial epicondyle proximally and the medial ulnar crest distally resulting in a distraction force applied across the medial column. This can translate into injuries of the medial epicondyle as well as the medial ulnar collateral ligament and its sites of attachment depending on the skeletal maturation of the patient.[42,43] Injury patterns to the medial elbow predicted by skeletal maturation are typically summarized as follows:

- In the skeletally immature player, injuries to the medial epicondyle apophysis prevail
- In the skeletally mature player, injures to the medial ulnar collateral ligament prevail

Note, however, that these injuries as described in more detail later in this article can occur concurrently, as skeletal maturation is a gradual evolving process.

Little league elbow in the prepubescent pitcher: medial epicondylitis/medial epicondyle apophysitis

In the skeletally immature, the physis at the base of the medial epicondyle apophysis is the weakest structure in the medial elbow.[42,43] Although variable, the medial epicondyle apophysis in male individuals typically begins to ossify at approximately 7 years of age and fuses at approximately 15 years of age (4 and 13 years, respectively in girls).[44] Most common in the younger throwing pitcher (typically <10 years old), the same pathophysiology that occurs in the proximal humeral physis in LLS also occurs across the open physis between the medial epicondyle and the distal humerus in prepubescent LLE. A better and more specific term is medial epicondylitis or medial epicondyle apophysitis.[43,45]

Diagnosis of medial epicondylitis can often be established by history and physical examination. Patients most commonly complain of medial elbow pain and tenderness. Radiographs may be normal, or reveal imaging findings reminiscent of physeal injuries elsewhere in the pediatric skeleton with widening and irregularity of the medial epicondylar physis.[2,39,43,46] Overgrowth of the medial epicondyle apophysis can also occur, but often a late finding related to chronic hyperemia[28,42,43,46] (**Fig. 8**). Although rarely necessary, MR imaging can confirm characteristic findings of physeal

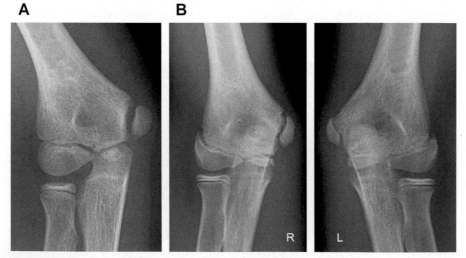

Fig. 8. (*A*) Classic AP radiographic findings of medial epicondyle physeal stress injury in a 10-year-old pitcher resulting in marked widening of the physis and mild fragmentation of the tip of the apophysis deep to the secondary physis. (*B*) Bilateral AP elbow radiographs in this right-hand–dominant pitcher demonstrate findings of chronic medial epicondyle apophyseal stress injury resulting in widening of the physis, apophyseal overgrowth, sclerosis, and peripheral fragmentation of the ossifying apophysis.

widening and irregularity of the medial epicondyle along its physeal border. Marrow edema in the apophysis as well as the adjacent humeral metaphyseal bone may also be evident on MR[2,13,43] (**Fig. 9**).

Little league elbow in the older pitcher: ligament bone avulsion injuries

As the pitcher nears skeletal maturation, the medial epicondyle strengthens with gradual physeal closure and fusion to the humerus. Vulnerability can then shift to the bone ligament interface of the medial epicondyle and medial ulnar collateral ligament, where endochondral ossification can be ongoing at the secondary physis (**Fig. 10**). The medial ulnar collateral ligament has a broad attachment to the inferior pole of the medial epicondyle. This can result in traction avulsion fractures, similar to those seen at the knee in Sinding Larsen Johannson and Osgood Schlatter.[2,42,43] Tears of the distal attachment of the medial ulnar collateral ligament on the sublime tubercle can be seen as well.[43]

This pattern of injury was corroborated by a study of 9 young pitchers (ages 8–13) with a clinical diagnosis of LLE. Imaging studies revealed a normal medial ulnar collateral ligament in all patients.[42] This led the authors to conclude that evaluation of MR did not change clinical management of "LLE." Lack of significant medial ulnar collateral ligament injury is predictable given the skeletal maturation of the included patients in this study. In this age group, it is likely that the medial epicondyle had not undergone fusion, and thus the medial epicondylar apophysis was most vulnerable to chronic repetitive stress rather than the ligament. After the onset of puberty, as the medial epicondyle apophysis fuses to the parent bone, the area of vulnerability shifts to the medial ulnar collateral ligament, common flexor/pronator tendon/muscles and the ulnar nerve.[2,43,47]

Following skeletal maturity, endochondral ossification ceases and the areas of weakness and subsequent injury shift yet again from the previously growing bone to the supporting soft tissue structures.[2] Tendons and ligaments now become the weakest structures of the joints, and in the medial elbow, continued distraction forces applied during throwing may result in significant tears of the medial ulnar collateral ligament itself following skeletal maturity.[13,43] Following complete fusion of the medial epicondyle, mid substance medial ulnar collateral ligament tears are most common.[43] Further, with chronic tears or laxity of the medial ulnar collateral ligament, the common flexor tendon may begin to fail.[2] In a recent study by Roedl and colleagues[47] from the group at Thomas Jefferson University Hospital, 53 of 144 baseball players (mean age 24.5 years) with medial elbow pain had medial ulnar collateral ligament tears, 48 of 144 had posteromedial elbow impingement with cartilage loss and osteophyte in the posterior ulnotrochlear joint, and 31 had ulnar neuritis. The study showed a combined imaging approach with MR arthrography and ultrasound (conventional and stress ultrasound) shows higher accuracy for the assessment of medial elbow pain than each modality alone. To predict medial ulnar collateral ligament tears with stress ultrasound alone, joint gapping of more than 1.5 mm compared with the contralateral elbow (>1.5 mm relative joint gapping) yields a sensitivity of 81% and a specificity of 91%. Combined with the direct visualization of the ligament tear on MR arthrography, the sensitivity increased to 96% and specificity to 99%.[47]

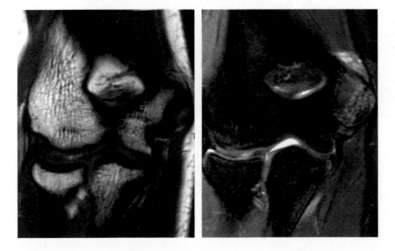

Fig. 9. Medial epicondylar "apophysitis" seen in this 15-year-old right-handed athlete. Coronal oblique T1-weighted and proton density fat-saturated images demonstrate delayed apophyseal closure, apophyseal overgrowth, and edema within the apophysis and the adjacent humeral metaphysis as well as in the overlying soft tissues. Partial thickness tear of the medial ulnar collateral ligament also noted involving the humeral attachment (*red arrow*).

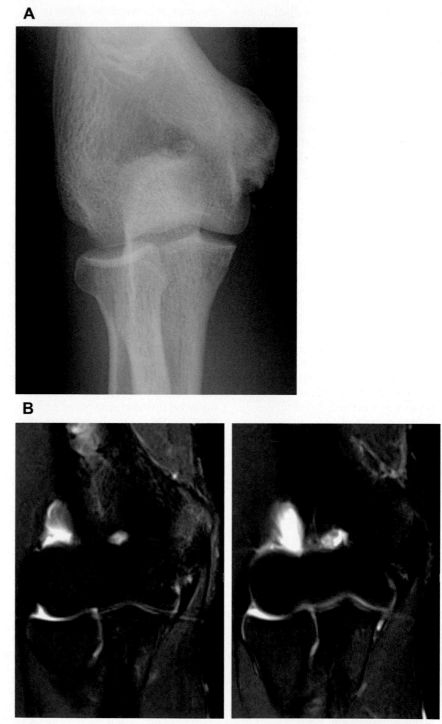

Fig. 10. Ligament bone avulsion injuries. A 17-year-old right-handed pitcher approaching skeletal maturity at the elbow. (*A*) AP radiograph demonstrates tell-tale findings of chronic medial epicondylitis with small fragments noted below the medial epicondyle. (*B*) Two consecutive coronal oblique fat-saturated proton density weighted images obtained at time of MR arthrography confirm central interstitial tear developing at the humeral attachment of the medial ulnar collateral ligament and the retained ossific fragments within the fibers of the ligament (*red arrow*). Note the persistent medial epicondylar edema despite near complete physeal closure.

Lateral Elbow Injuries: Juvenile Osteochondritis Dissecans

The complex dynamic forces of VEO during throwing are not limited to medial sided injuries, but simultaneously translate into compressive forces along the lateral aspect of the elbow. Repetitive compressive and shearing force to the lateral radiocapitellar joint predisposes to the development of osteochondritis dissecans (OCD). Juvenile OCD is an overuse injury to the chondroosseous junction occurring in pediatric patients before physeal closure. Typical age of presentation is 10 to 15 years old.[4] Although similar to its adult counterpart, juvenile OCD is associated with clinical, imaging, and prognostic features that are unique to the pediatric population.[11,48,49]

The pathophysiology predisposing skeletally immature patients to juvenile OCD likely mirrors that same pathophysiology discussed previously in primary physeal overuse injuries. Disruption of endochondral ossification along the secondary centers of ossification was first proposed by Laor and colleagues[11] as the etiology of juvenile OCD after anecdotally noting disruption of the secondary physis overlying juvenile OCD lesions. Chondroepiphyseal widening, subchondral marrow edema, and disruption of the secondary physis identified in juvenile OCD lesions in the knee by MR was noted to be reminiscent of the pathologic changes seen in primary physeal lesions such as LLS.[11] The edematous subchondral marrow in juvenile OCD lesions coined "metaphyseal equivalent" marrow corresponds to the newly ossified bone deep to the chondro-osseus junction within the secondary center of ossification of the developing epiphysis.[13]

Laor and colleagues[11] further proposed that the etiology for secondary physeal disruption in juvenile OCD may be related to its thinner and less organized morphology as compared with the primary physis, rending it more susceptible to injury. This may explain why younger patients are less susceptible to OCD and maintain a better prognosis than older patients, as their physes are thicker than those nearing skeletal maturity.

Experimental studies in animals and human cadavers have suggested that vascular injury to the epiphysis likely contributes to the development of juvenile OCD.[6,50] Compressive forces have been shown to inhibit normal cartilage growth and ossification.[6] In epiphyses, which are subjected to compressive forces, decreased perfusion pressure of subchondral vessels has been proposed.[6,11]

In the skeletally immature throwing athlete, OCD most frequently affects the capitellum; although less frequently reported sites include the radial head and trochlea.[13,51,52] The vascular anatomy of the capitellum and lateral trochlea make them more susceptible to ischemia.[51,53] The anterior or anterolateral aspect of the capitellum is most common site of OCD in baseball players secondary to the flexed posture of the elbow at the time of maximum valgus stress[13] (**Fig. 11**).

Stability of Elbow Osteochondritis Dissecans Lesions

Determining the stability of OCD lesions has prognostic and therapeutic implications. Application of adult MR knee OCD stability criteria may have high sensitivity but low specificity when applied to the pediatric population.[54,55] MR features of instability explicit to juvenile OCD favored to have high sensitivity and specificity include the following: rimlike hyperintense signal similar to joint fluid signal along the lesion-bone interface in addition to a second deeper linear margin of low signal and multiple sites of subchondral bone discontinuity.[48] The presence of multiple subchondral cysts or a single cyst larger than 5 mm associated with a lesion are imaging predictors of instability associated with low sensitivity but high specificity in juvenile OCD.[48] A study specific to the elbow assessing capitellar juvenile OCD lesions proposed that the position of the lesion within the capitellum may have prognostic implications as well. In a small cohort of skeletally immature patients with capitellar OCD, those lesions classified as "uncontained" (lesion extends beyond the lateral cartilage margin) were more likely to be associated with joint contractures on short-term follow-up.[56]

Posterior Elbow Injuries: Olecranon Stress Fractures

Olecranon stress fractures are relatively rare in the throwing athlete,[2,40,57] reported to occur in up to 5% of baseball players.[56] First described in javelin throwers,[58] olecranon stress fractures have been reported in a variety of other sports, including but not limited to baseball, softball, tennis, gymnastics, and diving.[57,59]

The olecranon apophysis normally fuses at approximately 15 to 17 years of age in boys[59]; physeal closure begins at the articular surface and extends to the dorsal surface.[57] The mechanism predisposing to olecranon overuse injury is somewhat controversial in the literature, with both valgus extension overload[40,57,60] and tension exerted by the triceps[2,43,59] playing a role. Increased medial elbow laxity predisposes to olecranon stress fractures, with medial ulnar collateral ligament injuries reported to be a

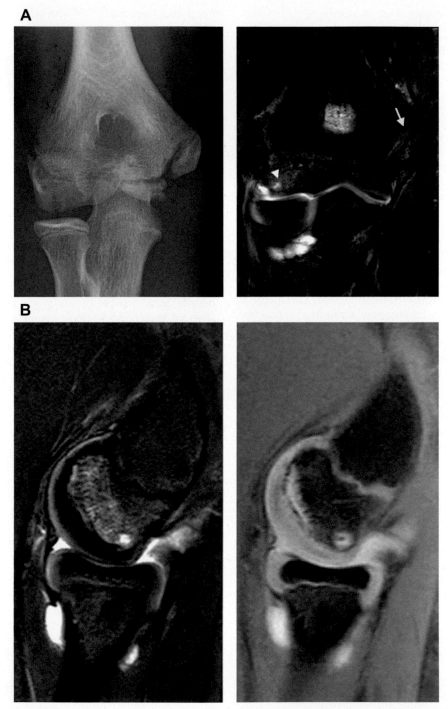

Fig. 11. The many faces of LLE in a 14-year-old pitcher. (*A*) AP radiograph and coronal oblique fat-saturated T2-weighted MR demonstrate features of chronic medial epicondyle stress injury (*yellow arrow*) as well as findings of capitellar osteochondritis dissecans (*white arrowhead*). Proximal medial ulnar collateral ligament edema/grade 1 sprain also noted at the humeral attachment (*red arrow*). (*B*) Sagittal short tau inversion recovery and fat-saturated T1-weighted MR arthrogram images emphasize the classic features of injury to the "metaphyseal equivalent" bone deep to the disorganized and obliterated secondary physis of the ossifying capitellum.

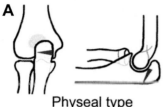

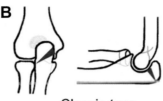

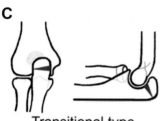

Physeal type
n = 101 (50.5%), 14.1 y

Classic type
n = 49 (24.5%), 18.6 y

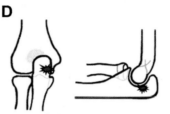

Transitional type
n = 26 (13.0%), 16.9 y

Sclerotic type
n = 19 (9.5%), 18.0 y

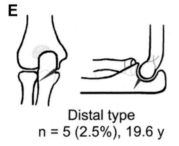

Distal type
n = 5 (2.5%), 19.6 y

Fig. 12. Olecranon stress fracture types. (*From* Furushima K, Itoh Y, Iwabu S, et al. Classification of olecranon stress fractures in baseball players. Am J Sports Med 2014;42(6): 1345; with permission.)

significant contributing risk factor.[40,57] A recent histologic study of olecranon physeal stress fractures confirmed by MR in 2 young baseball players (ages 14 and 15 years) demonstrated disorientation of chondral columns in the olecranon physis as well as hypocellularity and chondrocyte cluster formation on histologic examination.[61]

Classification of olecranon stress fractures into 5 types based on the orientation of the fracture line was recently proposed by Furushima and colleagues[57] after studying 200 baseball players (age range 13–27 years). The type of fracture was found to be directly related to the skeletal maturation of the patient at symptom onset. The "physeal type" defined as delayed closure or nonunion across the physis was most common in the youngest cohort (average age of 14.1 years) before expected physiologic fusion. The "transitional type" predominated closer to the time immediately following physeal closure, whereas "classic, sclerotic, and distal" occurred typically in the skeletally mature patient[57] (**Fig. 12**).

SUMMARY

The diagnosis of LLS and LLE in throwing athletes comprises a spectrum of specific injuries. The informed radiologist provides value by recognizing and reporting the distinct injuries within this spectrum. With a keen understanding of normal development and pathophysiologic stresses that occur during throwing, these unique pediatric injuries are often easily predicted based on the patient's skeletal maturation.

REFERENCES

1. Jaimes C, Chauvin NA, Delgado J, et al. MR imaging of normal epiphyseal development and common epiphyseal disorders. Radiographics 2014;34(2): 449–71.

2. Bedoya MA, Jaramillo D, Chauvin NA. Overuse injuries in children. Top Magn Reson Imaging 2015;24(2):67–81.

3. Dotter WE. Little leaguer's shoulder: a fracture of the proximal epiphysial cartilage of the humerus

due to baseball pitching. Guthrie Clin Bull 1953;
23(1):68–72.

4. Stein-Wexler R, Wootton-Gorges SL, Ozonoff MB.
Pediatric orthopedic imaging. Heidelberg, Baden-
Württemberg: Springer-Verlag; 2015.

5. Oestreich AE. The acrophysis: a unifying concept for
enchondral bone growth and its disorders. I. Normal
growth. Skeletal Radiol 2003;32(3):121–7.

6. Ytrehus B, Carlson CS, Ekman S. Etiology and pathogenesis of osteochondrosis. Vet Pathol 2007;44(4):
429–48.

7. Rivas R, Shapiro F. Structural stages in the development of the long bones and epiphyses: a study in
the New Zealand white rabbit. J Bone Joint Surg
Am 2002;84A(1):85–100.

8. Carter DR, Wong M. Modelling cartilage mechanobi-
ology. Philos Trans R Soc Lond B Biol Sci 2003;
358(1437):1461–71.

9. Trueta J, Amato VP. The vascular contribution to
osteogenesis. III. Changes in the growth cartilage
caused by experimentally induced ischaemia.
J Bone Joint Surg Br 1960;42B:571–87.

10. Yang L, Tsang KY, Tang HC, et al. Hypertrophic
chondrocytes can become osteoblasts and osteo-
cytes in endochondral bone formation. Proc Natl
Acad Sci U S A 2014;111(33):12097–102.

11. Laor T, Zbojniewicz AM, Eismann EA, et al. Juvenile
osteochondritis dissecans: is it a growth disturbance
of the secondary physis of the epiphysis? AJR Am J
Roentgenol 2012;199(5):1121–8.

12. Blumer MJ, Longato S, Fritsch H. Structure, formation and role of cartilage canals in the developing
bone. Ann Anat 2008;190(4):305–15.

13. Marshall KW. Overuse upper extremity injuries in the
skeletally immature patient: beyond Little League
shoulder and elbow. Semin Musculoskelet Radiol
2014;18(5):469–77.

14. Laor T, Jaramillo D. MR imaging insights into skeletal
maturation: what is normal? Radiology 2009;250(1):
28–38.

15. Jaramillo D, Laor T, Zaleske DJ. Indirect trauma to
the growth plate: results of MR imaging after epiphyseal and metaphyseal injury in rabbits. Radiology
1993;187(1):171–8.

16. Laor T, Hartman AL, Jaramillo D. Local physeal
widening on MR imaging: an incidental finding suggesting prior metaphyseal insult. Pediatr Radiol
1997;27(8):654–62.

17. Laor T, Wall EJ, Vu LP. Physeal widening in the knee
due to stress injury in child athletes. AJR Am J
Roentgenol 2006;186(5):1260–4.

18. Carson WG Jr, Gasser SI. Little Leaguer's shoulder.
A report of 23 cases. Am J Sports Med 1998;
26(4):575–80.

19. Zember JS, Rosenberg ZS, Kwong S, et al. Normal skeletal maturation and imaging pitfalls in the pediatric
shoulder. Radiographics 2015;35(4):1108–22.

20. Anton C, Podberesky DJ. Little League shoulder: a
growth plate injury. Pediatr Radiol 2010;
40(Suppl 1):S54.

21. Leonard J, Hutchinson MR. Shoulder injuries in skeletally immature throwers: review and current
thoughts. Br J Sports Med 2010;44(5):306–10.

22. Bishop JY, Flatow EL. Pediatric shoulder trauma.
Clin Orthop Relat Res 2005;(432):41–8.

23. Tullos HS, Fain RH. Little league shoulder: rotational
stress fracture of proximal epiphysis. J Sports Med
1974;2(3):152–3.

24. Meister K. Injuries to the shoulder in the throwing
athlete. Part two: evaluation/treatment. Am J Sports
Med 2000;28(4):587–601.

25. Adams JE. Little league shoulder: osteochondrosis
of the proximal humeral epiphysis in boy baseball
pitchers. Calif Med 1966;105(1):22–5.

26. May MM, Bishop JY. Shoulder injuries in young
athletes. Pediatr Radiol 2013;43(Suppl 1):S135–40.

27. Carson JT, McCambridge TM, Carrino JA, et al.
Case report: bilateral proximal epiphyseal clavicular
stress-related lesions in a male gymnast. Clin Orthop Relat Res 2012;470(1):307–11.

28. Ouellette H, Kassarjian A, Tetreault P, et al. Imaging
of the overhead throwing athlete. Semin Musculoskelet Radiol 2005;9(4):316–33.

29. Park JG, Lee JK, Phelps CT. Os acromiale associated with rotator cuff impingement: MR imaging of
the shoulder. Radiology 1994;193(1):255–7.

30. Roedl JB, Morrison WB, Ciccotti MG, et al. Acromial
apophysiolysis: superior shoulder pain and acromial
nonfusion in the young throwing athlete. Radiology
2015;274(1):201–9.

31. Pagnani MJ, Mathis CE, Solman CG. Painful os acromiale (or unfused acromial apophysis) in athletes.
J Shoulder Elbow Surg 2006;15(4):432–5.

32. Quinlan E, Bogar WC. Acromial apophysitis in a
13-year-old adolescent boy: a common condition
in an uncommon location. J Chiropr Med 2012;
11(2):104–8.

33. Morisawa K, Umemura A, Kitamura T, et al. Apophysitis of the acromion. J Shoulder Elbow Surg 1996;
5(2 Pt 1):153–6.

34. Mudge MK, Wood VE, Frykman GK. Rotator cuff
tears associated with os acromiale. J Bone Joint
Surg Am 1984;66(3):427–9.

35. Havranek P. Injuries of distal clavicular physis in children. J Pediatr Orthop 1989;9(2):213–5.

36. Eidman DK, Siff SJ, Tullos HS. Acromioclavicular lesions in children. Am J Sports Med 1981;9(3):150–4.

37. Cahill BR. Osteolysis of the distal part of the clavicle
in male athletes. J Bone Joint Surg Am 1982;64(7):
1053–8.

38. Roedl JB, Nevalainen M, Gonzalez FM, et al. Frequency, imaging findings, risk factors, and long-
term sequelae of distal clavicular osteolysis in young
patients. Skeletal Radiol 2015;44(5):659–66.

39. Brogdon BG, Crow NE. Little leaguer's elbow. Am J Roentgenol Radium Ther Nucl Med 1960;83:671–5.

40. Dugas JR. Valgus extension overload: diagnosis and treatment. Clin Sports Med 2010;29(4):645–54.

41. Wilson FD, Andrews JR, Blackburn TA, et al. Valgus extension overload in the pitching elbow. Am J Sports Med 1983;11(2):83–8.

42. Wei AS, Khana S, Limpisvasti O, et al. Clinical and magnetic resonance imaging findings associated with Little League elbow. J Pediatr Orthop 2010; 30(7):715–9.

43. Kijowski R, Tuite MJ. Pediatric throwing injuries of the elbow. Semin Musculoskelet Radiol 2010;14(4):419–29.

44. Patel B, Reed M, Patel S. Gender-specific pattern differences of the ossification centers in the pediatric elbow. Pediatr Radiol 2009;39(3):226–31.

45. Davis KW. Imaging pediatric sports injuries: upper extremity. Radiol Clin North Am 2010;48(6): 1199–211.

46. Klingele KE, Kocher MS. Little league elbow: valgus overload injury in the paediatric athlete. Sports Med (Auckland, NZ) 2002;32(15):1005–15.

47. Roedl JB, Gonzalez FM, Zoga AC, et al. Potential utility of a combined approach with US and MR arthrography to image medial elbow pain in baseball players. Radiology 2016;279(3):827–37.

48. Zbojniewicz AM, Laor T. Imaging of osteochondritis dissecans. Clin Sports Med 2014;33(2):221–50.

49. Bancroft LW, Pettis C, Wasyliw C, et al. Osteochondral lesions of the elbow. Semin Musculoskelet Radiol 2013;17(5):446–54.

50. Toth F, Nissi MJ, Ellermann JM, et al. Novel application of magnetic resonance imaging demonstrates characteristic differences in vasculature at predilection sites of osteochondritis dissecans. Am J Sports Med 2015;43(10):2522–7.

51. Marshall KW, Marshall DL, Busch MT, et al. Osteochondral lesions of the humeral trochlea in the young athlete. Skeletal Radiol 2009;38(5):479–91.

52. Janarv PM, Hesser U, Hirsch G. Osteochondral lesions in the radiocapitellar joint in the skeletally immature: radiographic, MRI, and arthroscopic findings in 13 consecutive cases. J Pediatr Orthop 1997;17(3):311–4.

53. Yamaguchi K, Sweet FA, Bindra R, et al. The extraosseous and intraosseous arterial anatomy of the adult elbow. J Bone Joint Surg Am 1997;79(11): 1653–62.

54. Kijowski R, Blankenbaker DG, Shinki K, et al. Juvenile versus adult osteochondritis dissecans of the knee: appropriate MR imaging criteria for instability. Radiology 2008;248(2):571–8.

55. Krause M, Hapfelmeier A, Moller M, et al. Healing predictors of stable juvenile osteochondritis dissecans knee lesions after 6 and 12 months of nonoperative treatment. Am J Sports Med 2013;41(10): 2384–91.

56. Shi LL, Bae DS, Kocher MS, et al. Contained versus uncontained lesions in juvenile elbow osteochondritis dissecans. J Pediatr Orthop 2012;32(3): 221–5.

57. Furushima K, Itoh Y, Iwabu S, et al. Classification of olecranon stress fractures in baseball players. Am J Sports Med 2014;42(6):1343–51.

58. Waris W. Elbow injuries of javelin-throwers. Acta Chir Scand 1946;93(6):563–75.

59. Parr TJ, Burns TC. Overuse injuries of the olecranon in adolescents. Orthopedics 2003;26(11):1143–6.

60. Charlton WP, Chandler RW. Persistence of the olecranon physis in baseball players: results following operative management. J Shoulder Elbow Surg 2003;12(1):59–62.

61. Enishi T, Matsuura T, Suzue N, et al. Cartilage degeneration at symptomatic persistent olecranon physis in adolescent baseball players. Adv Orthop 2014;2014:545438.

Imaging Injuries in Throwing Sports Beyond the Typical Shoulder and Elbow Pathologies

Paul J. Read, MD*, William B. Morrison, MD

KEYWORDS

- Athlete • Injury • Bone • Tendon • Muscle • Ligament • Nerve • Vessel

KEY POINTS

- Several injuries may occur in athletes that fall out of the category of typical for their activity but may be just as debilitating as their more common counterparts.
- Awareness of these injuries allows for accurate, timely diagnosis, and appropriate management.
- Some of these injuries are not always fully imaged because they may occur in regions that are not entirely included in standard fields of view of routine MR imaging. Recognition of these injuries may allow customization of imaging protocols to fully evaluate degree of injury.

BONE INJURIES

The hamate is an irregularly shaped bone located in the ulnar aspect of the distal carpal row. From its volar margin, it has a hooklike bony projection, the hamulus, which is susceptible to direct compression injuries. As seen in **Fig. 1**, fractures are usually seen in athletes participating in racket sports, golf, and baseball. The typical presentation in the acute setting is point tenderness over the fracture with ecchymosis. It is not uncommon for fractures to present after a delay from the initial injury, and symptoms may include persistent pain with palpation, gripping or resisted flexion, and ulnar nerve parathesias/weakness given the proximity of the ulnar nerve as it travels through Guyon canal.[1] Imaging initially consists of a standard radiographic series of the hand. Norman and colleagues[2] described 3 signs as indicative of fracture: absence of the hook of the hamate; sclerosis of the hook; and lack of cortical density (ie, a barely visible outline) of the hamulus.

Radiographs are insensitive, however, for this diagnosis. A study by Kato and colleagues[3] demonstrated a sensitivity of only 31% for these fractures with a standard posteroanterior view. Additional views (carpal tunnel and supine oblique) increased sensitivity to 80%; CT demonstrated 100%. If the initial radiographs do not demonstrate a fracture and the clinical suspicion is high, CT should be the next step in the imaging algorithm. Management of these injuries may consist of an initial period of immobilization or surgical excision. Fractures managed conservatively typically require a long period of immobilization (>10 weeks) and may progress to nonunion. Resection of the hamate typically allows for return to activity in a much shorter time frame (6 weeks).[4]

MUSCLE/TENDON INJURIES

The latissimus dorsi is a large, fan-shaped muscle that has its origins from the T7-L5 spinous processes, thoracolumbar fascia, iliac crest, the

Disclosures: Nothing to disclose (P.J. Read). Consultant: Zimmer-Biomet. Co-patent holder: Apriomed Inc. Royalties: Elsevier (W.B. Morrison).
Division of Musculoskeletal Radiology and Interventions, Department of Radiology, Thomas Jefferson University Hospital, 132 South 10th Street, Philadelphia, PA 19107, USA
* Corresponding author.
E-mail address: paul.read@jefferson.edu

Radiol Clin N Am 54 (2016) 857–864
http://dx.doi.org/10.1016/j.rcl.2016.05.001

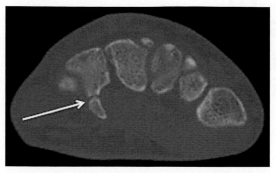

Fig. 1. A 55-year-old golfer with sudden onset of dull wrist pain after striking the ground with club. CT image demonstrates a nondisplaced fracture of the hook of the hamate (*arrow*).

inferior 3 or 4 ribs, and the inferior scapula. It inserts on the intertubercular groove of the humerus and functions to adduct, extend, and internally rotate the humerus. The teres major muscle similarly has its origin from the inferior scapula inserts on the intertubercular groove of the humerus and functions to adduct and internally rotate the humerus. Although each muscle has its own insertion, studies have shown that they are intimately associated[5,6] and electromyographic data show these muscles typically function as one unit.[7] During the throwing motion, the latissumus is most active during the late cocking and acceleration phases.[8] At the time of injury, patients typically describe an acute pain posteriorly along the axilla, usually with no significant preceding symptoms.[9,10] As seen in **Figs. 2** and **3**, MR imaging demonstrates high signal intramuscular edema and fluid consistent with strain involving the myotendinous unit. In the setting of an intramuscular hematoma, a well-defined mass with heterogeneous T1 shortening is seen related to methemoglobin. An additional example is seen in **Fig. 4**, which nicely illustrates the concept of initial incomplete evaluation of an injury due to limitations of a standard field of view. Awareness of injury patterns in these athletes, however, led to calling patients back for additional imaging, resulting in better characterization of the extent of tear (**Fig. 5**). These injuries are treated nonoperatively, with a majority of athletes returning to preinjury level competition within 3 months.[11]

Injury to the extensor tendons at the distal interphalangeal joints of the fingers is referred to as *mallet finger* or *baseball finger*. This injury is characterized by disruption of the terminal attachment of the extensor tendon to the distal phalanx, with or without an osseous avulsion fragment. The typical clinical history is forced flexion of an extended finger, and the patient presents

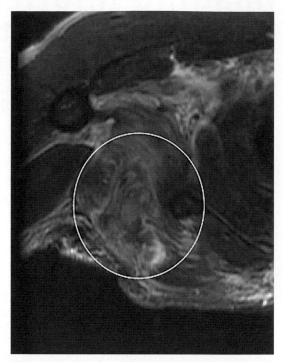

Fig. 2. A 30-year-old professional baseball pitcher with sudden-onset chest wall pain in dominant arm while pitching. Water-sensitive axial MR images show intramuscular edema and fluid within the latissimus dorsi muscle belly (*circle*) compatible with grade 2 strain.

with inability to actively extend the distal interphalangeal joint as well as pain and swelling.[12] If the lesion is purely tendinous, pain may be minimal. From an imaging standpoint, radiographs are

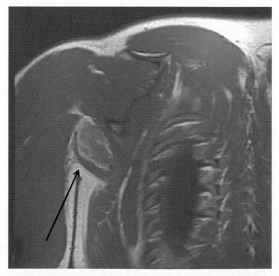

Fig. 3. Same patient, short interval follow-up. T1 coronal MR imaging shows organized intramuscular collection with intrinsic T1 shortening consistent with hematoma (*arrow*). T1 shortening is related to breakdown of oxyhemoglobin to methemoglobin.

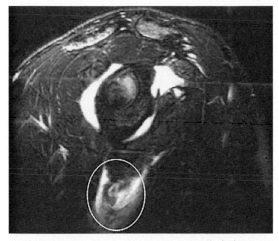

Fig. 4. A 25-year-old professional baseball pitcher with shoulder pain. Clinical concern for labral tear. Direct MR arthrography was performed. Water-sensitive sagittal imaging shows fluid within the glenohumeral joint related direct contrast injection. No intra-articular abnormality was found. Intramuscular edema was noted within the teres major muscle belly (*circle*). This area was only partially included in the field of view of the standard shoulder protocol.

used to assess bony involvement, because this is the main determinant to treatment. Purely soft tissue injuries are treated conservatively with splinting for approximately 6 to 8 weeks.[13] Lesions with bone fragments involving greater than one-third of the articular surface, chronic injuries/failures of conservative therapy, or the inability to work with hand in splint (**Fig. 6**) are treated with surgical fixation.[14]

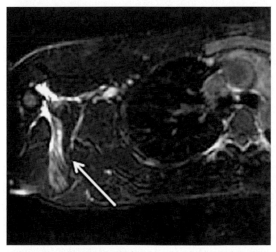

Fig. 5. Same patient, returns for additional imaging. Water-sensitive axial MR imaging with an expanded field of view shows intramuscular edema and fluid within the teres major muscle belly (*arrow*), consistent with a grade 2 strain.

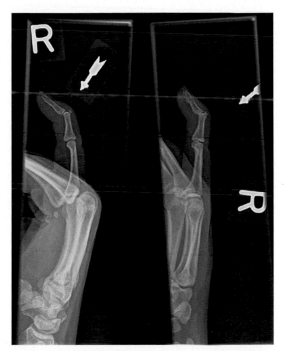

Fig. 6. A 23-year-old baseball catcher with inability to extend digit after catching a pitch. Lateral (*left*) and oblique (*right*) radiographs demonstrate flexion deformity at the distal interphalangeal joint on each view with a dorsal avulsion fragment, consistent with mallet finger.

An isolated injury to the brachialis muscle is a rare injury that can be seen in the setting of elbow dislocation.[15] The brachialis has its origin from the anterior margin of the distal humerus and inserts on the coronoid process of the ulna; its function is flexion at the elbow, independent of pronation/supination. Injury as a result of posterior dislocation is thought to be due to the anterior translation of the humerus, but complete tear is rare. Recently, at the authors' institution, a teenage lacrosse player presented with significant pain in the arm primarily used for cradling. No precipitating trauma was noted and the pain was reported only with and exacerbated by the cradling motion. A reasonable hypothesis is that this injury may represent a type of exertional compartment syndrome, with pain resulting from swelling of the muscle due to overuse. Whether due to trauma or overuse, the imaging features of brachialis muscle injury include edema with or without frank disruption of the muscle fibers (**Fig. 7**). Given the rarity of brachialis injury, specific guidelines for treatment are lacking. In the case of the complete tear secondary to elbow dislocation, surgical repair was performed.[15] The presumed overuse injury was managed conservatively by rest and avoidance of the inciting activity.

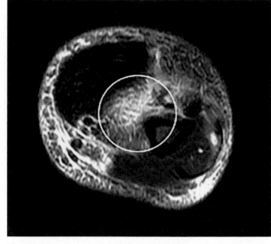

Fig. 7. A 15-year-old lacrosse player with arm pain, worsened with cradling. Water-sensitive axial MR imaging demonstrates marked edema within the substance of the brachialis muscle belly (*circle*).

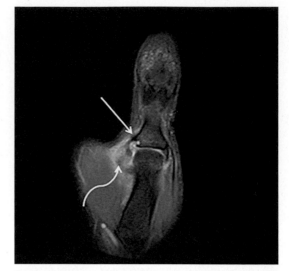

Fig. 8. A 30-year-old recreational softball player with thumb pain and instability after sliding into a base. Coronal water-sensitive MR imaging images show a complete tear of the ulnar collateral ligament of the thumb (*curved arrow*), with retraction of several millimeters. The position of the adductor aponeurosis (*white arrow*) inhibits conservative healing of the ligament, the Stener lesion.

LIGAMENT INJURIES

Injury to the ulnar collateral ligament at the metacarpal phalangeal joint of the thumb has historically been referred to as *gamekeeper's thumb* but more recently has been referred to as *skier's thumb* to reflect the activity that now more commonly results in injury. The ulnar collateral ligament proper and with the radial collateral ligament proper and their accessory ligaments are the main stabilizers of the metacarpal phalangeal and interphalangeal joints of the thumb.[16] The ulnar collateral ligament is reinforced by the aponeurosis of the adductor pollucis tendon, which sits immediately superficial. In the setting of a forced abduction/hyperextension injury, the ulnar collateral ligament may tear, retract, and displace superficially, resulting in the interposition of the adductor aponeurosis. This is referred to as the Stener lesion[17] and this interposition prevents ligament healing by conservative treatment. Surgical intervention is required to reattach. The initial imaging study to evaluate for a Stener lesion should be radiographs to assess for an osseous avulsion injury. Better delineation of the ligamentous injury is provided by MR imaging (**Fig. 8**), which has been shown effective in assessing both tear of the ulnar collateral ligament and displacement,[18] the latter important clinically because a full-thickness, displaced (greater than 3 mm) tear requires surgery whereas nondisplaced or minimally displaced tears may be managed conservatively.[19]

NERVE INJURIES

Nerve injuries at the shoulder in the throwing athlete occur at multiple locations: at the thoracic outlet in thoracic outlet syndrome, the long thoracic nerve along the chest wall, the axillary nerve in the quadrilateral space, and the suprascapular nerve at the glenoid.

Thoracic outlet syndrome is a compressive phenomenon that occurs at the superior thoracic aperture as the brachial plexus and subclavian artery/vein pass between the anterior and middle scalene muscles. This discussion focuses on the neurogenic entity; the vascular variant is discussed later. The brachial plexus is composed of the C5-T1 nerve roots as they exit the neural foramina and course between the scalene muscles, inferior to the clavicle and above the first rib to travel to the upper extremity. A combination of an anatomically constricted space and the shoulder hyperabduction/depression[20] that occurs during the throwing motion can result in thoracic outlet syndrome. Additional predisposing factors include hypertrophy of the scalene muscles, fibrous bands, and the presence of a cervical rib.[21] The neurologic variant is the most common type, accounting for approximately 95% of cases of thoracic outlet syndrome.[22] Diagnosis may be problematic, because the clinical presentation is often nonspecific: pain, paresthesias, and fatigue, usually centered at the elbow but often radiating centrally to the shoulder, neck, or face and distally to the fingers.[20] Imaging consists of radiographs to assess osseous anatomy/cervical rib; cross-sectional imaging with MR imaging may help assess the brachial plexus and any local mass or mass effect.[23] Treatment is initially conservative with rest and physical therapy; surgery may be considered in cases of a cervical rib as the cause or when conservative management fails.[24]

The long thoracic nerve has its origin from the ventral roots of C5-C7 of the brachial plexus. It exits anterior to the posterior scalene muscle and runs deep to the clavicle and inferiorly along the chest wall in the midaxillary line, providing innervation to the serratus anterior muscle. During the throwing motion, with the head flexed, rotated, and tilted laterally away from involved shoulder, the nerve is displaced anteriorly and medially, and a repetitive traction neuropathy may develop.[25] The athlete often presents with the insidious onset of pain and weakness, exacerbated by repetitive overhead activity. Scapular winging may be present.[24] The injury usually resolves with conservative management within 9 months.[25] Occasionally, atrophy of the serratus anterior muscle may result. Imaging usually consists of radiographs to exclude other obvious causes, like a cervical rib.[24] Cross-sectional imaging has a limited role but may document muscle atrophy in long standing cases, as seen in **Fig. 9**.

Quadrilateral space syndrome refers to an entrapment neuropathy of the axillary nerve that occurs in the quadrilateral space of the shoulder. The axillary nerve consists of contributions of C5 and C6 fibers of the brachial plexus. It travels peripherally, posterior to the axillary artery and anterior to the subscapularis muscle, and through the quadrilateral space, an anatomic space consisting of the subscapularis muscle as the anterior border, teres minor posteriorly, long head of triceps medially, and the surgical neck of the humerus laterally to provide innervation to the teres minor and deltoid muscles. Within this space, the axillary nerve and posterior circumflex humeral artery may be constricted by fibrous bands,[26] paralabral cyst,[27] or hypertrophy of the adjacent musculature,[28] resulting in an axillary neuropathy. An athlete typically presents with point tenderness over the quadrilateral space and pain, numbness, and weakness with hyperabduction and external rotation of the arm.[29] MR imaging demonstrates selective fatty atrophy of the teres minor and deltoid muscles[30]; the cause may also be shown, as in the case of a paralabral cyst causing axillary nerve compression. The fibrous bands often seen at surgery are not able to be resolved with MR imaging (**Fig. 10**). Treatment initially consists of rehabilitation focusing on strength and range of motion of the shoulder girdle muscles. Exploratory surgery should be considered if there is no improvement in 3 to 6 months.[31]

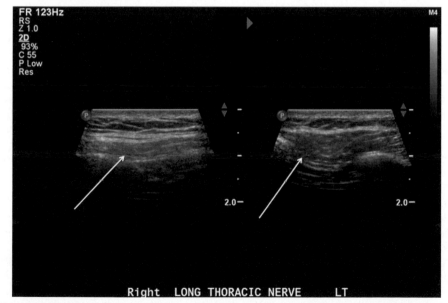

Fig. 9. A 47-year-old former volleyball player with dominant-side chest wall pain and weakness. Ultrasound imaging of the dominant right serratus anterior muscle belly (*arrow [left]*) shows diminished bulk and increased echogenicity compared with the left (*arrow [right]*) in keeping with fatty atrophy in the setting of a chronic long thoracic nerve palsy.

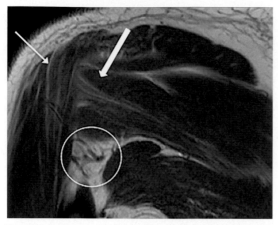

Fig. 10. A 28-year-old football quarterback with shoulder pain and weakness in throwing arm. T1 coronal MR imaging shows streaky T1 shortening within the infraspinatus (*thick arrow*) and deltoid (*thin arrow*) muscle bellies, compatible with quadrilateral space syndrome. The contents of the quadrilateral space (*circle*) are within normal limits, and findings are presumably related to crossing fibrous bands.

In the throwing athlete, suprascapular neuropathy may result from several causes, including compression, traction, friction, repetitive microtrauma, and direct injury.[32] From a radiologic perspective, the most commonly encountered cause is compression. Suprascapular nerve compression occurs in 2 locations: the suprascapular and spinoglenoid notches of the scapula. The nerve itself has it origin from the C5-C6 fibers of the brachial plexus. It traverses the posterior triangle of the neck and runs along the superior border of the scapula, through the suprascapular notch below the superior transverse scapular ligament, and into the supraspinous fossa where branches provide innervation to the supraspinatus muscle. The nerve then continues inferiorly and laterally through the spinoglenoid notch into the infraspinous fossa where branches provide innervation to the infraspinatus muscle. A common scenario for a throwing athlete is a tear of the labrum with an associated paralabral cyst. These cysts may extend away from the glenoid, into the suprascapular and/or spinoglenoid notch, and result in compression of the suprascapular nerve. Cysts in the suprascapular notch result in edema and atrophy of both the supraspinatus and infraspinatus muscles. Cysts in the spinoglenoid notch result in infraspinatus atrophy alone.[33] Additionally, the nerves may appear enlarged and have intrinsic high signal on water-sensitive sequences peripheral to the cyst due to compression.[34] Clinically, the presentation can vary. Patients early in the course of disease may have nonspecific pain and

little functional deficit. Advanced disease can result in weakness in external rotation and abduction with overhead activity and obvious asymmetry of the musculature due to atrophy.[32] Treatment is initially nonoperative; however, if the neuropathy is due to a cyst, nonoperative therapy is less effective and ultrasound-guided aspiration or surgery to resect the cyst can be considered.[35]

VASCULAR INJURIES

Similar to the neurologic counterpart, described previously, the subclavian vein and artery may be exposed to compressive injury as part of thoracic outlet syndrome. The predisposing factors are the same: anomalous/cervical rib, muscle hypertrophy, and fibrous bands related to microtrauma. The arterial variant with the development of aneurysm and distal embolization is exceedingly rare; a 12-year review by Chandra and colleagues[36] at Stanford did not include a single case. The venous compression syndrome; however, is a well-recognized entity. The hyperabduction of the arm during the throwing motion, often in combination with the predisposing factors described previously, may result in injury to the subclavian vein. Over time, intimal damage may result in effort thrombosis, referred to as Paget-Schroetter syndrome. Typical presentation is that of gradual onset of arm heaviness or tiredness, with swelling developing over the course of 2 to 7 days. The affected arm may also be slightly discolored, with nonspecific parasthesias and palpable axillary cords.[37] In addition to radiographs to assess for osseous abnormality, ultrasound provides assessment of the extent of thrombosis, and MR imaging with MR angiography/venography can help assess the degree and location of obstruction[11] (**Figs. 11–13**). Treatment consists of an initial course of anticoagulation, possibly also with catheter-directed venography and thrombolysis (more effective in the acute setting). After a period of anticoagulation, definitive therapy is performed: decompression with first rib resection with possible venous reconstruction. Good outcomes are seen in 80% to 90% of patients with anticoagulation and delayed decompression and 90% to 95% with immediate thrombolysis and reconstruction.[38]

In summary, there are several clinical entities that do not fall into the classic injuries seen in the overhead-throwing athlete. There are means, however, of accurately diagnosing and treating these less common conditions. Clinicians should be aware of these injuries when the clinical picture is nonspecific or a patient does not improve with

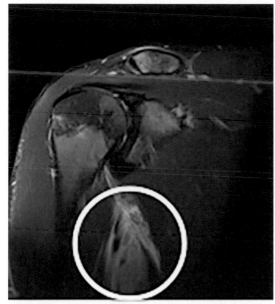

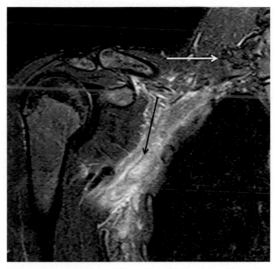

Fig. 13. Same patient. Water-sensitive coronal imaging shows the expanded; thrombus filled subclavian vein (*black arrow*). A cervical rib is the source of the subclavian vein impingement (*white arrow*).

Fig. 11. An 18-year-old high school baseball player with insidious onset of pain and weakness in the throwing arm. Water-sensitive coronal MR images using a standard shoulder protocol show edema along the axillary neurovascular bundle (*circle*). The remainder of the study was normal. Based on this finding, patient was asked to return for additional imaging.

rest and therapy. Radiologists should be aware of these injuries as well because quick recognition allows for additional optimal imaging and helps plan future treatment.

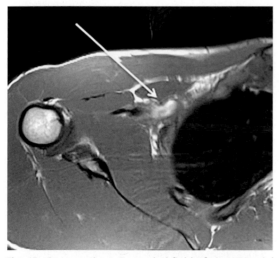

Fig. 12. Same patient. Expanded field of view T1 axial MR imaging shows T1 shortening within the lumen of the subclavian vein (*arrow*), consistent with thrombus in the setting of Paget-Schroetter syndrome. The normal flow void within the adjacent subclavian artery is preserved.

REFERENCES

1. Suh N, Ek ET, Wolfe SW. Carpal fractures. J Hand Surg Am 2014;39(4):785–91.
2. Norman A, Nelson J, Green S. Fractures of the the hook of hamate: radiographic signs. Radiology 1985;154(1):49–53.
3. Kato H, Nakamura R, Horii E, et al. Diagnostic imaging for the hook of the hamate fracture. Hand Surg 2000; 5(1):19–24.
4. Devers BN, Douglas KC, Naik RD, et al. Outcomes of hook of hamate fracture excision in high-level amateur athletes. J Hand Surg Am 2013;38(1):72–6.
5. Morelli M, Nagamori J, Gilbart M, et al. Latissimus dorsi tendon transfer for massive irreparable cuff tears: an anatomic study. J Shoulder Elbow Surg 2008;17(1):139–43.
6. Beck PA, Hoffer MM. Latissimus dorsi and teres major tendons: separate or conjoint tendons? J Pediatr Orthop 1989;9(3):308–9.
7. Pearl ML, Perry J, Torburn L, et al. An electromyographic analysis of the shoulder during cones and planes of arm motion. Clin Orthop Relat Res 1992; 284:116–27.
8. DiGiovine N, Jobe F, Pink M, et al. An electromyographic analysis of the upper extremity in pitching. J Shoulder Elbow Surg 1992;1:15–25.
9. Malcolm PN, Reinus WR, London SL. Magnetic resonance imaging appearance of teres major tendon injury in a baseball pitcher. Am J Sports Med 1999;27(1):98–100.
10. Turner J, Stewart MPM. Latissimus dorsi tendon avulsion: 2 case reports. Injury Extra 2005;36(9):386–8.
11. Schickendantz MS, Kaar SG, Meister K, et al. Latissimus dorsi and teres major tears in professional

baseball pitchers: a case series. Am J Sports Med 2009;37(10):2016–20.

12. McMurtry JT, Isaacs J. Extensor tendon injuries. Clin Sports Med 2015;34:167–80.

13. Simpson D, McQueen MM, Kumar P. Mallet deformity in sport. J Hand Surg Br 2001;26(1):32–3.

14. Bendre AA, Hartigan BJ, Kalainov DM. Mallet finger. J Am Acad Orthop Surg 2005;13(5):336–44.

15. Krych AJ, Kohen RB, Rodeo SA, et al. Acute brachialis muscle rupture caused by closed elbow dislocation in a professional American football player. J Shoulder Elbow Surg 2012;21(7):1–5.

16. Hirschmann A, Sutter R, Schweizer A, et al. MRI of the thumb: anatomy and spectrum of findings in asymptomatic volunteers. Am J Roentgenol 2014; 202(4):819–27.

17. Stener B. Displacement of the ruptured ulnar collateral ligament of the metacarpophalangeal joint of the thumb. J Bone Joint Surg Br 1962;44:869–79.

18. Hinke DH, Erickson SJ, Chamoy L, et al. Ulnar collateral ligament of the thumb: MRI findings in cadavers, volunteers, and patients with ligamentous injury (gamekeeper's thumb). Am J Roentgenol 1994;163:1431–4.

19. Milner CS, Manon-Matos Y, Thirkannad SM. Gamekeeper's thumb-a treatment oriented magnetic resonance imaging classification. J Hand Surg Am 2015;40(1):90–5.

20. Strukel RJ, Garrick JG. Thoracic outlet compression in athletes: a report of four cases. Am J Sports Med 1978;6:35–9.

21. Demondion X, Herbinet P, Van Sint Jan S, et al. Imaging assessment of thoracic outlet syndrome. Radiographics 2006;26(6):1735–50.

22. Fugate MW, Rotellini-Coltvet L, Freischlag JA. Current management of thoracic outlet syndrome. Curr Treat Options Cardiovasc Med 2009;11(2):176–83.

23. Esposito MD, Arrington JA, Blackshear MN, et al. Thoracic outlet syndrome in a throwing athlete diagnosed with MRI and MRA. J Magn Reson Imaging 1997;7(3):598–9.

24. Safran MR. Nerve injury about the shoulder in the athlete, part 2: long thoracic nerve, spinal accessory nerve, burners/stingers, thoracic outlet syndrome. Am J Sports Med 2004;32(4):1063–76.

25. Gregg JR, Labosky D, Harty M, et al. Serratus anterior paralysis in the young athlete. J Bone Joint Surg Am 1979;6(6):825–32.

26. Cahill BR, Palmer RE. Quadrilateral space syndrome. J Hand Surg 1983;8:65–9.

27. Sanders TG, Tirman PF. Paralabral cyst: an unusual cause of quadrilateral space syndrome. Arthroscopy 1999;15(6):632–7.

28. Paladini D, Dellantonio R, Cinti A, et al. Axillary neuropathy in volleyball players: report of two cases and literature review. J Neurol Neurosurg Psychiatry 1996;60:345–7.

29. Redler MR, Ruland LJ, McCue FC. Quadrilateral space syndrome in a throwing athlete. Am J Sports Med 1986;14(6):511–3.

30. Linker CS, Helms CA, Fritz RC. Quadrilateral Space Syndrome: findings at MR imaging. Radiology 1993; 188:675–6.

31. Perlmutter GS. Axillary nerve injury. Clin Orthop 1999;368:28–36.

32. Safran M. Nerve injury about the shoulder in athletes, part 1: suprascapular nerve and axillary nerve. Am J Sports Med 2004;32(3):803–19.

33. Fritz RC, Helms CA, Steinbach LS, et al. Suprascapular nerve entrapment: evaluation with MR imaging. Radiology 1992;182(2):437–44.

34. Bencardino JT, Rosenberg ZS. Entrapment neuropathies of the shoulder and elbow in the athlete. Clin Sports Med 2006;25(3):465–87.

35. Cummins CA, Messer TM, Nuber GW. Current concepts review-suprascapular nerve entrapment. J Bone Joint Surg Am 2000;82(3):415–24.

36. Chandra V, Little C, Lee JT. Thoracic outlet syndrome in high performance athletes. J Vasc Surg 2014;60(4):1012–8.

37. DiFelice GS, Paletta GA, Phillips BB, et al. Effort thrombosis in the elite throwing athlete. Am J Sports Med 2002;30(5):708–12.

38. Illig KA, Doyle AJ. A comprehensive review of Paget-Schroetter syndrome. J Vasc Surg 2010; 51(6):1538–47.

Imaging Athletic Groin Pain

Annu Chopra, MRCS, FRCR[a], Philip Robinson, MRCP, FRCR[a,b,*]

KEYWORDS

• Groin pain • Athlete • Inguinal disruption • Adductor injury • Imaging

KEY POINTS

• Outlining the diagnostic challenges of groin pain in athletes.
• Describing the 4 main entities of groin pain based on clinical findings.
• Describing the key imaging features of the 4 clinical entities.

INTRODUCTION

Sports hernia, athletic pubalgia, Gilmore's groin, hockey groin, and osteitis pubis are just some of the terms used interchangeably to describe groin pain in athletes. This reflects the difficulty radiologists encounter when reporting the pathology in this area. This is in part explained by the very complex anatomic area of the body, where soft tissue and bony structures are intimately related. The lack of a consensus on pathologic findings and terminology poses a real difficulty for allowing a clear discourse with clinicians about patient management options and comparative research. In an attempt to define this complex condition and unify diagnostic terms across different clinical disciplines, leading experts in this field met in the first world conference on groin pain. The key aspect of this conference was to agree on terminology and definitions of groin pain.[1] First, 'groin pain in athletes' was agreed as the preferred term for this group of conditions. They defined 4 clinical 'entities' for groin pain in athletes to reflect the recognizable pattern of symptoms and signs exhibited by the athlete. Therefore, the entities are primarily based on history and clinical examination and not imaging findings. The 4 defined entities are (**Fig. 1**):

• Adductor-related groin pain,
• Pubic-related groin pain,
• Inguinal-related groin pain, and
• Iliopsoas-related groin pain.

The athlete's history should include groin pain worsening with exercise. The clinical examination should comprise palpation, resistance testing, and stretching of the specific affected muscle groups.[1] Based on the injury pattern on imaging, the radiologist will help in deciding which of the 4 patterns or combination of patterns is present. The expert group also agreed that pain from the hip joint should always be considered as a possible cause of groin pain. When there is clinical suspicion of hip-related pain, the patient should be accordingly referred and managed.

This article outlines each separate clinical entity, with a description of the corresponding functional anatomy and imaging findings. The imaging has been described mainly in terms of MR imaging findings, because this is the principal imaging modality used to investigate groin pain, although plain radiographs and ultrasound can be very useful adjuncts in specific circumstances, especially if an alternative pathology needs to be excluded.

Conflicts of Interests: None declared.
[a] X-Ray department, Musculoskeletal Centre, Leeds Teaching Hospitals, Chapel Allerton Hospital, Chapeltown Road, Leeds LS7 4SA, UK; [b] Leeds Musculoskeletal Biomedical Research Unit, Leeds Teaching Hospitals, Chapel Allerton Hospital, Chapeltown Road, Leeds LS7 4SA, UK
* Corresponding author.
E-mail address: Philip.robinson10@nhs.net

Radiol Clin N Am 54 (2016) 865–873
http://dx.doi.org/10.1016/j.rcl.2016.04.007

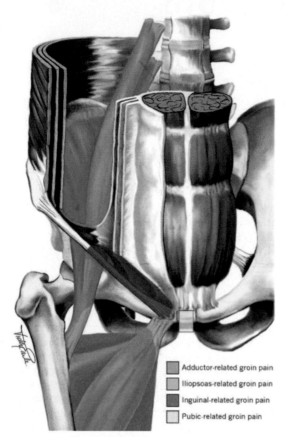

Adductor-related groin pain

Iliopsoas-related groin pain

Inguinal-related groin pain

Pubic-related groin pain

Fig. 1. Defined clinical entities for groin pain. Adductor-related groin pain: Adductor tenderness AND pain on resisted adduction. Iliopsoas-related groin pain: Iliopsoas tenderness and more likely if pain on resisted hip flexion AND/OR pain on hip flexor stretching. Inguinal-related groin pain: Pain in inguinal canal region AND tenderness of the inguinal canal. No palpable inguinal hernia is present. More likely if aggravated with abdominal resistance OR Valsalva/cough/sneeze. Pubic-related groin pain: Local tenderness of the pubic symphysis and the immediately adjacent bone. No particular resistance tests to test specifically for pubic-related groin pain. (*From* Weir A, Brukner P, Delahunt E, et al. Doha agreement meeting on terminology and definitions in groin pain in athletes. Br J Sports Med 2015;49:768–74; with permission.)

FUNCTIONAL ANATOMY OF THE CLINICAL ENTITIES OF GROIN PAIN

The groin is a very complex anatomic region and it is accepted that often the clinical/imaging findings will not be able to diagnose a discrete entity since multiple groin pathologies may coexist. Another contributing factor to diagnostic confusion is the variable nerve supply of the groin. The lumbar plexus is formed by the ventral rami of L1 to L5 and is located posteromedial to the psoas muscle and anterior to the lumbar vertebrae. The branches of the lumbar plexus provide innervation to the

groin and thigh. A detailed anatomic description of the nerve supply to the groin is beyond the scope of this article, but it should be appreciated that any variation in the neural anatomy will cause variation in symptoms, even when produced by the same pathology. Also any involvement of a nerve close to the area of pathology will cause referred pain as well as local symptoms, again causing diagnostic confusion.

Adductor-Related Groin Pain

The hip adductor muscles are composed of the short adductors: pectineus, adductor brevis, and adductor longus and the long adductors (gracilis and adductor magnus); (**Fig. 2**). The adductors originate on the pubis and ischial bones and insert onto the posteromedial femur with the exception of gracilis, which inserts onto the medial tibia. The pectineus is innervated by the femoral nerve, whereas all the other adductor muscles are innervated by branches of the obturator nerve (L2-L4). The main function of this muscle group is to adduct the hip and stabilize the pelvis during the swing phase of gait. With regard to sport, they are important in any sport that requires fast changes in direction and rapid leg movements against resistance, such as kicking a ball. It is the adductor longus muscle that is chiefly implicated in adductor-related groin pain. The adductor longus is the most anterior of the adductor muscles and it has a tendinous origin from the anterior pubic body. This tendon has a characteristic triangular shape and it meets and blends with the

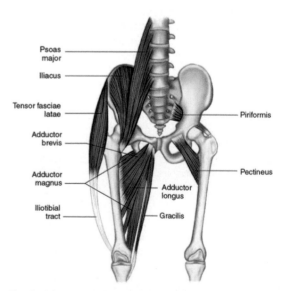

Psoas major

Iliacus

Tensor fasciae latae

Adductor brevis

Adductor magnus

Iliotibial tract

Piriformis

Pectineus

Adductor longus

Gracilis

Fig. 2. Diagrammatic representation of the adductor muscle anatomy and their relationship to surrounding structures.

contralateral adductor longus tendon across the midline. The proximal myotendinous origin also attaches to the capsular tissues of the pubic symphysis. It is here, at the capsular insertion, that the adductor longus is continuous with the inferior rectus abdominis fibers and pyramidalis that attach to the pubic crest and pubic symphysis capsular tissues and disc[2] (**Fig. 3**). This close anatomic relationship is an important consideration when interpreting adductor-related symptoms and imaging findings.

Adductor-related groin injury is particularly prevalent amongst soccer players.[3] Their presenting complaint is typically medial thigh pain and clinical examination demonstrates tenderness at the adductor enthesis and reproducible pain on passive adductor stretching and resisted adduction of the thigh.[1]

Pubic-Related Groin Pain

The pubic symphysis is an amphiarthrodial secondary cartilaginous joint between the 2 pubic bones. The joint is reinforced by 4 strong pubic ligaments—the superior, inferior, anterior and posterior—and through their review of cadaveric dissection and MR imaging, Robinson and colleagues[2] described an intimate relationship between the symphysis pubis and the anterior parasymphyseal soft tissues. These authors found that the joint capsule and fibrocartilagenous disc receive contributions from the adductor longus tendon and rectus abdominis tendon via an aponeurosis (**Fig. 4**). The central fibrocartilage disc cushions against compressive loads across the symphysis and acts to dissipate impaction forces, akin to a shock absorber. The articular disc often develops a central nonsynovialized 'primary cleft' by late teens reflecting increasing functional demands across the symphysis with increasing loads and greater transitional motion. The pubic symphysis is vulnerable to both degeneration and injury, particularly in athletes where it is repetitively subjected to high torsional and shear loads, especially seen in soccer players.

According to the consensus agreement,[1] patients considered to have pubic-related groin pain should have local tenderness of the pubic symphysis and the immediately adjacent bone. This condition has been described previously under the term *osteitis pubis*—inflammation of the symphysis pubis. However, this term is no longer favored because it is merely descriptive without implying an underlying pathology. The term osteitis pubis could encompass many etiologies, including trauma, inflammatory arthropathies,

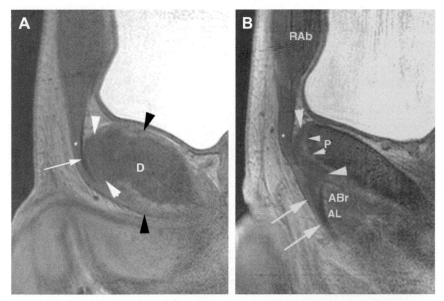

Fig. 3. Sagittal T1-weighted fast-field echo MR images of a male athlete show the normal anatomy. Image *A* shows the edge of the fibrocartilage disc (D) with interdigitating hyaline cartilage and pubic bone (*black arrowheads*). Anteriorly, capsular tissues (*white arrowheads*) merge with the disk and rectus abdominis tendon (*arrow*). Pyramidalis is present anteriorly (*asterisk*). Image *B* is lateral to *A* and shows pubic marrow and cortex (P) with a thin layer of hyaline cartilage (*small arrowheads*) closely applied to anterior capsular tissues (*between large arrowheads*). Merging with this tissue are rectus abdominis muscle (RAb), pyramidalis (*asterisk*), adductor longus tendon (*arrows*) and muscle (AL) and adductor brevis (ABr) muscle. (*From* Robinson P, Salehi F, Grainger AJ, et al. Cadaveric and MRI study of the musculotendinous contributions to the capsule of the symphysis pubis. AJR Am J Roentgenol 2007;188:440–5; with permission.)

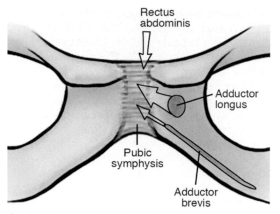

Fig. 4. Diagrammatic illustration of relative position of tendinous attachments with direction (*arrows*) of involvement over symphyseal capsular tissues.

pregnancy, and childbirth, as well as high levels of athletic activity. Fricker and colleagues[4] used the term 'osteitis pubis in athletes' and recognized it to be most commonly attributed to mechanical causes (seen in 48 of 59 patient records reviewed).

Inguinal-Related Groin Pain

The inguinal canal is essentially a passageway between the abdominal wall and perineum that transmits the spermatic cord in males and round ligament in females, along with neurovascular structures. Its boundaries are made up from continuations of the anterior abdominal wall muscles (**Fig. 5**):

- Anterior wall—aponeurosis of the external oblique, reinforced laterally by the internal oblique muscle;
- Posterior wall—transversalis fascia and reinforced medially by the lowermost fibers of the internal oblique and transversis abdominis muscles;
- Roof—transversalis fascia, internal oblique and transversus abdominis; and
- Floor—inguinal ligament (rolled-up edge of the external oblique aponeurosis).

- Two openings:
  - Deep inguinal ring—round opening in transversalis fascia found 1 cm above inguinal ligament and lateral to the inferior epigastric vessels; and
  - Superficial inguinal ring—a V-shaped opening in the external oblique aponeurosis just above the pubic tubercle and marks the end of the inguinal ligament.

Based on the consensus agreement, the clinical findings of groin pain and tenderness in the inguinal canal region in the absence of a palpable hernia describe inguinal-related groin pain. This diagnosis was more likely if the pain was aggravated with resistance testing of the abdominal muscles or on Valsalva/cough/sneeze.[1] Patients classified into this entity do not have a true inguinal hernia, but instead it is believed they have an acquired inguinal wall deficiency/dysfunction through overuse. For ease of disruption Koulouris[5] has subdivided this as either involving the anterior inguinal wall, the posterior wall or both.

Anterior inguinal wall deficiency

Anterior inguinal wall deficiency arises as a consequence of degeneration and tear of the external oblique muscle and aponeurosis resulting in a dehiscence between the inguinal ligament and leading to dilatation of the superficial inguinal ring. Positive imaging findings are rarely seen in this group and therefore this is primarily a clinical diagnosis.

Posterior inguinal wall deficiency

Posterior inguinal wall deficiency is due to degeneration of the transversis abdominis and internal oblique muscles resulting in weakness of the posterior inguinal wall, which becomes lax and can protrude into the inguinal canal causing a mass effect during straining. With ongoing injury, this can potentially in turn lead to complete disruption of the posterior wall resulting in a direct inguinal hernia.

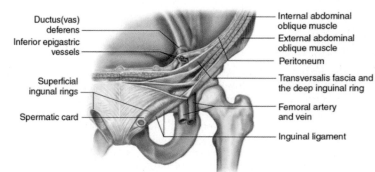

Fig. 5. Diagrammatic representation of inguinal canal anatomy.

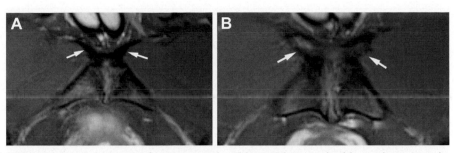

Fig. 6. Axial T2 Fat Saturated images of a young male athlete with normal adductor longus tendon insertions (*white arrows*) (*A*) and another with bilateral adductor longus tendinopathy (*white arrows*) (*B*).

Iliopsoas-Related Groin Pain

The iliopsoas muscle is formed by the combination of the iliacus and psoas major muscles within the abdomen and these unite to form a conjoined tendon, which inserts onto the lesser trochanter (see **Fig. 2**). The psoas major takes its origin from the lateral surfaces of the vertebral bodies of T12 to L5 and the iliacus originates from the inner surface of the iliac fossa. The 2 muscles unite at the level of the inguinal canal and cross anterior to the hip joint to insert into the lesser trochanter. The iliopsoas is the most powerful hip flexor and plays a major role in posture, walking, and running and also contributes to external rotation of the femur.

The iliopsoas bursa is the largest bursa in the body and is situated beneath the musculotendinous portion of the iliopsoas muscle, anterior to the hip joint capsule and lateral to the femoral vessels. The iliopsoas bursa directly communicates with the hip joint in approximately 15% of individuals.[6]

In relation to athletes, acute injury and chronic overuse injuries are the 2 main causes of iliopsoas pathology. The acute injuries typically involve an eccentric contraction or direct trauma, whereas overuse injuries occur in activities involving repeated hip flexion or external rotation of the thigh, for example, running, soccer, and gymnastics. Iliopsoas-related groin pain is more likely if there is pain on resisted hip flexion and/or pain on stretching of the hip flexors.[1]

IMAGING FINDINGS OF GROIN PAIN

Adductor-Related Groin Pain

Branci and colleagues[7] performed a critical literature search to evaluate the radiologic findings in adductor-related groin pain. They found 4 main radiologic findings that consistently occurred in this patient group: pathology at the adductor origin, pubic bone marrow edema, the secondary cleft sign, and remodeling changes at the pubic symphyseal joint.

Adductor origin

The rectus abdominis–adductor aponeurosis acts as a dynamic stabilizer of the pubic symphysis and is thought to be the site of injury in adductor-related groin pain.[8] Based on targeted entheseal pubic injections in competitive athletes, Schilders and colleagues[9] also concluded that the pathology of adductor-related groin pain is at the adductor enthesis. The imaging features of adductor-related groin pain are those of tendinopathy around the rectus abdominis–adductor aponeurosis (**Fig. 6**). MR imaging reveals diffuse high signal intensity at the adductor enthesis with more focal fluid signal areas representing tendon tears.[5] In **Fig. 7**, the MR imaging shows

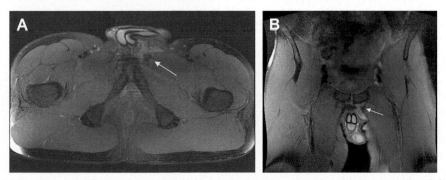

Fig. 7. Axial (*A*) & Coronal (*B*) T2 Fat Saturated MR images in a young male with longstanding left groin pain show an acute-on-chronic full-thickness tear in a tendinopathic left adductor longus tendon (*white arrow*).

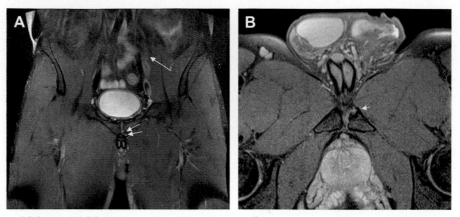

Fig. 8. Coronal (*A*) & Axial (*B*) T2 Fat Saturated MR images of a young male athlete with left groin pain show a left secondary cleft sign (*white arrows*).

an acute-on-chronic injury with a full-thickness tear in a tendinotic adductor longus tendon. Although not used commonly, a study using contrast enhanced MR imaging in adductor-related groin pain demonstrated that enhancement of the enthesis and anterior pubic region significantly and reproducibly correlated with site of the athletes' symptoms.[10]

Secondary cleft sign

This sign was described originally as an arthrographic finding after injection of the symphysis pubis and discovering an inferior extension of the contrast from the central symphyseal cleft. The MR imaging equivalent is seen as a curvilinear area of high signal between the pubic body and common adductor–rectus abdominis insertion (**Fig. 8**). It is thought to represent a tenoperiosteal avulsion that occurs at the tendon attachment to the inferior border of the symphyseal fibrocartilage that extends to involve the enthesis. This tear can be partial or complete. It causes extension of the physiologic or primary symphyseal cleft and formation of the secondary cleft around the inferior margin of the pubis.[11,12]

Pubic bone marrow edema and degenerative changes of the pubic symphysis

Other associated findings commonly encountered are degenerative changes of the pubic symphysis and pubic bone marrow edema (**Fig. 9**). Branci and colleagues[13] reported these osseous findings to be significantly more prevalent in symptomatic soccer players with adductor groin pain than asymptomatic players. They also reported a much higher incidence of these osseous MR imaging findings in soccer players in general when compared with nonsoccer players. However, as described below, significant pubic bone edema

is also seen with pubic-related groin pain as well as degenerative changes of the pubic symphysis. Pubic marrow edema is therefore not a highly specific finding and needs to be interpreted in the context of the other imaging findings and correlated with the clinical history and examination.

Pubic-Related Groin Pain

Pubic bone edema is the overriding imaging finding in this group. It is evident that this very complex junctional anatomic area between the torso and lower limbs is subjected to significant mechanical stress. In young patients, the physis is often weaker than the surrounding ligaments and tendons and the preferred site of stress resulting with some authors developing the term "apophysitis" in this patient group.[14] The pubic marrow edema in athletes reflects an osseous stress response related to the mechanical overload of the symphysis pubis. The main diagnostic conundrum with is that the bone marrow edema occurs in isolation as well as with some of the

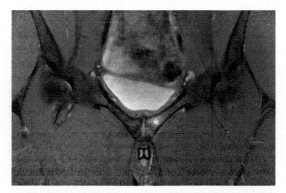

Fig. 9. Coronal T2 Fat Saturated image shows unilateral left sided pubic marrow oedema (*asterisk*).

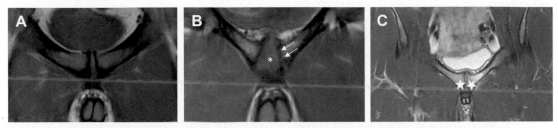

Fig. 10. Coronal T1 MR images of a young male athlete show (*A*) normal MR appearances of the symphysis pubis, (*B*) MR image of a degenerative pubic symphysis with joint irregularity and resorption (*white arrows*) & fluid signal within the pubic symphysis (*asterisk*) and Coronal T2 MR images (*C*) shows bilateral pubic marrow oedema (*star*).

other entities of groin pain. It is, therefore, imperative to take a clear history and thorough examination. The diagnosis of pubic-related groin pain should be made only when the imaging features are concordant with the clinical signs. Pubic bone edema is also seen frequently in asymptomatic athletes, again questioning its value as a discriminating imaging finding.[15] However, studies have shown that symptomatic athletes have a higher incidence of more 'extensive' bone marrow edema than the asymptomatic group.[15,16] More specifically, Verrall and colleagues[17] found that, as athletes became more symptomatic, the degree of bone marrow edema also increased. In this study, they used umpires as there control group, because they run but in general are not involved with any twisting or cutting motions. They found that no individual in the control group had 'significant' pubic bone edema. Kunduracioglu and colleagues[18] also analyzed the correlation between MR imaging findings (**Fig. 10**) with clinical features of osteitis pubis and found that subchondral pubic marrow edema, fluid within the symphysis pubis joint, and periarticular edema were the most reliable MR imaging findings of osteitis pubis if the history of pain was less than 6 months.

Subchondral sclerosis, subchondral resorption, and pubic osteophytes were the most reliable MR findings of chronic disease in those with a history of longer than 6 months. Similar findings of superior pubic bone spurs, pubic symphysis joint irregularity, and fluid signal in the pubic symphysis disc were reported by Verrall and colleagues[17] in athletes with a past history of groin pain. This finding supports the theory of pubic-related groin pain as a mechanical entity that is on a spectrum between pubic stress response that can be seen in asymptomatic athletes to established degenerative changes in chronic cases.

Inguinal-Related Groin Pain

Inguinal-related groin pain is best assessed initially with ultrasound to exclude the presence of a true inguinal or femoral hernia and then to make a dynamic assessment of the posterior inguinal wall looking for incompetence or disruption.[19] The patient is asked to strain (with Valsalva) and the inguinal canal is scanned both in long axis and short axis. The test of posterior wall incompetence is thought to be positive if there is bulging of the posterior wall into the inguinal canal (**Fig. 11**).

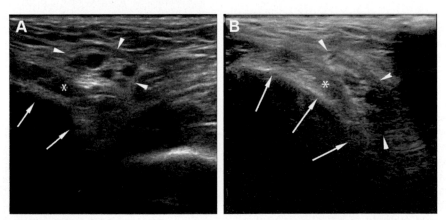

Fig. 11. Sagittal US images of the right groin. At rest (*A*) show normal short axis anatomy of the inguinal canal and (*B*) with increased intra-abdominal pressure show ballooning of the posterior inguinal wall causing distortion of the inguinal canal. Peritoneum (*white arrows*), pre-peritoneal fat (*asterisk*) & margins of the inguinal canal (*arrowheads*).

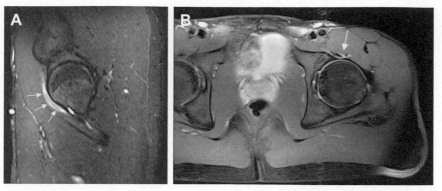

Fig. 12. T2 Fat Saturated MR images of a young male athlete with left groin pain. Sagittal image (*A*) shows fluid distension of the left iliopsoas bursa (*white arrows*) anterior to the hip joint capsule. Axial image (*B*) shows fluid surrounding the iliopsoas tendon (*white arrows*) anterior to the hip joint capsule and lateral to the femoral vessels - incidentally the iliacus and psoas major tendons have not united in this patient.

The ilioinguinal nerve travels in the distal part of the inguinal canal once it has pierced through the internal oblique muscle and emerges through the superficial inguinal ring. Thereby, an incompetent posterior wall can cause irritation of the ilioinguinal nerve and subsequent groin pain. The ultrasound findings were shown to be more specific when occurring bilaterally and with advancing age. However, they also occurred commonly in asymptomatic patients and a subsequent study corroborated that overall this finding is neither sensitive nor specific.[15,19,20]

The main role of MR imaging in this group of patients is to exclude an alternative diagnosis such as inguinal canal masses. Occasionally, injury to the aponeurotic structures can be identified as areas of hyperintensity.

ILIOPSOAS-RELATED GROIN PAIN

Iliopsoas bursitis is caused by overuse and friction as the iliopsoas tendon rides over the iliopectineal eminence of the pubis. Iliopsoas bursitis is characterized by deep groin pain, which is sometimes referred to the anterior hip or thigh. The normal iliopsoas bursa is collapsed and thus is not visualized. In iliopsoas bursitis, MR images reveal a thin walled homogenously hypointense mass on T1 and hyperintense on T2 sequences (**Fig. 12**). However, if the bursitis becomes chronic, the bursa wall can become thicker and the bursa content complex. MR imaging allows comprehensive evaluation of the iliopsoas tendon, its bursa, and the surrounding soft tissues. Owing to its multiplanar capabilities and superior soft tissue delineation, MR imaging is the most accurate imaging modality to assess the bursal size and whether or not it communicates with the hip joint.[21] Ultrasound

imaging can be used to assess for snapping iliopsoas tendon syndrome.

REFERENCES

1. Weir A, Brukner P, Delahunt E, et al. Doha agreement meeting on terminology and definitions in groin pain in athletes. Br J Sports Med 2015;49:768–74.
2. Robinson P, Salehi F, Grainger AJ, et al. Cadaveric and MRI study of the musculotendinous contributions to the capsule of the symphysis pubis. AJR Am J Roentgenol 2007;188:440–5.
3. Holmich P. Long-standing groin pain in sportspeople falls into three primary patterns, a "clinical entity" approach: a prospective study of 207 patients. Br J Sports Med 2007;41:247–52.
4. Fricker PA, Taunton JE, Ammann W. Osteitis pubis in athletes. Infection, inflammation or injury? Sports Med 1991;12:266–79.
5. Koulouris G. Imaging review of groin pain in elite athletes: an anatomic approach to imaging findings. AJR Am J Roentgenol 2008;191:962–72.
6. Allen WC, Cope R. Coxa saltans: the snapping hip revisited. J Am Acad Orthop Surg 1995;3:303–8.
7. Branci S, Thorborg K, Nielsen MB, et al. Radiological findings in symphyseal and adductor-related groin pain in athletes: a critical review of the literature. Br J Sports Med 2013;47(10):611–9.
8. Zoga AC, Kavanagh EC, Omar IM, et al. Athletic pubalgia and the "sports hernia": MR imaging findings. Radiology 2008;247(3):797–807.
9. Schilders E, Bismil Q, Robinson P, et al. Adductor-related groin pain in competitive athletes. The role of adductor enthesis, magnetic resonance imaging and entheseal pubic cleft injections. J Bone Joint Surg Am 2007;89:28–33.
10. Robinson P, Barron D, Parsons W, et al. Adductor-related groin pain in athletes: correlation of MR

imaging with clinical findings. Skeletal Radiol 2004; 33:451–7.

11. Cunningham PM, Brennan D, O'Connell M, et al. Patterns of bone and soft tissue injury at the symphysis pubis in soccer players; observation at MRI. AJR Am J Roentgenol 2007;188:W291–6.

12. Brennan D, O'Connell MJ, Rayan M, et al. Secondary cleft sign as a marker of injury in athletes with groin pain: MR image appearance and interpretation. Radiology 2005;235:162–7.

13. Branci S, Thorborg K, Bech BH, et al. MRI findings in soccer players with long-standing adductor-related groin pain and asymptomatic controls. Br J Sports Med 2015;49(10):681–91.

14. Sailly M, Whiteley R, Read JW, et al. Pubic apophysitis: a previously undescribed clinical entity of groin pain in athletes. Br J Sports Med 2015; 49(12):828–34.

15. Robinson P, Grainger AJ, Hensor EMA, et al. Do MRI and ultrasound of the anterior pelvis correlate with, or predict, young football players' clinical findings? A 4-year prospective study of elite academy soccer players. Br J Sports Med 2015; 49:176–82.

16. Lovell G, Galloway H, Hopkins W, et al. Osteitis pubis and assessment of bone marrow edema at the pubic symphysis with MRI in an elite junior male soccer squad. Clin J Sport Med 2006;16:117–22.

17. Verrall GM, Slavotinek JP, Fon GT. Incidence of pubic bone marrow oedema in Australian rules football players: relation to groin pain. Br J Sports Med 2001; 35:28–33.

18. Kunduracioglu B, Yilmaz C, Yorubulut M, et al. Magnetic resonance findings of osteitis pubis. J Magn Reson Imaging 2007;25:535–9.

19. Orchard JW, Read JW, Neophyton J, et al. Groin pain associated with ultrasound finding of inguinal canal posterior wall deficiency in Australian Rules footballers. Br J Sports Med 1998;32:134–9.

20. Steele P, Annear P, Grove JR. Surgery for posterior inguinal wall deficiency in athletes. J Sci Med Sport 2004;7:415–21.

21. Wunderbaldinger P, Bremer C, Schellenberger E, et al. Imaging features of iliopsoas bursitis. Eur Radiol 2002;12:409–15.

Ultrasound-guided Interventions for Core and Hip Injuries in Athletes

Eoghan McCarthy, MD[a], Tarek M. Hegazi, MD, MBBS, FRCPC[a,b],
Adam C. Zoga, MD[a], William B. Morrison, MD[a], William C. Meyers, MD[c],
Alex E. Poor, MD[c], Mika T. Nevalainen, MD[a], Johannes B. Roedl, MD, PhD[a,*]

KEYWORDS

- Core muscles • Hip • Ultrasonography guided • Athletic pubalgia • Percutaneous needle tenotomy
- Platelet-rich plasma

KEY POINTS

- MR imaging remains the primary modality for imaging core muscle and hip injuries, but ultrasonography-guided diagnostic and therapeutic procedures play a substantial role in the management of these conditions.
- If properly performed and with the right indication, ultrasonography-guided procedures can get the athlete through the season. Surgery can often be performed in the off-season.
- In chronic tendinosis and mild, chronic rectus abdominis–adductor aponeurosis/plate injuries, ultrasonography-guided percutaneous tenotomy shows promising results, but studies are warranted to determine the clinical value. For acute or high-grade injuries, surgery is the treatment of choice at this point.

PART I: GENERAL CONCEPTS

General Procedure Steps and Needle Placement

Before any ultrasonography-guided musculoskeletal procedure, an ultrasonography examination is performed to determine the best approach for the intervention. Color images are used to identify and avoid vessels, such as the femoral artery in iliopsoas or hip joint injections, the inferior epigastric arteries in rectus abdominis trigger point injections, or superior/inferior gluteal arteries in piriformis injections. An in-plane approach should be used around the pelvis/hips to visualize the entire needle at all times. Once the correct probe position is found, a line is drawn with a surgical marker at the edge of the transducer indicating the skin entry site and the transducer orientation. Sterile gloves are worn and the skin at the procedure site is cleaned and prepped with chlorhexidine and sterile towels. The skin is then anesthetized with local anesthetic using a 25-G needle and while the anesthetic takes effect, a sterile cover is placed over the ultrasound probe and the medications are drawn up. The appropriate needle is subsequently advanced to the required position. In sensitive patients, instilling a small amount of local anesthetic while advancing the needle might reduce pain. However, a larger amount of anesthetic might be more painful then effective because of the burning sensation and

The authors have nothing to disclose.
[a] Division of Musculoskeletal Imaging and Interventions, Department of Radiology, Jefferson Medical College, Thomas Jefferson University Hospital, Thomas Jefferson University, 132 South 10th Street, Suite 1096, 1087 Main Building, Philadelphia, PA 19107, USA; [b] Department of Radiology, University of Dammam, PO Box 2114, Dammam 31451, Saudi Arabia; [c] General Surgery, Vincera Institute, 1200 Constitution Avenue, Philadelphia, PA 19112, USA
* Corresponding author.
E-mail address: Johannes.Roedl@jefferson.edu

Radiol Clin N Am 54 (2016) 875–892
http://dx.doi.org/10.1016/j.rcl.2016.04.008
0033-8389/16/$ – see front matter © 2016 Elsevier Inc. All rights reserved.

local mass effect of the anesthetic. The needle should be kept as perpendicular as possible to the sound beam, meaning as parallel to the skin surface as possible. This orientation creates a strong reverberation artifact, making the needle echogenic and visible. In addition, manufactures have recognized the difficulties associated with sonographic guidance and have added echogenicity-enhancing features to their needles,[1-3] which might help when starting with ultrasonography-guided procedures. Jiggling the needle gently while slowly moving the transducer from side to side over the projected needle path helps to find the needle when lost.[4,5]

Corticosteroid and Local Anesthetic Injections

Indications

Tendinosis is initially treated conservatively with rest, physical therapy, and nonsteroidal antiinflammatory drugs (NSAIDs). About 60% to 80% of patients respond to conservative management. If these measures are unsuccessful, then more invasive treatment should be considered and a corticosteroid injection is often the initial step of the interventional therapy. Corticosteroid injections in inflammatory joints, bursitis, and tenosynovitis are well accepted and reduce the inflammatory response, including the local blood flow and local leukocytes.[6,7] This alleviates pain, albeit with often only temporary relief.[8] Corticosteroid treatment of tendon and muscular injuries is controversial. Although corticosteroid injections in muscles have been shown to reduce pain and facilitate return to preinjury activity in limited retrospective evaluations,[9,10] the long-term benefit from repeated corticosteroid injections in chronic tendinopathies is questionable.[11] There have been studies showing that the intratendinous injection of corticosteroids increases the risk of tendon rupture.[12-14] However, a study published in *The Lancet* by Coombes and colleagues[11] could not confirm this: only 1 of 991 patients receiving an intratendinous corticosteroid injection subsequently had a tendon rupture. The adductor longus is the only adductor that has a short intramuscular tendon at its origin, which is surrounded by muscle fibers. The other adductors (brevis, magnus, pectineus, gracilis) have muscular origins without tendons. In experienced hands and with the right indication, a small amount of corticosteroid injected around or in the adductor longus tendon occasionally helps with the tightness and has a similar effect to a surgical partial tendon release. A partial tear of some fibers of the tendon is a welcome side effect from the injection in that case and might help release the tightness without substantially impairing function. The risk of rupture is very low because the short adductor longus tendon is surrounded by the adductor longus muscle. However, studies are warranted to prove the clinical value of these ultrasonography-guided procedures. This concept can also be applied to snapping iliopsoas tendon disorder and to some degree to iliotibial band (ITB) syndrome. Instead of a surgical release of the iliopsoas tendon or ITB, a partial release with percutaneous tenotomy and small amount of corticosteroid in the thick iliopsoas tendon or ITB might be an alternative treatment option. Intratendinous corticosteroid injection should be used with caution in other tendons around the hips and pelvis, including hamstring, rectus femoris, sartorius, and gluteus medius and minimus tendons, in which a partial tendon release is contraindicated.

Corticosteroid agents

The corticosteroid agent most commonly used for musculoskeletal injections in the United States is triamcinolone acetonide (eg, Kenalog 10 mg/mL or 40 mg/mL) with duration of action of about 14 days, followed by methylprednisolone acetate (eg, Depo-Medrol 40 mg/mL or 80 mg/mL) with duration of action of about 8 days.[15,16] A typical dose for a hip jôint injection is 40 mg for both Kenalog and Depo-Medrol.

Mixture with local anesthetic

In general, corticosteroids are mixed with local anesthetic agents to add volume to the injectate and to relieve procedure-related pain. Local anesthetics inhibit the sodium-specific ion channels of the nerve cell membranes, thus preventing the propagation of an action potential. The most frequently used local anesthetic preparations are the amide agents, including lidocaine, bupivacaine, and ropivacaine. Epinephrine, a vasoconstrictor, can be added to enhance the anesthetic and reduce the systemic effect by concentrating the agent in the vicinity of the neuron. Lidocaine comes in 1% (10 mg/mL) and 2% (20 mg/mL) preparations with a maximum dose recommendation of 4.5 mg/kg up to 300 mg in the United States (30 mL of 1%), onset of action in 1 to 2 min, and duration of action between 80 and 120 minutes. Using lidocaine and epinephrine mixtures increases the maximum dose to 7.5 mg/kg up to 500 mg. Bupivacaine comes in 0.25% (2.5 mg/mL) and 0.5% (5 mg/mL) preparations with a maximum dose recommendation for an average adult male patient of 150 mg. However, this is patient weight and dose dependent; for an average-weight male patient up to 50 mL of 0.25% and up to 25 mL of

0.5% bupivacaine can be used, the onset of duration is 30 minutes and duration of action between 180 and 360 minutes (for both 0.25% and 0.5%). Ropivacaine has duration of action between 140 and 200 minutes and the maximum dose recommondation is 375 mg.[15,17,18] For diagnostic and therapeutic purposes, the authors frequently inject multiple sites in 1 setting. For this reason, we prefer to mix the corticosteroid with 0.25% bupivacaine because a total of up to 60 mL of bupivacaine can be given safely. Corticosteroid crystals might aggregate when mixed with lidocaine containing preservative. Therefore, preservative-free lidocaine should be used (as indicated on the vial) or bupivacaine, which generally is preservative free. Iodinated contrast material does not lead to aggregation/precipitation of corticosteroid and might be used to confirm intra-articular placement with fluoroscopy after an ultrasonography-guided hip joint injection.[15,19]

Injections used as diagnostic tests

Before and after any injection, a physical examination eliciting the patient's pain should be performed. The patient is asked to describe the severity of the pain on an analog 10-point pain scale before and after the injection. Once the target has been injected, the relief of pain by the local anesthetic agent is used as a diagnostic test. The patient should be informed that the pain is likely to return in several hours once the numbing medication wears off. The pain should then improve again once the corticosteroid takes effect in about 3 to 5 days after the injection. However, studies to verify the clinical value of diagnostic ultrasonography-guided injections around the core are needed.

Corticosteroid side effects

The most common side effect of a corticosteroid injection is the so-called steroid flare phenomenon (2%–10% of injections).[20–22] In a steroid flare, the pain gets paradoxically worse, often within hours of the injection. Transient facial flushing is another fairly common complication (1%–10%). Patients with diabetes should be warned about temporary hyperglycemia and patients with glaucoma about a transient increase of intraocular pressure secondary to the corticosteroid. Diabetic patients should be cognizant of their glucose readings and may require alterations to their medications during the hyperglycemia effect, which lasts about 5 to 21 days.[8] Loss of skin pigmentation and atrophy of subcutaneous fat are side effects in superficial injections, but are not concerning in the hip/pelvis area secondary to the increased depth of most injections.

The main side effects of local anesthetic overdoses are cardiac arrhythmias, nausea, dizziness, and metallic taste. There have been controversial reports that local anesthetics are toxic to both skeletal muscle and to chondrocytes in very high doses.[23–27] However, the doses used in musculoskeletal injections are much lower than those used in these studies.

Percutaneous Tenotomy, Prolotherapy, and Platelet-rich Plasma

Percutaneous needle tenotomy and prolotherapy

In percutaneous needle tenotomy (PNT), a needle (typically 20 G or 18 G) is advanced to the area of tendon disorder (tendinosis) under ultrasonography guidance. Local anesthetic (typically lidocaine) is injected in the tendon with separation of tendon fibers (hydrodissection). Needling (percutaneous tenotomy) is then performed to further loosen up the pathologic tendon tissue and to induce bleeding in and around the stimulated tendon. The bleeding recruits platelets and other cells that release growth factors and cytokines. This process induces healing and restores normal tendon fibers. Housner and colleagues[28] showed an improvement in patients' symptoms after ultrasonography-guided percutaneous tenotomy in a mixture of tendons, including the proximal gluteus medius, proximal iliotibial tract, proximal rectus femoris, and proximal hamstring tendons.

The injected local anesthetic (lidocaine or bupivacaine) also functions as a proliferant therapy altering the chemical environment and assisting healing. Other proliferants, like hyperosmolar dextrose, can be injected.[29,30] This procedure has been termed prolotherapy. Corticosteroids are not instilled with needle tenotomy because needling incites a local inflammatory reaction, which would be inhibited by corticosteroids.[31]

Platelet-rich plasma: mechanism of action

To enhance the inflammatory healing response of the percutaneous tenotomy, platelet-rich plasma (PRP) can be injected together with the needling. PRP is blood plasma that has been enriched with platelets via centrifugation. The platelets collected in PRP induce the release of the growth factors. Growth factors recruit cells and vessels to the site and stimulate healing of tendon and muscle injuries. Released growth factors include:

- Platelet-derived growth factor
- Transforming growth factor beta
- Fibroblast growth factor

Platelet rich plasma: preparation

Venous blood is drawn from the patient. With centrifugation, 3 layers of blood are separated with a kit: PRP, platelet-poor plasma, and packed red blood cells. The PRP is aspirated with a syringe. In humans, the typical baseline whole-blood platelet count is approximately 200,000/μL. Therapeutic PRP concentrates the platelets by roughly 5-fold to about 1,000,000/μL.

Platelet rich plasma: procedure and postprocedure care

Under sterile conditions and local anesthetic, the needle (typically 20 G) is advanced to the area of tendon disorder. The authors always perform needling (percutaneous tenotomy) first to loosen up the tendon tissue and create space for the PRP. The PRP is then injected in the tendon. There is an expected transient increase in pain in the first few days after the procedure secondary to the acute inflammatory effect of the needling and PRP. This pain can be treated with paracetamol preparations.[32] Antiinflammatory pain medications (NSAIDs and steroids) should be avoided before and after injection. Immobilization is advised for 24 hours, with mobilization thereafter, as soon as tolerated. Physical therapy can usually begin 2 days after the procedure, with gradual increase in intensity. In most cases, only 1 treatment session is necessary; however, occasionally a second procedure is performed after 6 months if the pain does not subside.

Platelet rich plasma: clinical evidence

PRP has a good safety profile without any substantial side effects published at the time of writing. However, in patients who underwent PRP injections in the adductors, the authors anecdotally have seen foci of heterotopic ossification. In lateral epicondylitis at the elbow (common extensor tendinosis), there is limited level I evidence showing inferior short-term but superior long-term (after 1 year) outcomes for PRP versus corticosteroid injections.[33] Other studies also showed good results in treating lateral epicondylitis with PRP[34,35] but mixed outcomes for Achilles tendinosis[34,36] (and disappointing outcomes for patellar tendinosis).[34] A recent (2013) Cochrane Review concluded that the available evidence is insufficient to support the use of PRP. That review described a minor benefit of PRP in managing pain in the short term (up to 3 months) but no difference in function in the short, medium, or long terms. The investigators concluded that current evidence was of low quality and there was vast heterogeneity between studies in the preparation of the PRP.[37] In our daily clinical practice, the authors perform percutaneous tenotomies without PRP in most patients. From our experience, the addition of PRP adds little additional value but also no additional side effects or disadvantage. In the presence of tendon tears within the tendinosis, we often add PRP and it might improve outcome. In adductor and rectus abdominis–adductor aponeurosis/plate injuries, we avoid PRP because of our observation that PRP might predispose to heterotopic ossification in these injuries. However, more randomized clinical studies are warranted using PRP, especially for other tendons, like hamstring, rotator cuff, common flexor tendons at the elbow, and ankle tendons.

It is important to know when treating athletes that the World Anti-Doping Agency has confirmed that PRP itself is permitted, although some of the growth factors released from PRP individually are banned.[38]

PART 2: CONDITIONS
Core Muscle Injuries

Core muscles include muscles at the trunk from the lower rib cage to the midthighs. A narrower definition includes muscles that have attachments to the pubic bone.[39–42] The 2 most important core muscles are the rectus abdominis and adductor longus (Fig. 1A), which are contiguous and merge in a rectus abdominis–adductor aponeurosis/plate overlying the pubic tubercle (Figs. 1B and 2). This aponeurosis/plate can detach anteriorly from the pubic tubercle creating a defect/tear. Symptoms include pubic and groin pain, and proximal adductor and distal rectus abdominis pain. In the past this clinical presentation of pubalgia was thought to be related to a hernia and the term sports hernia was erroneously coined. After a dedicated MR imaging protocol was developed, the rectus abdominis–adductor aponeurosis/plate detachment could be visualized and it became clear that it was not a sports hernia, but a core muscle injury.[43,44]

On ultrasonography, the rectus abdominis–adductor aponeurosis/plate is best visualized by placing the probe in a slightly oblique, caudal-cranial plane centered over the pubic tubercle (see Fig. 1A for scanning of the left rectus abdominis–adductor aponeurosis/plate). It helps to have the patient in a slight frog-leg position with the knee flexed and the hip abducted. On both MR imaging and ultrasonography, the aponeurosis/plate is seen as a triangular structure on the sagittal images with confluence of the adductor muscle group toward the aponeurosis/plate from caudal (Fig. 1C, D). The rectus abdominis joins the aponeurosis/plate from cranial

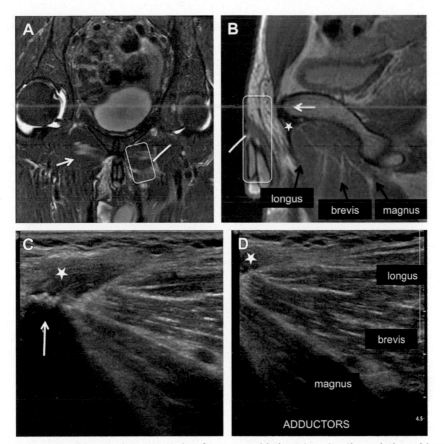

Fig. 1. Rectus abdominis–adductor plate. Coronal T2 fat saturated (FS) MR imaging through the pubic symphysis (*A*) shows the ideal orientation of the ultrasound probe (*rectangle*) for scanning the left adductor origins. There are grade 1 muscle strains of the left proximal adductors underlying the ultrasound probe and similar contralateral strains on the right side (*white arrow*). The corresponding sagittal MR imaging (proton density [PD], non-FS) shows the sagittal probe orientation and sagittal anatomy of the proximal adductor muscles (*B*), which line up from anterior to posterior as adductor longus, brevis, and magnus. The adductor longus and brevis blend anteriorly into a triangular-shaped hy-pointense plate (*white star*), the rectus abdominis–adductor plate, which is also known as the rectus abdominis–adductor aponeurosis. This plate is located just anterior to the pubic tubercle (*white arrow*) and is cranially contiguous with the distal rectus abdominis muscle. The correlating ultrasonography images in *C* and *D* show the proximal adductors and the confluence of the adductor origins at the rectus abdominis–adductor plate (*white star*) at the level of the pubic tubercle (*white arrow* in *C*).

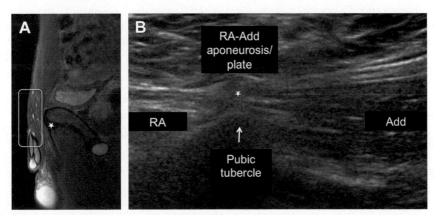

Fig. 2. Rectus abdominis–adductor plate. The sagittal MR imaging (PD, non-FS) in (*A*) shows the probe orientation (*rectangle*) of the corresponding ultrasonography image in (*B*). The ultrasonography image shows the proximal adductor muscles (Add), which blend in the rectus abdominis–adductor plate/aponeurosis (*white star*) with fibers from the distal rectus abdominis muscle (RA). The RA-Add plate is located anterior to the pubic tubercle (*white arrow*).

(see **Figs. 1**B and **2**). No literature has been published on detecting aponeurosis/plate injuries on ultrasonography. However, from our experience, small aponeurosis/plate detachments cannot be seen on ultrasonography. A large detachment is seen as a hypoechoic cleft between the pubic tubercle and the aponeurosis/plate. MR imaging remains the modality of choice for diagnosing core muscle injuries. Adductor tendinosis is identified on ultrasonography as heterogeneity and thickening of the adductor longus tendon. The tendon origin is contiguous with the triangular aponeurosis/plate. For interventions, the authors favor a caudal-cranial needle approach. A diagnostic/therapeutic local anesthetic/steroid injection or percutaneous needle can be performed for treating both the aponeurosis/plate itself and the adductor origins. A 22-G spinal needle is used and the needle is manually bent to get access to the adductor longus tendon and the aponeurosis/plate. A recent publication by Jose and colleagues[9] reviewed the outcome of ultrasonography-guided corticosteroid injection for so-called athletic pubalgia in a cohort of 12 patients. All 12 patients had focused preprocedural ultrasonography examinations showing either partial or complete tears around the insertion of the rectus abdominis and/or the adductor longus origin. Six weeks following successful ultrasonography-guided steroid injection, all subjects had returned to their preinjury activity levels. Furthermore, during the follow-up (ranging from 6 to 19 months), no patients opted for surgical repair.[9] However, a randomized controlled trial in 2011 showed the superiority of surgery compared with noninterventional conservative therapy. Ninety percent of the operative group returned to activity at 3 months versus 27% of the nonoperative group; 23% of the nonoperative cohort eventually elected to undergo surgical intervention.[45] The largest series of patients with surgical core muscle repairs was published by Meyers and colleagues[46] with excellent results. To date, there have been no studies evaluating the outcome of ultrasonography-guided tenotomy for rectus abdominis–adductor aponeurosis/plate injuries. Anecdotally, the authors have found this procedure beneficial with excellent outcome in patients with chronic low-grade injuries who want to avoid surgery during the season and also in a group of patients with persistent groin pain and adductor tightness after surgery. However, dedicated studies are warranted to validate these observations.

Hip Joint

Hip joint injections with local anesthetic and with or without corticosteroids and with or without gadolinium contrast (before hip MR arthrogram) are among the most common procedures in the pelvic region. The authors perform a detailed hip physical examination before and after the procedure to assess pain relief from the injection. Pain relief indicates an intraarticular cause of the pain, including labral tears, femoroacetabular impingement, and/or cartilage defects. Pain with passive hip flexion, adduction, and internal rotation typically indicates an underlying cam-type femoroacetabular impingement with associated anterosuperior labral tears. It is important to wait at least for 10 minutes with lidocaine and at least 45 minutes with bupivacaine to assess pain relief after the hip joint injection because of the delayed onset of the local anesthetic effect. If patients get an MR arthrogram, the authors assess pain relief after the completion of the MR imaging. If corticosteroids were injected, patients are also instructed to self-assess pain relief about 5 days after the injection to evaluate relief from the steroid effect. The authors usually inject 40 mg of Kenalog (40 mg/mL) and either 4 mL of 1% lidocaine or 6 mL of 0.25% bupivacaine in hip joints. If the setup allows, the correct intraarticular needle placement with ultrasonography guidance can be confirmed with a single fluoroscopic image, as shown in **Fig. 3**A.

With ultrasonography guidance, the hip can be approached from an anterior longitudinal (sagittal) caudal-cranial needle approach, as shown in **Fig. 3**A, C. With this approach, the needle is guided to the femoral neck until bone is reached (**Fig. 3**B). MR arthrogram is the modality of choice for diagnosing labral tears, cartilage defects, and cam-type femoroacetabular impingement morphology. On sonography, the osseous bump in cam-type femoroacetabular morphology can often be seen (**Fig. 4**A, C). The anterior labrum can also be visualized on ultrasonography (**Fig. 4**B) and detached (full-thickness) tears are often depicted, but clinicians should not rely on ultrasonography for the diagnosis of labral tears. A synovial herniation pit at the anterosuperior femoral head-neck junction is an indirect imaging sign of femoroacetabular impingement. **Fig. 5** depicts a synovial herniation on 3 modalities: MR imaging (see **Fig. 5**A), ultrasonography (see **Fig. 5**B), and a Dunn lateral radiograph (see **Fig. 5**C).

Paralabral Cysts

Full-thickness (detached) labral tears are often associated with paralabral cysts that fill with joint fluid and often extend cranially, deep to the iliacus muscle or just lateral to the rectus femoris origin.

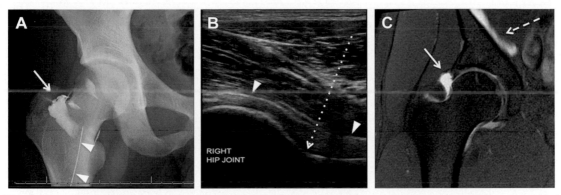

Fig. 3. Hip joint injection. The fluoroscopic image (*A*) of the right hip is taken after an ultrasonography-guided intra-articular injection (*B*) of iodinated and MR contrast via a long-axis approach. Contrast outlines the femoral neck (*white arrow* in *A*) and the spinal needle is identified by the arrowheads. The needle path (*dotted arrow* in *B*) is aimed toward the femoral neck. The white arrowheads point out the anterior hip joint capsule. The coronal T1 FS MR arthrogram image (*C*) shows MR contrast both in the hip joint (*arrow*) and contrast decompressed in the iliopsoas bursa deep to the iliacus muscle (*dashed arrow*). The anatomic variant of a communication between the hip joint and the iliopsoas bursa is seen in about 10% of patients.

These cysts can become very big and complex, mimicking a large iliopsoas bursitis and occasionally can even compress anterior hip structures such as the femoral nerve.[47] Ultrasonography is an effective modality for the diagnosis and treatment of paralabral cysts.[48–50] Under ultrasonography guidance, the cysts can be aspirated (usually with a 20-G or 18-G needle), the cyst wall fenestrated, and a small amount of undiluted corticosteroid injected (**Fig. 6**). Sometimes, the cysts are so complex and thick (gel-like) that aspiration is not possible. In these cases, the cyst wall fenestration helps to decompress the cyst. Most patients report excellent pain relief. Similar to other ultrasonography-guided procedures, this technique often gets an athlete through the season. Definite treatment of the underlying cause (in this case the labral tear) can be performed in the off-season.

Iliopsoas Tendon/Bursa

Aside from hip joint disorders and rectus abdominis–adductor core muscle injuries, the iliopsoas tendon is a common cause of groin pain. The most common iliopsoas-related abnormalities are iliopsoas tendinosis, iliopsoas bursitis, iliopsoas muscle atrophy, and snapping iliopsoas tendon. Dynamic (stress) ultrasonography is an emerging modality in musculoskeletal radiology[51] and is accurate for the diagnosis of snapping iliopsoas tendon. The snapping of the iliopsoas tendon is seen while the patient performs a straight leg raise. The iliopsoas bursa surrounds the iliopsoas tendon at the level of the acetabulum. The hip joint communicates with the iliopsoas bursa in about 15% of the healthy population. In patients with hip disorders, about 40% of hip joints communicate and decompress into the iliopsoas bursa,

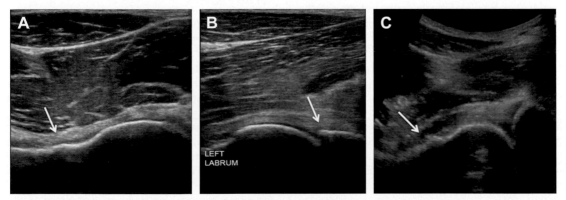

Fig. 4. Femoroacetabular impingement (FAI) morphology on ultrasonography: Long-axis ultrasonography image (with a 15-MHz probe) of the anterior femoral head-neck junction (*A*) shows a cam-type FAI osseous bump (*white arrow*). Scanning further toward the femoral head (*B*) shows a normal labrum (*white arrow*). (*C*) Another patient with a cam-type FAI bony prominence at the femoral head-neck junction (*white arrow*) is imaged with a 5-MHz probe.

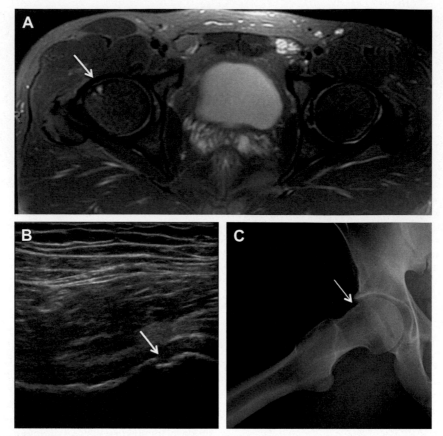

Fig. 5. Synovial herniation pits on ultrasonography. Axial T2 FS MR imaging (*A*) with a synovial herniation pit at the right femoral head-neck junction (*white arrow*). This defect is also shown on ultrasonography (*B*) and a Dunn lateral radiograph (*C*).

similar to a Baker cyst in patients with intraarticular knee disorders. Iliopsoas bursitis is therefore either secondary to an associated hip disorder or caused by a primary iliopsoas tendon disorder such as tendinosis, tear, or snapping iliopsoas tendon. The primary function of the bursa is to prevent friction between the iliopsoas tendon and the underlying acetabulum and between the tendon and the surrounding iliopsoas muscle. The bursa can be aspirated via an axial approach at the level of the acetabulum just cranial to the hip joint from a lateral to medial needle approach (**Fig. 7**). The needle passes just anterior to the anterior inferior iliac spine (AIIS) and then extends deep between the iliopsoas tendon and the acetabulum (see **Fig. 7**). After aspiration, corticosteroid (eg, 20 mg of Kenalog) is injected to reduce inflammation and avoid recurrence. A recently published study of patients undergoing fluoroscopy-guided iliopsoas bursa injection for suspected iliopsoas tendinopathy showed symptomatic improvement at 1 month and significant reduction of pain as soon as 15 minutes after the injection.[52] Iliopsoas bursitis can be complex, mimicking a soft tissue mass (**Fig. 8**). Ultrasonography-guided PNT can be performed for snapping iliopsoas tendon or moderate/severe tendinosis with tendon thickening.

Rectus Femoris

The rectus femoris tendon origin has 2 heads: The direct head, which arises directly from the AIIS, and the indirect head, which originates just lateral and caudal to the AIIS from the superolateral rim of the acetabulum. In absolute numbers, rectus femoris disorders are not as common as iliopsoas injuries, but they are fairly common at the dominant leg of soccer players or football kickers. Chronic tendinosis of the rectus femoris tendon origin presents on ultrasonography as tendon thickening at the dominant leg compared with the contralateral side. On axial ultrasonography, the rectus femoris can be found just lateral to the iliopsoas tendon originating from the AIIS (**Fig. 9**A, B). For ultrasonography-guided injections, an axial (lateral to medial) needle approach

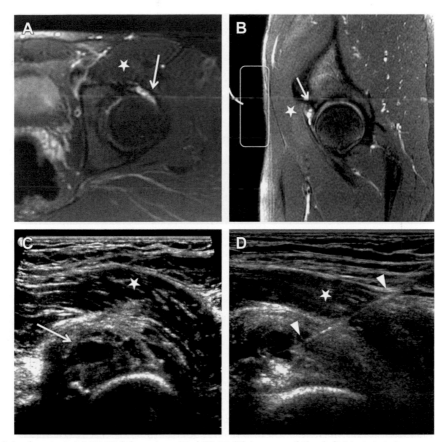

Fig. 6. Paralabral cyst. Axial T2 FS (*A*) and sagittal T2 FS (*B*) images of the left hip joint show a paralabral cyst (*white arrow*) originating from the anterosuperior labrum and located deep to the left iliopsoas muscle (*white star*). The probe orientation (*rectangle* in *B*) is depicted for the corresponding ultrasonography images (*C* and *D*). (*C*) The partially complex, multiloculated paralabral cyst (*white arrow*) is shown deep to the iliopsoas muscle (*white star*). Needle aspiration (*arrowheads* in *D*), wall fenestration, and subsequent steroid aspiration in the area of the decompressed cyst.

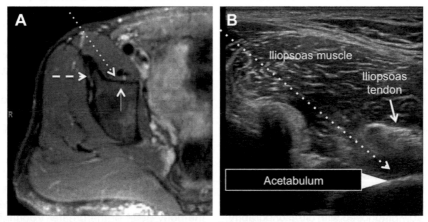

Fig. 7. Iliopsoas bursa. Axial T2 FS image (*A*) shows the MR anatomy of a typical right iliopsoas bursa injection under ultrasonography (*B*) at the level of the anterior inferior iliac spine (AIIS; *dashed arrow* in *A*) and acetabulum (*white arrow* in *B*). On the MR image (*A*), the dotted white arrow shows the ideal needle course through the iliopsoas muscle with the needle tip at a small hyperintense focus of iliopsoas bursitis between the acetabulum and the iliopsoas tendon. The ultrasonography image (*B*) after the injection of local anesthetic shows that the iliopsoas tendon (*white arrow*) is slightly lifted off the acetabulum by the injection of fluid in the bursa between the acetabulum (*white arrowhead*) and the tendon. The dotted white arrow represents the needle course.

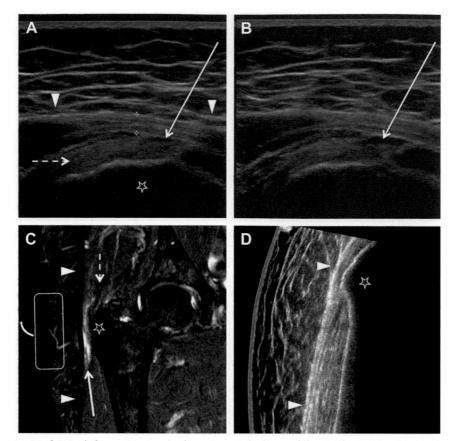

Fig. 10. Greater trochanteric bursa. Long-axis ultrasonography image (*A*) over the greater trochanter (*white star*) shows the iliotibial band (*arrowheads*), which is thickened (calipers measure 5.5 mm, normal value <5 mm). There is mild greater trochanteric bursitis (*white arrow*) between the iliotibial band and the gluteal tendons (*dashed arrow*). After injection of local anesthetic and steroid (*B*), the volume of fluid within the bursa has increased (*white arrow*). The white arrow also depicts the needle course slightly oblique from caudal to cranial. The correlating MR imaging anatomy in (*C*) shows the probe orientation, iliotibial band (*white arrowheads*) and the bursitis (*white arrow*) between the gluteal tendon (*dashed arrow*) and the greater trochanter (*white star*). (*D*) An extended panorama view of the iliotibial band (*arrowhead*) over the greater trochanter (*white star*) and proximal femur.

ultrasonography-guided percutaneous tenotomy should be considered. The preferred scanning approach is a longitudinal probe orientation, as shown in **Fig. 11**C, D, and a needle approach from caudal to cranial. The sciatic nerve runs lateral to the hamstring origin (immediately lateral to the ischial tuberosity). To ensure the safety of the sciatic nerve, the medial edge of the hamstring origin (the conjoint tendon of biceps femoris and semitendinosus) should be targeted first, and then the clinician should carefully work the needle laterally toward the semimembranosus origin. PRP can also be injected together with the percutaneous tenotomy in the management of chronic tendinopathy. A double-blind study with ultrasonography-guided injection with either PRP or whole blood in chronic proximal hamstring tendinopathy resulted in significant functional improvement for both groups.[62]

Ultrasonography plays little role in the treatment of an acute, complete avulsion of the hamstring origin.

Ischiofemoral Impingement

Narrowing of the distance between the ischial tuberosity and the lesser trochanter of less than 18 mm (normal mean value is 13 mm with a standard deviation of 5 mm) can result in impingement and resultant painful edema of the quadratus femoris muscle with atypical posterior hip/buttock pain.[63] Backer and colleagues[64] recently evaluated the role of ultrasonography-guided corticosteroid injection into the quadratus femoris muscle in a small cohort of patients with symptoms and MR imaging findings suggestive of ischiofemoral impingement. There was a statistically significant improvement in pain between the

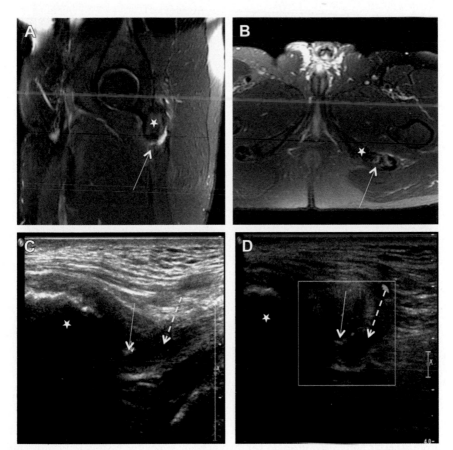

Fig. 11. Hamstring origin. High-grade partial tear (*white arrows* in *A* and *B*) of the left hamstring origin at the ischial tuberosity (*white star*) on sagittal (*A*) and axial (*B*) T2 FS images. Corresponding longitudinal gray-scale (*C*) and color Doppler (*D*) ultrasonography images show a calcific deposit (*white arrow*) within the area of the hypoechoic high-grade partial tear (*dashed arrow*) of the hamstring origin (at the ischial tuberosity, *white star*). There is also increased vascularity at the site of the tear indicating acuity of the injury. The calcium deposits suggest underlying mild calcific tendinosis.

injected and control groups. All of the injections provided at least mild relief, with 73% providing good relief. One significant limitation of this study was a follow-up end point of only 2 weeks.[64]

Piriformis Syndrome

The piriformis muscle mainly originates from the anterior sacrum, then extends through the greater sciatic foramen and inserts on the greater trochanter. For scanning, a 5-MHz probe is used and the starting point is at the iliac bone in an axial orientation. The probe is then moved caudally until the iliac bone disappears and the greater sciatic foramen shows (**Fig. 12**). The piriformis muscle becomes apparent in the greater sciatic notch deep to the gluteal musculature. The piriformis is flanked in the greater sciatic foramen cranially by the superior gluteal artery and caudally by the inferior gluteal artery, which should be identified with color ultrasonography before injection. The piriformis is

an external hip rotator and passive internal and external rotation of the hip during scanning also helps identify the muscle. The piriformis injection is done from a lateral-to-medial needle approach. Piriformis syndrome occurs when a spastic or abnormally sized (atrophied or hypertrophied) piriformis muscle irritates the sciatic nerve, resulting in buttock pain and often sciatica. Posttraumatic piriformis syndrome with hematoma and myositis ossificans resulting in mass effect on the sciatic nerve is also a recognized entity,[65,66] especially in athletes performing contact sports. Piriformis syndrome may be a contributing factor in 6% to 8% of the general population with lower back pain.[67] In 17% of the population, the common peroneal nerve portion of the sciatic nerve courses through the piriformis muscle, which predisposes to piriformis syndrome. Corticosteroid and local anesthetic or botulinum toxin can be injected into the piriformis muscle for both diagnosis and treatment if physical therapy fails.[68] Fluoroscopic, computed tomographic,

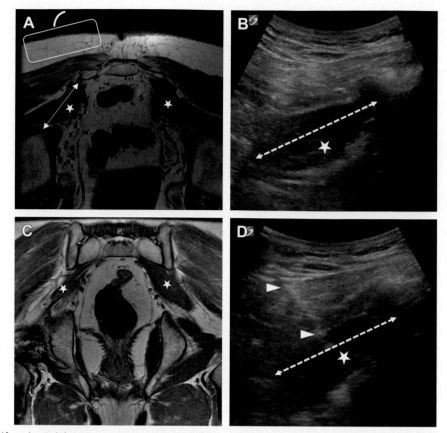

Fig. 12. Piriformis. Axial T1 non-FS MR imaging (*A*) with normal, symmetric bilateral piriformis muscles (*white star*), which occupy the greater sciatic foramen (*dashed white arrow*). The gluteal musculature is superficial to the piriformis muscle with an ultrasound probe icon showing a plane/orientation for sonographic evaluation. Ultrasonography image (*B*) shows the corresponding anatomy on ultrasonography of the right piriformis muscle (*white star*) in the greater sciatic notch (*dashed white arrow*). (*C*) Asymmetry of the piriformis muscles is shown (right atrophied compared with left), which clinically presented as piriformis syndrome. Trigger point injection (*D*) in the right piriformis muscle (*white star*) with the needle track (*arrowheads*) through the overlying gluteal musculature. Greater sciatic foramen (*dashed arrow*) between the sacrum and ischial spine is shown.

MR imaging, and electrophysiologic guidance techniques have all been described in the literature for piriformis injections.[69,70] However, in our opinion, ultrasonography is radiation free and is the easiest, quickest, cheapest, and safest injection technique because the gluteal arteries can be monitored with color ultrasonography. Relief of pain after instillation of local anesthetic is diagnostic of piriformis syndrome. A double-blinded, randomized controlled study (57 patients) showed that local anesthetic injections were clinically effective in the treatment of piriformis syndrome, but saw no additional benefit when adding corticosteroids to the local anesthetic.[71]

Selected Nerves

Ilioinguinal/iliohypogastric nerve
The ilioinguinal and iliohypogastric nerves are best visualized with ultrasonography between the internal oblique and transverse abdominis muscles at the level of the ASIS or iliac crest. Athletes with these nerve injuries may present with pain and paresthesia traveling from the flank to the inguinal ligament, medial groin, medial thigh, or scrotum/labia. Most common reasons for nerve irritations are abdominal/flank contusions or nerve injury from inguinal hernia repair. **Fig. 13** explains the probe orientation and steps of the combined nerve block.

Pudendal nerve
Pudendal nerve injuries present as pain and paresthesia at the penis/lower vagina, scrotum/vulva, perineum, or anorectal region. Chronic irritation and injury of the nerve is seen with prolonged sitting, and long-distance cyclists are often affected.

The pudendal nerve enters the gluteal region through the greater sciatic notch, curves around

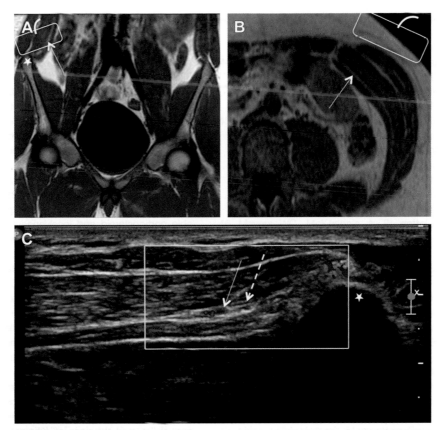

Fig. 13. Ilioinguinal/iliohypogastric nerve. The ultrasound probe orientation for imaging the ilioinguinal/iliohypogastric nerves (*white arrow*) is depicted in coronal T1 non-FS (*A*) and axial T1 non-FS (*B*) images. The probe is positioned just cranial to the ASIS (*white star*) and pointed toward the umbilicus. The lateral abdominal wall consists of 3 muscle layers: the external oblique, internal oblique, and transverse abdominis muscles (from superficial to deep). The ilioinguinal/iliohypogastric nerves run in the plane between the internal oblique and the transverse abdominis muscles (*white arrow* in *B*). The corresponding ultrasonography images (*C*) at the level of the ASIS (*white star*) show the ilioinguinal/iliohypogastric nerves and corresponding vessels (*white arrow*) in the plane between the internal oblique and transverse abdominis muscles (*dashed arrow*).

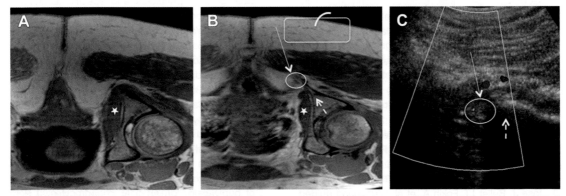

Fig. 14. Pudendal nerve. Upside-down/flipped axial T1 non-FS image (*A*), just cranial to the left hamstring origin at the level of the obturator internus muscle (*white star*). Image (*B*) is 1 slice cranial to (*A*), at the level of the ischial spine (*dashed white arrow*). At that level, the pudendal nerve, accompanying artery, and 2 veins can be found just medial to the ischial spine (*white circle*). The white arrow indicates the needle course for a pudendal nerve block under ultrasonography. The orientation of the probe is also shown. The ultrasonography image (*C*) at the level of the ischial spine (*dashed white arrow*) also shows the needle course (*white arrow*) pointing to the pudendal nerve (within the *white circle*), which is often not directly seen, but located between the ischial spine and the pudendal vessels.

56. Strauss EJ, Nho SJ, Kelly BT. Greater trochanteric pain syndrome. Sports Med Arthrosc 2010;18: 113–9.

57. Klauser AS, Martinoli C, Tagliafico MD, et al. Greater trochanteric pain syndrome. Semin Musculoskelet Radiol 2013;17:43–8.

58. Long SS, Surrey DE, Nazarian LN. Sonography of greater trochanteric pain syndrome and the rarity of primary bursitis. AJR Am J Roentgenol 2013; 201:1083–6.

59. Brinks A, van Rijn RM, Bohnen AM, et al. Corticosteroid injections for greater trochanteric pain syndrome: a randomized controlled trial in primary care. Ann Fam Med 2011;9:226–34.

60. McEvoy JR, Lee KS, Blankenbaker D, et al. Ultrasound-guided corticosteroid injections for the treatment of greater trochanteric pain syndrome: greater trochanteric bursa versus subgluteus medius bursa. AJR Am J Roentgenol 2013;201:W313–7.

61. Hamilton B, Tol JL, Almusa E, et al. Platelet-rich plasma does not enhance return to play in hamstring injuries: a randomized controlled trial. Br J Sports Med 2015;49:943–50.

62. Davenport KL, Campos JS, Nguyen J, et al. Ultrasound-guided intratendinous injections with platelet-rich plasma or autologous blood for treatment of proximal hamstring tendinopathy: a double blind randomized controlled trial. J Ultrasound Med 2015;34:1455–63.

63. Torriani M, Souto SCL, Thomas BJ, et al. Ischiofemoral impingement syndrome: an entity with hip pain and abnormalities of the quadratus femoris muscle. AJR Am J Roentgenol 2009;193:186–90.

64. Backer MW, Lee KS, Blankenbaker D, et al. Correlation of ultrasound-guided corticosteroid injection of the quadratus femoris with MRI findings of ischiofemoral impingement. AJR Am J Roentgenol 2014;203:589–93.

65. Benson ER, Schutzer SF. Posttraumatic piriformis syndrome: diagnosis and results of operative treatment. J Bone Joint Surg Am 1999;81:941–9.

66. Beauchesne RP, Schutzer SF. Myositis ossificans of the piriformis muscle: an unusual case of piriformis syndrome. A case report. J Bone Joint Surg Am 1997;79:906–10.

67. Hallin R. Sciatic pain and the piriformis muscle. Postgrad Med 1983;74:69–72.

68. Hopayian K, Song F, Riera R, et al. The clinical features of the piriformis syndrome: a systematic review. Eur Spine J 2010;19:2095–109.

69. Fishman S, Caneris O, Bandman T, et al. Injection of the piriformis muscle by fluoroscopic and electromyographic guidance. Reg Anesth Pain Med 1998; 23:554–9.

70. Fanucci E, Masala S, Sodani G, et al. CT guided injection of botulinic toxin for percutaneous therapy of piriformis muscle syndrome with preliminary MRI results about denervative process. Eur Radiol 2001; 11:2543–8.

71. Misirliogu TO, Akgun K, Palamar D, et al. Piriformis syndrome: comparison of the effectiveness of local anesthetic and corticosteroid injections: a double-blinded, randomized controlled study. Pain Physician 2015;18:163–71.

72. Hough DM, Wittenberg KH, Pawlina W, et al. Chronic perineal pain caused by pudendal nerve entrapment: anatomy and CT guided perineural injection technique. AJR Am J Roentgenol 2003;181: 561–7.

73. Shafik A, el-Sherif M, Youssef A, et al. Surgical anatomy of the pudendal nerve and its clinical implications. Clin Anat 1995;8:110–5.

Core Injuries Remote from the Pubic Symphysis

Jeffrey A. Belair, MD[a],*, Tarek M. Hegazi, MD, MBBS, FRCPC[a,b],
Johannes B. Roedl, MD, PhD[a], Adam C. Zoga, MD[a], Imran M. Omar, MD[c]

KEYWORDS

• Core • Muscle • Injury • Athlete • Imaging • MRI • Ultrasound

KEY POINTS

- The *core* refers to the central musculoskeletal system of the torso (including the lower thorax, abdomen, pelvis, thoracolumbar spine, and proximal thighs) and plays an essential role in both static stabilization and dynamic function.
- Core injuries remote from the pubic symphysis are important, potentially overlooked considerations in both athletes and active nonathletes.
- MR imaging is often the modality of choice for assessing core injuries given its superior soft tissue contrast. Specialized imaging protocols tailored to the area of interest should be used when assessing for core injury.
- Large field-of-view (FOV) MR imaging of both the affected and unaffected sides may increase conspicuity of subtle edema or asymmetry, whereas focused small FOV images of the affected side provide improved spatial resolution to better characterize an abnormality.
- Ultrasound often plays an adjunctive role in evaluating and potentially treating core injuries.

INTRODUCTION

The *core* in most general terms refers to the central musculoskeletal system of the torso and plays an essential role in both static stabilization and dynamic function. Anatomically, the core includes the musculoskeletal structures of the lower thorax, abdomen, pelvis, thoracolumbar spine, and proximal thighs. The importance of the midline pubic plate and rectus abdominis-adductor aponeurosis for core stability and function has been previously described.[1,2] Core injuries remote from the pubic symphysis, however, are additional, potentially overlooked considerations in both athletes and active nonathletes and are often similar in presentation and pathophysiologic mechanism. This article presents an overview of commonly encountered injuries involving the core anatomy remote from the pubic symphysis.

MR imaging is often the modality of choice for assessing core injuries given its superior soft tissue contrast. Specialized imaging protocols tailored to the area of interest should be used when assessing for core injury. For most injuries involving the central core, it is prudent to use imaging in 3 planes using both traditional fluid-sensitive sequences, including short tau inversion recovery (STIR) and T2 fat-suppression (FS), and anatomic sequences, including T1 and proton-density (PD) non-FS. As another general guideline, large FOV imaging of both the affected and unaffected sides should be included, which may increase conspicuity of subtle edema or

Disclosures: The authors have nothing to disclose.
[a] Division of Musculoskeletal Imaging and Interventions, Department of Radiology, Jefferson Medical College, Thomas Jefferson University Hospital, Thomas Jefferson University, 132 South 10th Street, Suite 1096, 1087 Main Building, Philadelphia, PA 19107, USA; [b] Department of Radiology, University of Dammam, PO Box 2114, Dammam 31451, Saudi Arabia; [c] Department of Radiology, Northwestern Memorial Hospital, 676 North Saint Clair Street, Suite 800, Chicago, IL 60611, USA
* Corresponding author.
E-mail address: jeff.belair@gmail.com

Radiol Clin N Am 54 (2016) 893–911
http://dx.doi.org/10.1016/j.rcl.2016.04.009

asymmetry. Focused small FOV images of the affected side provide improved spatial resolution to better characterize the abnormality. As with all imaging studies, each MR imaging examination should be tailored to a patient's specific clinical scenario. In addition to MR imaging, ultrasound often plays an adjunctive role in evaluating and potentially treating core injuries. Initial work-up for many injuries often includes standard radiographs to evaluate for acute osseous pathology. The utility of each modality as it relates to particular core injuries is described in greater detail in each subsection.

In addition to reviewing core musculotendinous injuries away from the pubic symphysis, this article covers several specific clinical syndromes and their relevant imaging features. Although core injuries may be found in all patient populations, they are most relevant in young, active individuals and athletes. The importance of core strengthening and conditioning for both performance and injury prevention is of great interest to athletes and trainers and is the subject of entire books and physiatry programs.

MUSCULOTENDINOUS INJURIES

The most commonly encountered core injury in clinical practice is a muscle strain in the torso or proximal thighs. Muscles in the lower thorax susceptible to injury include the intercostal, serratus anterior, and proximal external oblique muscles. The major muscles of the abdominal wall include the rectus abdominis, transversus abdominis, internal oblique, and external oblique muscles. Important muscles about the lower spine include the quadratus lumborum, multifidus, erector spinae, and psoas major, among other paraspinal muscles. Muscles in the proximal thigh are manifold and can be subdivided into groups based on

function, including hip flexion, extension, adduction, abduction, internal rotation, and external rotation.

The most commonly used grading system for muscle strains among radiologists includes 3 grades of injury based on characteristic MR imaging features.[3] Grade 1 strains are characterized histopathologically by mild inflammatory cell infiltration, edema, and swelling, possibly with disruption of the endomysium or perimysium connective tissues. MR imaging findings of grade 1 strains include interstitial muscle edema with or without associated hemorrhage but with preservation of normal muscle architecture (**Figs. 1** and **2**). Grade 2 and grade 3 strains are characterized by partial or complete tears of the musculotendinous unit, respectively, with possible defect or retraction of torn muscle fibers (**Figs. 3–6**). Higher-grade muscle strains frequently demonstrate associated intramuscular hemorrhage by imaging. Acute muscle strains tend to occur at the myotendinous junction, where the muscle-tendon complex is weakest and there is higher concentration of tensile forces.[3–5] Complete musculotendinous avulsions occur at origin or insertion attachment sites to the bones.

Acute muscle strains are almost invariably managed conservatively. Although standard therapy once focused on rest, ice, compression, and elevation (RICE) therapy, the benefits of immobilization, compression, and elevation are uncertain. Some clinicians now advocate for early mobilization and rehabilitation for low-grade muscle strains, which may reduce scarring and accelerate healing response. Management has also been expanded to include nonsteroidal anti-inflammatory drugs (NSAIDs) and other adjunctive therapies.[6] Direct intramuscular injections of NSAIDs and corticosteroids have been used with success in high-level athletes, providing

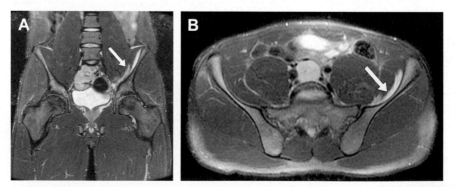

Fig. 1. Iliacus muscle strain in a 16-year-old male soccer player with left groin pain. (*A*) Coronal STIR and (*B*) axial T2 FS MR images demonstrate feathery edema within the left iliacus muscle belly without disruption of muscle fibers (*arrows* [*A*, *B*]), consistent with a grade 1 strain.

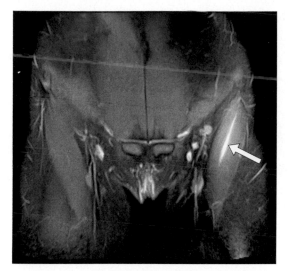

Fig. 2. Sartorius muscle strain in a 41-year-old female cyclist with left thigh pain. Coronal STIR MR image demonstrates feathery edema within the left sartorius muscle belly without disruption of muscle fibers (*arrow*), consistent with a grade 1 strain.

symptomatic relief and allowing faster return to play.[7,8] Injection of platelet-rich plasma is also increasingly used for the treatment of musculotendinous injuries, although the data supporting the use of this technique remain inconclusive.[9] The typical recovery period for low-grade muscle strains ranges from a few days to weeks, although reinjury or high-grade strains often require longer

convalescence.[10,11] High-grade and complete muscle tears or musculotendinous avulsions may benefit from surgical intervention.[12–14]

Acute muscle contusion is another consideration in individuals involved in contact sports or who sustain direct trauma. Whereas acute muscle strains have a propensity for the myotendinous junction, muscle contusions may occur anywhere in the muscle belly. On MR imaging, muscle contusions are characterized by a region of muscle edema and overlying soft tissue swelling at the site of direct trauma, although they may be indistinguishable from an acute muscle strain. Contusion is often accompanied by intramuscular hemorrhage, which may be infiltrative or present as a discrete hematoma (**Fig. 7**). Correlation with clinical history is paramount given significant overlap in imaging features of intramuscular hematoma and soft tissue neoplasms. Large intramuscular hematomas are often painful and may warrant aspiration, particularly in high-level athletes where such interventions may allow earlier return to play.[15] Important potential complications of severe muscle contusion include compartment syndrome in the acute phase and delayed development of scarring/fibrosis, atrophy, or myositis ossificans.[3,6]

Finally, delayed-onset muscle soreness (DOMS) is an acute overuse phenomenon typically encountered in individuals performing new activities or activities different from those to which they are accustomed. Intense, typically eccentric

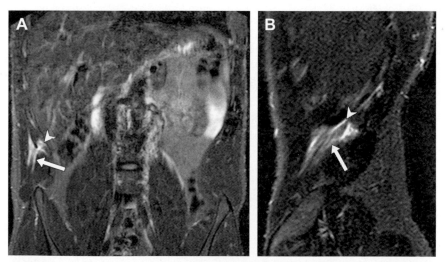

Fig. 3. External oblique muscle strain in a 22-year-old male ice hockey player after an abdominal twisting injury. (*A*) Coronal STIR MR image of the lower chest wall demonstrates edema within the right external oblique muscle (*arrow*). Edema is also noted within the internal oblique muscle (*arrowhead*). (*B*) Sagittal STIR MR image again shows interstitial edema (*arrow*) and partial disruption of the external oblique muscle fibers at the proximal attachment on the inferior margin of the anterolateral right 11th rib (*arrowhead*), which have an anteroinferior course.

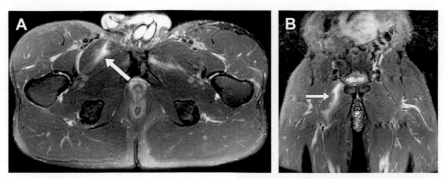

Fig. 4. Pectineus muscle strain in a 37-year-old ice hockey player with right groin pain while skating. (*A*) Axial T2 FS and (*B*) coronal STIR MR images demonstrate edema centered in the right pectineus muscle belly with a small tear defect filled with fluid/hemorrhage (*arrows* [*A*, *B*]), consistent with a grade 2 strain.

muscle exertion leads to muscle edema, cellular inflammatory response, and development of muscle pain, usually peaking at 24 to 72 hours.[3,16,17] Muscle edema may be diffuse and/or bilateral (**Fig. 8**), although findings are often indistinguishable from acute muscle strain by MR imaging. Clinical history and laboratory findings of elevated serum creatine kinase may be helpful in differentiating these entities. DOMS is a self-limited diagnosis without risk for permanent muscle damage and is treated symptomatically with RICE, NSAIDs, and massage.[18]

SIDE STRAIN, ROWER'S RIB, AND SLIPPING RIB SYNDROME

Side strain refers to a muscle strain of the internal oblique at its insertion, typically encountered in athletic activities requiring prolonged, repetitive upper body movements.[19] The internal oblique muscle originates from the iliac crest, inguinal ligament, and thoracolumbar fascia. It fans out superomedially to insert on the inferior margin of the 9th through 12th ribs and costal cartilages and blend with the internal intercostal muscles. Proximally, the internal oblique muscle is bordered superficially by the external oblique muscle and deep by the transversus abdominis muscle. Internal oblique muscle strains were first described in elite rowers and cricket fast bowlers, although they may also be encountered in ice hockey, baseball, golfing, and other throwing sports. Such players may also develop strains of the serratus anterior, external oblique, or transversus abdominis muscles, which may have a similar presentation.

Rower's rib is a related diagnosis in which repetitive muscular loading on the rib cage during rowing results in rib stress response or stress fracture.[20] Such injuries have also been described in golfers, baseball pitchers, and weight lifters.[21–23] Stress fractures result from abnormal, excessive loading on normal bones, and the ribs are commonly affected non–weight-bearing bones in athletes. High-impact sports, such as American football and hockey, may also result in acute fracture or contusion due to direct trauma. In addition to rib fractures,

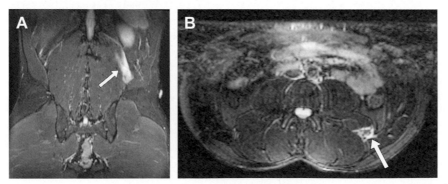

Fig. 5. Quadratus lumborum muscle strain in a 29-year-old male baseball player with left flank pain after a game. (*A*) Coronal STIR MR image of the lower posterior abdominal wall demonstrates asymmetric edema within the left quadratus lumborum muscle belly (*arrow*). (*B*) Axial TS FS image shows intramuscular edema and partial disruption of muscle fibers of the left quadratus lumborum muscle (*arrow*), consistent with a grade 2 strain.

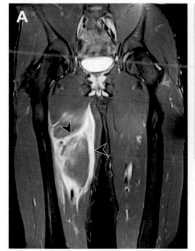
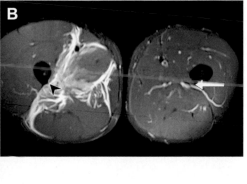

Fig. 6. High-grade adductor muscle strain in a 23-year-old football kicker with acute, severe medial right thigh pain and history of right adductor muscle strain several weeks prior. (*A*) Coronal STIR MR image demonstrates extensive edema within the adductor compartment, particularly within the right adductor magnus muscle, with fluid and hemorrhage extending along the fascial planes (*arrowheads*). (*B*) Axial STIR image confirms complete disruption of the right adductor magnus muscle from its distal insertion on the linea aspera (*arrowhead*), consistent with a grade 3 strain. The left adductor magnus muscle inserts normally (*arrow*).

fractures of the costal cartilage or costochondral junction may be encountered, which can be difficult to diagnosis and typically require longer recovery times.

Slipping rib syndrome is occasionally encountered in athletes, characterized by hypermobility of the costal cartilages of the vertebrochondral (8th through 10th) ribs. Repeated anterior subluxation of the affected rib may lead to localized soft tissue inflammation, irritation of the intercostal nerve, intercostal muscle strain, or costal cartilage stress response.[24] A positive hooking sign is a clinical finding of this syndrome, whereby reproducible pain or clicking is elicited by applying an anteriorly directed force at the lower costal margin.

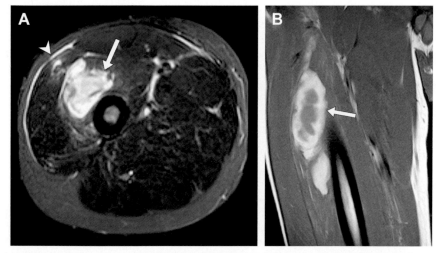

Fig. 7. Quadriceps contusion with intramuscular hematoma in a 17-year-old male football player with contact trauma to the right anterior thigh. (*A*) Axial T2 FS MR image through the proximal right thigh demonstrates edema within the right vastus intermedius muscle belly with an associated T2-hyperintense intramuscular hematoma (*arrow*). There is mild edema within overlying vastus lateralis muscle and fluid/edema extending along the muscular fascia (*arrowhead*), consistent with soft tissue contusion. (*B*) Coronal T1 MR image better demonstrates a heterogeneous intramuscular hematoma within the vastus lateralis containing T1-hyperintense blood products (*arrow*).

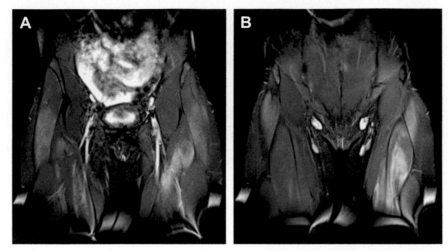

Fig. 8. DOMS in a 24-year-old woman after recently taking a spin class. (*A, B*) Two sequential coronal STIR MR images of the proximal thighs demonstrate bilateral multicompartment interstitial edema within the quadriceps, adductor, and tensor fascial lata musculature, consistent with DOMS in keeping with the clinical history.

Clinically, it is difficult to distinguish between these related chest wall injuries, given overlap in patient history and presentation. MR imaging is the preferred imaging modality given its ability to demonstrate both osseous and soft tissue pathology. A chest wall protocol should be used, with acquisition of large FOV images and small FOV images focused on the affected side. Given respiratory motion and potential artifacts related to inhomogenous FS, the authors typically rely on STIR sequences acquired in multiple planes to identify soft tissue or bone marrow edema. Internal oblique strains are characterized by intramuscular edema, typically localized to the proximal attachment margin on the inferior ribs or costal cartilages (**Fig. 9**). Additional findings may include a fluid-filled gap in muscle fibers, intramuscular

hematoma, or intermuscular hematoma dissecting along the anterolateral chest wall. The internal oblique muscle fibers have a normal anterosuperior orientation, which can be discerned from the external oblique muscle fibers, which have a nearly perpendicular anteroinferior course.[19] In the setting of rib fracture, initial work-up typically includes rib series radiographs, which may demonstrate subtle periosteal reaction, callus formation, or a nondisplaced fracture line. MR imaging demonstrates focal marrow edema with an associated fracture line (**Fig. 10**). In patients with normal radiographs who cannot tolerate MR imaging or for whom MR imaging is contraindicated, imaging with technetium Tc 99m–methylene diphosphonate scintigraphy or single-photon emission computed tomography (SPECT)/CT

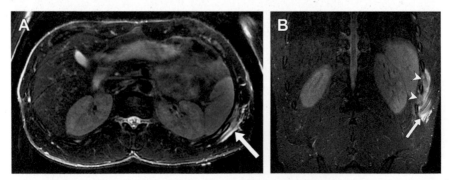

Fig. 9. Side strain injury in a 24-year-old ice hockey player after violent twisting injury while being checked during a game. (*A*) Axial T2 FS and (*B*) coronal STIR MR images of the anterolateral chest wall demonstrate edema and loss of normal muscle fiber architecture within the left internal oblique muscle at its proximal margin (*arrows* [*A, B*]), consistent with a grade 2 side strain. There is a concomitant grade 2 strain of the adjacent external oblique muscle, which has a perpendicular orientation, and is best demonstrated on (*B*) the coronal image. Additional grade 1 strains of the intercostal muscles between the 9th and 10th and 10th and 11th ribs are noted (*arrowheads* [*B*]).

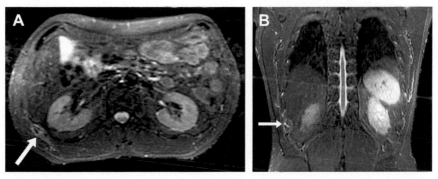

Fig. 10. Subacute rib fracture in a 38-year-old male weight lifter with right chest wall pain and a clicking sensation, without history of antecedent trauma. (A) Axial STIR MR image of the chest demonstrates a hyperintense fracture cleft at the posterior right 11th rib with surrounding periostial soft tissue edema (*arrow*), consistent with nondisplaced subacute stress fracture. (B) Coronal STIR MR image also demonstrates the nondisplaced fracture (*arrow*).

may be considered to evaluate for rib fracture. Ultrasound may have a limited role in these diagnoses but can demonstrate soft tissue hematoma in the setting of muscle strain or cortical discontinuity or callus formation in the setting of rib fracture. Ultrasound may be particularly helpful in diagnosing costal cartilage fracture, evidenced by disruption of the smooth cartilage surface.[25] In the setting of slipping rib syndrome, dynamic ultrasound may demonstrate abnormal mobility of the costal cartilages of the affected vertebrochondral rib during Valsalva maneuver and contraction of the rectus abdominis muscles (**Fig. 11**).[26]

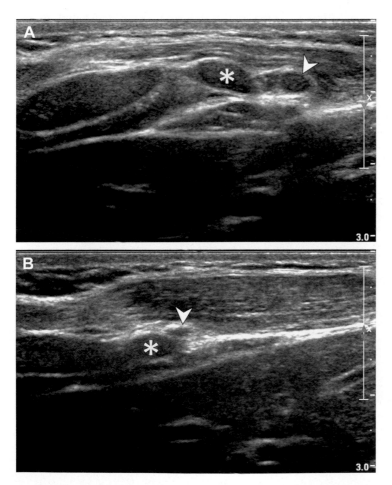

Fig. 11. Slipping rib syndrome in a 30-year-old woman with left anterior lower rib pain and occasional "popping" sensation during physical activity. Sequential dynamic longitudinal ultrasound images (A) before and (B) after contraction of the abdominal wall musculature demonstrate abnormal slipping of the right 8th rib costal cartilage (*arrowheads* [A, B]) on top of the right 7th anterior rib (*asterisks* [A, B]).

Treatment of both side strain and rib fracture is conservative, but differentiating between the 2 can be useful for anticipating return to play because rib fractures typically require longer convalescence. Slipping rib syndrome is also typically treated initially with conservative measures, although rib resection has been performed in refractory cases.[24,27]

HOCKEY GOALIE/BASEBALL PITCHER SYNDROME

Hockey goalie/baseball pitcher (HGBP) syndrome was initially described by Meyers and colleagues[28] as a reproducible injury pattern seen in such position players, characterized by a tear of the proximal adductor longus epimysium with myofascial herniation. Players often present with chronic, intermittent pain localized to the adductor longus muscle belly, which may be acutely exacerbated due to temporary entrapment of muscle fibers. As its name suggests, this injury may be related to similar body mechanics during goaltending and the stride phase of pitching.

MR imaging is the preferred imaging modality for evaluating adductor longus muscle pathology. MR imaging may demonstrate focal edema in the adductor longus muscle belly with herniation or bulging of muscle fibers through a fascial defect (**Fig. 12**). In cases of intermittent myofascial herniation, however, MR imaging findings may be limited to intramuscular and perifascial edema without visible defect. In such situations, the diagnosis of HGBP syndrome may be suggested on MR imaging if muscle edema is centered within the muscle belly several centimeters distal to the pubic symphysis, whereas edema at the myotendinous junction favors an acute muscle strain.[1] Ultrasound can be complementary in making the diagnosis of true myofascial herniation, demonstrating focal bulging of muscle tissue, which may be more conspicuous during resisted adduction. Additionally, patients can direct a sonographer to the site of pain for targeted interrogation.

Muscle fiber entrapment results in delayed healing and unremitting pain, which may ultimately require surgical release via fasciotomy and débridement.[1,28] This diagnosis should not be confused with a simple adductor longus muscle strain, which would be treated conservatively.

HOCKEY GROIN SYNDROME

Hockey groin syndrome, also referred to colloquially as slap shot gut, has been described in professional ice hockey players as a tear of the external oblique aponeurosis with associated ilioinguinal nerve entrapment.[29] The ilioinguinal nerve, a branch of the first lumbar nerve (L1), arises at the posterolateral edge of the psoas muscle and extends obliquely along the anterolateral abdominal wall, piercing the transversus abdominis and internal oblique muscles at the level of the iliac crest. The ilioinguinal nerve then enters the superficial inguinal ring, ultimately supplying sensory fibers to the superomedial thigh, base of the penis, and upper scrotum in male athletes and labium majora and root of the clitoris in female athletes. A tear in the external oblique aponeurosis below the level of the iliac crest may allow entrapment of the ilioinguinal nerve prior to entering the inguinal canal.

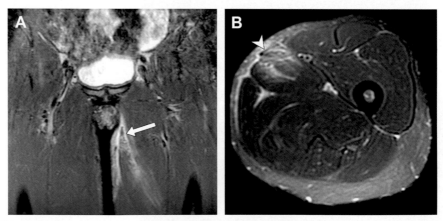

Fig. 12. HGBP syndrome in a 42-year-old figure skater with intermittent left groin pain for several months. (*A*) Coronal STIR MR image demonstrates intramuscular edema within the left adductor longus centered several centimeters distal to the pubic symphysis (*arrow*). (*B*) Axial T2 FS MR image shows edema within the adductor longus muscle with subtle bulging of the muscle belly anteriorly (*arrowhead*) and associated fascial edema. The diagnosis of HGBP syndrome with myofascial herniation was suggested by imaging and confirmed at surgery.

This syndrome is a clinical diagnosis made predominantly in elite athletes. Clinical criteria include persistent groin pain typically exacerbated by sudden movements requiring contracture of the core musculature or Valsalva maneuver and failure to improve with conservative measures.[29,30] There may also be a palpable gap in the external oblique aponeurosis near the inguinal ring. In ice hockey players, symptoms are often exacerbated during the push-off phase of skating or while taking a slap shot. This entity has also been described in other high-level athletes, including those participating in rugby, American football, cycling, marathon running, and cricket.[30] Ilioinguinal neuropathy may also occur after hernia repair due to entrapment by mesh or scar tissue.

Imaging studies have traditionally been insufficient for making this diagnosis. In 1 of the largest operative series, presented by Irshad and colleagues,[29] only 1 of 22 National Hockey League players with surgically proved external oblique aponeurosis tears had imaging findings supporting the diagnosis. In that particular case, MR imaging demonstrated a tear defect in the external oblique aponeurosis. Thus, MR imaging may be useful in supporting the diagnosis, although lack of imaging evidence should not preclude ruling it out. If this syndrome is suspected clinically, the MR imaging protocol should be tailored to image the anterior abdominal wall and include large FOV imaging for side-to-side comparison. Although not previously reported in the literature, the diagnosis of ilioinguinal nerve entrapment may be suggested by ultrasound in the setting of a focally tender and enlarged ilioinguinal nerve (Fig. 13). Ultrasound-guided anesthetic block of the ilioinguinal nerve may also be useful diagnostically to determine if symptoms abate after injection. Those patients meeting clinical criteria for the diagnosis have been shown to benefit from surgical repair of the aponeurotic defect using mesh combined with ilioinguinal resection or neurolysis.[29,30]

GREATER TROCHANTERIC PAIN SYNDROME

Greater trochanteric pain syndrome is a clinical diagnosis characterized by lateral hip pain and focal tenderness over the greater trochanter on palpation. This diagnosis represents the common clinical manifestation of several underlying causes. Usually symptoms are attributable to underlying pathology of the distal gluteus minimus and medius tendons, the hip abductors, which are sometimes collectively referred to as the rotator cuff of the hip.[31,32] Although traditionally diagnosed in middle-aged women, this entity is increasingly diagnosed in athletes, in particular runners and dancers.[33]

Both the gluteus minimus and gluteus medius tendons arise from the external iliac fossa and attach on the greater trochanter, with the gluteus minimus inserting on the anterior facet and the gluteus medius on the lateral and superoposterior facets.[34] A complex of 3 bursae about the greater trochanter has been described, including the subgluteus minimus bursa, subgluteus medius bursa, and greater trochanteric (subgluteus maximus) bursa.[35] The greater trochanter bursa is the largest of the 3, lying superficial to the posterior facet and deep to the gluteus maximus muscle belly. Although the term, greater trochanteric bursitis, is often applied to patients with greater trochanteric pain syndrome, this may not accurately reflect the underlying pathology.

Repetitive overuse of the hip abductors results in tendinosis, tendon microtears, adjacent soft tissue inflammation, and secondary fluid accumulation in their respective bursae.[36–40] Low-grade tendon injuries may ultimately progress to high-grade partial or full-thickness tendon tears. Injuries of the gluteus minimus and medius tendons occur with nearly equal frequency and often

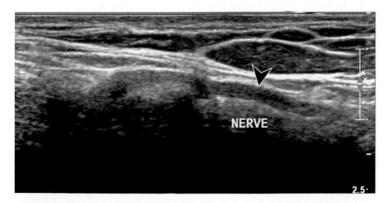

Fig. 13. Ilioinguinal nerve entrapment in a 41-year-old man with right scrotal pain and history of prior inguinal hernia repair several years earlier. Longitudinal ultrasound image demonstrates marked thickening of the left ilioinguinal nerve (*arrowhead*) just deep to the external oblique aponeurosis with focal tenderness, suggesting entrapment related to prior hernia repair. Diagnostic nerve block with local anesthetic alleviated patient symptoms.

in combination. MR imaging and ultrasound are both useful in the assessment of greater trochanteric pain syndrome. MR imaging may demonstrate tendon thickening and/or increased intrinsic signal (tendinosis), interstitial tearing, peritendinous edema (peritendinitis), or abnormal bursal fluid (bursitis) (**Fig. 14**). Complete tendon tear or avulsion from the greater trochanter creates a gap defect filled with fluid, hematoma, or granulation tissue.[37] Incidental bursal effusions or peritrochanteric edema on MR imaging may be encountered with high frequency in asymptomatic patients, in particular in those who are overweight, and findings may not always correlate with clinical symptoms. Ultrasound is useful both for diagnostic purposes and image-guided intervention. By ultrasound, gluteal tendinosis may be characterized by tendon thickening, heterogeneity, or hypoechogenicity that may be focal or diffuse. Enthesopathy may be seen as bony irregularity and spurring at the tendinous insertions on the greater trochanter facets. Partial or full-thickness tendon tears are manifest by anechoic defects or focal, abrupt tendon narrowing (**Fig. 15**). Abnormal fluid may be identified in the bursae, although it is only present in a minority of patients.[41] Ultrasound may also demonstrate peritendinitis, characterized by peritendinous hyperemia on color Doppler interrogation. As in the shoulder, calcific tendinosis is occasionally encountered in the gluteal tendons, with characteristic findings on radiography, ultrasonography, and MR imaging.

Greater trochanteric pain syndrome is usually managed conservatively, with surgery reserved for patients with high-grade tendon tear or avulsion.[32,36] Available ultrasound-guided therapeutic measures include bursal injection with corticosteroid (typically into the greater trochanteric bursa), percutaneous tenotomy, or platelet-rich plasma injection. Such interventions are most effective when combined with tailored physiotherapy.[38,42]

APOPHYSITIS AND APOPHYSEAL INJURIES

Apophyses are normal non–weight-bearing secondary ossifications centers in the developing skeleton that serve as musculotendinous attachment sites, also known as traction epiphyses. Although most physes in the body are fused by age 20, several apophyses in the pelvis may not be fully mature until age 25 years or older.[43,44] In children, the hyaline cartilage of the physis is weaker than the attaching tendon or adjacent bone and is, therefore, susceptible to injury.[43,45–47] Two patterns of injury occur at apophyses: a sudden, strong muscular contraction may cause an acute separation of the physeal plate resulting in a Salter-Harris type 1 avulsion fracture; or, repetitive traction on an apophysis may lead to chronic microtrauma and associated reparative inflammation, a condition termed *apophysitis*.[43,48]

Core apophyseal injuries occur most commonly in the bony pelvis, frequently associated with running sports and gymnastics. Typical sites of apophyseal injury include the ischial tuberosity,

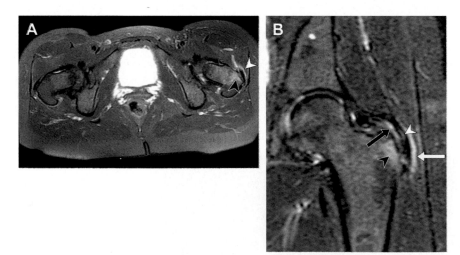

Fig. 14. Gluteus minimus insertional tendinosis with bursitis in a 38-year-old woman with lateral hip pain during yoga when sitting cross-legged. (*A*) Axial T2 FS MR image through the hips demonstrates left gluteus minimus insertional tendinosis with subentheseal marrow edema (*black arrowhead*) and peritendinitis (*white arrowhead*). (*B*) Coronal STIR MR image shows gluteus minimus tendon thickening with interstitial tearing (*white arrowhead*) and subentheseal marrow edema (*black arrowhead*). Subgluteus minimus bursitis (*black arrow*) and greater trochanteric bursitis (*white arrow*) are also seen.

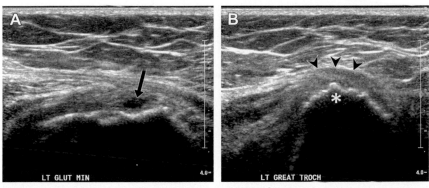

Fig. 15. Gluteus minimus tendon interstitial tearing in a 32-year-old female marathon runner with lateral hip pain. (A) Longitudinal ultrasound image of the lateral hip demonstrates thickening of the gluteus minimus tendon with an interstitial tear near its insertion on the greater tronchanter (arrow). (B) Transverse ultrasound image at the level of the greater trochanter demonstrates thickening and heterogeneity of the gluteus minimus tendon (arrowheads). Bony irregularity at the greater trochanter (asterisk) is consistent with enthesopathy.

anterior superior iliac spine (ASIS), anterior inferior iliac spine (AIIS), and iliac crest.[43,48] Patients often present with localized pain and focal tenderness over the affected apophysis. Patients with apophyseal avulsions frequently present with a history of an acute inciting event, whereas those presenting with apophysitis often have a more insidious onset of pain exacerbated by activity. Undiagnosed and untreated apophyseal injuries may lead to prolonged symptoms, delayed return to play, and injury progression. Apophyses of the bony pelvis away from the pubic symphysis and their associated tendon attachments include

- Ischial tuberosity: common hamstring tendon
- Iliac crest: external oblique, internal oblique, transversus abdominis, gluteus medius, tensor fascial lata, quadratus lumborum
- ASIS: sartorius and tensor fascia lata
- AIIS: rectus femoris

Initial imaging for suspected apophyseal injury should include a standard anteroposterior radiograph of the pelvis. In the setting of an acute apophyseal avulsion injury, an avulsed fracture fragment is typically evident if the apophysis is ossified. If the apophyseal ossification center has not yet begun to ossify, initial radiographs may be normal and patients should be further evaluated with MR imaging dedicated to the bony pelvis. Radiographs likewise are often normal in the setting of apophysitis, although they may demonstrate apophyseal irregularity, fragmentation, or subtle widening of the physeal plate.[43,44] On MR imaging, acute apophyseal avulsions are characterized by displacement of the cartilaginous or ossified apophysis, fluid-equivalent signal in the separated physis, and associated marrow and periosseous edema (Fig. 16).[48,49] In apophysitis, MR imaging

typically demonstrates bone marrow edema spanning the physis and adjacent soft tissue edema (Fig. 17).[43,45] Ultrasound has been used in assessing apophyseal injuries, and findings include regional hypoechogenicity, widening of the hypoechoic physis, or hyperemia on Doppler color flow interrogation.[50,51] Side-to-side comparison is useful to detect subtle unilateral injury.

Treatment of apophysitis is conservative, including NSAIDs, activity modification, and physiotherapy. Nondisplaced avulsion fractures and avulsion fractures that are displaced less than 2 cm are usually treated conservatively; however, the duration of rest is usually longer than that required for apophysitis. Avulsion fractures that are displaced more than 2 cm or result in development of painful fibrous nonunion may require surgery.[46]

ILIOPSOAS TENDINITIS AND BURSITIS, SNAPPING HIP SYNDROME, AND ILIOPSOAS IMPINGEMENT

The paired iliopsoas muscles connect the spine directly to the lower extremities, serving as the primary hip flexors and also playing an important role in maintaining upright posture and core balance. The iliopsoas muscle comprises the psoas major and iliacus muscles proximally, which merge to form a single muscle belly distally. The psoas muscle origin spans the lateral aspect of the T12 through L5 vertebrae, intervertebral discs, and ventral surfaces of the transverse processes. The iliacus muscle origin has a broad origin along the iliac fossa. The psoas major and iliacus musculotendinous units converge to form a single tendinous insertion on the lesser trochanter. Distal fibers of the iliacus muscle also insert directly onto the proximal femur, anterolateral to the

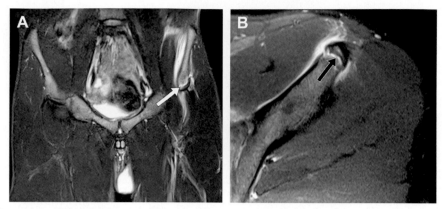

Fig. 16. AIIS apophyseal avulsion in a 14-year-old male lacrosse athlete with acute onset of left hip pain after suddenly stopping from sprinting. (*A*) Coronal STIR MR image demonstrates acute avulsion of the left AIIS apophysis, the attachment site of the proximal rectus femoris tendon. Mild physeal widening (*arrow*), adjacent soft tissue edema, and associated grade 1 strains of the left iliacus and proximal rectus femoris muscles are noted. (*B*) Small FOV axial PD FS MR image demonstrates fluid-equivalent signal in the ASIS physis (*arrow*) with surrounding edema and fluid/hemorrhage.

tendinous insertion.[52] The iliopsoas bursa is large, extending from the iliac fossa to the lesser trochanter, and normally does not contain any visible quantity of fluid by imaging. The iliopsoas bursa may communicate with the hip joint in up to 15% of normal individuals, and significant joint effusion or intra-articular instillation of contrast may decompress into the bursa.[53]

The iliopsoas muscles are normally symmetric in bulk and signal. Psoas muscle atrophy is uncommon in athletes unless there is a history of hip joint replacement. Iliopsoas strains typically occur at the myotendinous junction and are usually related to acute injury. Chronic overuse injuries include tendinosis, partial tendon tear, peritendinitis, and iliopsoas bursitis. Complete tendon tears are uncommon and usually occur in elderly patients. Activities requiring sudden or repetitive hip flexion, including running and kicking sports, gymnastics,

ballet dancing, and rowing, are commonly associated with iliopsoas pathology.[54]

Iliopsoas pathology is best evaluated by pelvic or hip MR imaging. Myotendinous strains exhibit characteristic intramuscular edema on fluid-sensitive sequences and may be isolated to either the psoas major or iliacus muscles or may involve the entire iliopsoas muscle complex. Iliopsoas bursitis is characterized by any amount of fluid identified within the iliopsoas bursa (**Fig. 18**), usually detected at the level of the acetabular rim. Bursitis may be graded as mild, moderate, or severe, depending on the quantity of fluid and complexity. Ultrasound can be useful for detecting iliopsoas bursitis and peritendinitis and may be used for image-guided injection of corticosteroid into the bursa.

Snapping hip syndrome, also known as coxa saltans or dancer's hip, is clinically evident as a palpable or audible snapping associated with hip

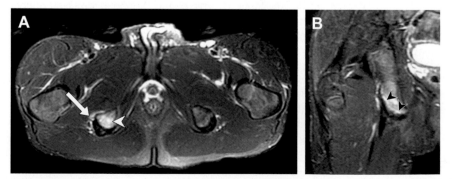

Fig. 17. Hamstring origin apophysitis in a 15-year-old male wrestler with persistent right buttocks pain. (*A*) Axial T2 FS MR image demonstrates pronounced subentheseal marrow edema in the right ischial tuberosity (*arrowhead*) and peritendinous edema about the right hamstring tendon origin (*arrow*). (*B*) Coronal STIR MR image shows marked edema in the right ischial tuberosity and within the physis (*arrowheads*), consistent with apophysitis.

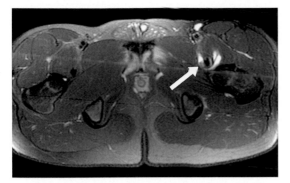

Fig. 18. Iliopsoas bursitis in an 18-year-old male football player with bilateral groin and left hip pain. Axial T2 FS MR image demonstrates thickening of the left iliopsoas tendon just below the hip joint with a large amount of fluid in the bursa (*arrow*), consistent with iliopsoas tendinosis and bursitis. Concomitant left worse than right proximal adductor strains and acute-on-chronic osteitis pubis are also noted.

flexion and extension. Extra-articular causes are either anterior (internal), resulting from snapping of the iliopsoas tendon over the iliopectineal eminence or iliacus muscle belly, or lateral (external), related to snapping of the iliotibial band over the greater trochanter.[55–57] Repetitive trauma due to snapping may result in tendinosis, peritendinitis, or bursitis (**Fig. 19**). Dynamic ultrasound is useful for demonstrating sudden displacement of the iliopsoas tendon or iliotibial band with provocative hip maneuvers. Dynamic or stress ultrasound is one of the emerging techniques in musculoskeletal radiology adding substantial value in addition to MR imaging.[58] Although treatment is usually conservative, iliotibial band or iliopsoas tendon release may be beneficial in recalcitrant cases given the mechanical etiology of symptoms.[59,60]

Iliopsoas impingement is an entity postulated to result from a tight or scarred iliopsoas tendon. Increased traction results in abnormal friction on the anterior acetabular labrum, ultimately resulting in an anterior labral tear. The diagnosis may be suggested on MR imaging or magnetic resonance arthrography in the setting of a directly anterior labral tear (3-o'clock position) as opposed to the more commonly encountered anterosuperior location (**Fig. 20**).[61] In such situations, the iliopsoas tendon is often adherent to the anterior joint capsule at arthroscopy. If iliopsoas impingement is suspected, iliopsoas tendon release at time of labral repair may be effective.[62]

OSSEOUS STRESS INJURIES

Osseous stress injuries in the core may be encountered in high-level athletes and active individuals. Common sites of involvement include the femoral neck, acetabulum, pubic rami, sacrum, and ribs. In young athletes with low back pain, pars interarticularis stress fractures are an additional important consideration.[63] Stress fractures,

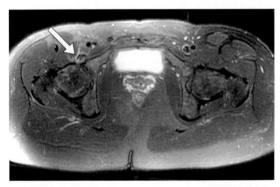

Fig. 19. Snapping hip syndrome in a 36-year-old female runner with anterior right hip "clicking" during active flexion. Axial T2 FS MR image demonstrates thickening of the right iliopsoas tendon with associated iliopsoas bursitis and peritendenous edema extending along the adjacent iliacus muscle (*arrow*). Findings are suggestive of snapping hip syndrome given the clinical history. Subsequently performed ultrasound (not shown) revealed snapping of the right iliopsoas tendon over the iliacus muscle belly with active hip flexion.

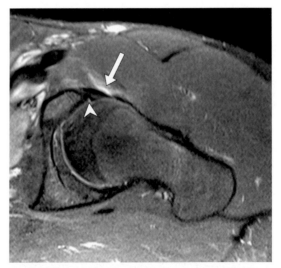

Fig. 20. Iliopsoas impingement in a 15-year-old male lacrosse player with left hip pain. Axial PD FS MR image (nonarthrogram) demonstrates left iliopsoas bursitis (*arrow*) immediately overlying a left anterior labral tear (*arrowhead*), suggestive of iliopsoas impingement syndrome. The iliopsoas tendon was adherent to the anterior joint capsule at arthroscopy and iliopsoas tendon release was performed in addition to labral repair.

or more accurately fatigue fractures, are part of a pathologic continuum. Abnormal, repetitive stresses applied to normal bone result in bony remodeling, with osteoblastic new bone formation lagging behind osteoclastic activity and resulting in mechanical weakening. Bony remodeling is subverted by trabecular microfracture and eventually frank cortical break.[64,65] A stress fracture begins as an incomplete fracture but may progress to a complete fracture if subjected to continued biomechanical loading. Completed fractures portend a longer recovery period, and fractures with a large cortical defect or displacement may require internal fixation.[66,67]

Stress fractures involving the hips are most commonly encountered in long-distance and competitive runners. A majority of femoral stress fractures involve the medial femoral neck at the site of compressive stresses, although they may also occur at the lateral femoral neck (tension stress fracture), intercondylar region, or proximal femoral diaphysis.[68] Radiographs or CT may demonstrate cortical disruption, periosteal reaction, or endosteal sclerosis. These findings are not consistently seen, however, and often lag behind clinical presentation.[69–71] Characteristic MR imaging features include focal intense marrow edema at the fracture site on fluid-sensitive sequences with associated linear hypointensity that represents the developing fracture line (**Fig. 21**).[64,68,71–73] Osseous stress

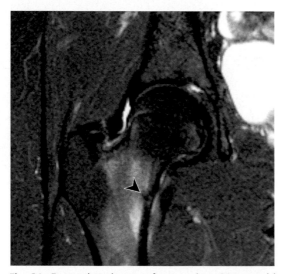

Fig. 21. Femoral neck stress fracture in a 29-year-old female runner with deep aching right groin pain while training for a marathon. Small FOV coronal T2 FS MR image of the right hip demonstrates marked marrow edema centered at the medial aspect of the femoral neck with associated hypointense fracture line (*arrowhead*), consistent an incomplete femoral neck stress fracture.

injury, or osseous stress response, is the imaging precursor to stress fracture. MR imaging findings of endosteal marrow edema, periostitis, and reactive soft tissue edema correspond to trabecular microfracture, osteoclastic resorption, and associated inflammatory response.[64,65] It has been suggested, however, that the term, *stress fracture*, be used in the femur even in cases of a discrete fracture line not seen by MR imaging, due to the high risk of progression to complete fracture if athletic activity is continued.[64] Stress fractures in the femur are treated conservatively with non–weight-bearing, rehabilitation, and gradual return to activity.[65] Optimal recovery time and return to full play is highly variable and dependent on severity of the injury, sometimes requiring upwards of 20 to 30 weeks in higher-grade stress injuries.[74]

Adductor insertion avulsion syndrome, commonly referred to as thigh splints, is analogous to medial tibial stress syndrome (shin splints) and results from chronic, repetitive avulsive stress of the adductors along their insertion on the posterior femur. This entity has been described primarily in athletes participating in running-intense sports. Patients typically present with posteromedial thigh pain after heavy physical activity, which is relieved by rest. MR imaging demonstrates periosteal edema along the posteromedial cortex of the mid-femoral diaphysis. Additional findings may include endosteal and intramedullary marrow edema in more advanced cases (**Fig. 22**).[75] Radiographs may demonstrate subtle cortical thickening or periosteal reaction, although these findings are insensitive. Adductor insertion avulsion syndrome was first described in patients with increased radiotracer uptake in characteristic location on bone scintigraphy, and radionuclide imaging may be performed on patients in whom MR imaging is contraindicated.[76]

ISCHIOFEMORAL IMPINGEMENT AND PIRIFORMIS SYNDROMES

Although not core injuries per se, ischiofemoral impingement and piriformis syndromes are alternative considerations in patients presenting with hip, thigh, or buttocks pain. Ischiofemoral impingement syndrome has a strong female predominance, whereas piriformis syndrome is encountered in male athletes and female athletes with similar frequency.[77,78] Neither is thought to result from activity-related injury, although both are nonetheless occasionally encountered in athletes.[79]

In ischiofemoral impingement syndrome, narrowing of the ischiofemoral and quadratus femoris spaces results in impingement of the quadratus femoris muscle belly. Sensitive and specific MR imaging findings include an ischiofemoral space measuring

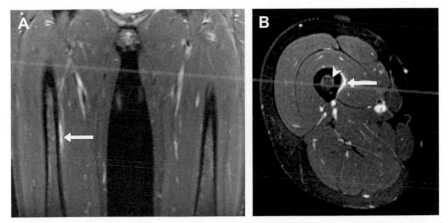

Fig. 22. Adductor insertion avulsion syndrome (thigh splints) in a 26-year-old female marathon and trail runner with right midthigh pain. (*A*) Coronal STIR MR image of the thighs demonstrates focal, asymmetric periosteal edema at the medial aspect of the right mid femoral diaphysis (*arrow*). (*B*) Small FOV axial T2 FS MR image of the right thigh demonstrates focal periosteal edema (*arrow*) and subtle endosteal marrow edema (*arrowhead*) at the adductor magnus attachment site, consistent with adductor insertion avulsion syndrome.

less than 1.5 cm, quadratus femoris space measuring less than 1.0 cm, and characteristic focal quadratus femoris intramuscular edema on fluid-sensitive sequences (**Fig. 23**).[78,80] Management of ischiofemoral impingement syndrome is usually conservative, although recent patient series suggest ultrasound-guided injection of corticosteroid is a safe and effective treatment option.[81]

Piriformis syndrome is characterized by leg or buttocks pain attributable to entrapment of the sciatic nerve by the piriformis muscle at the level of the greater sciatic notch. Clinical features of piriformis syndrome include buttocks pain exacerbated by sitting, tenderness over the greater sciatic notch, and reproduction of pain with maneuvers requiring contraction of the piriformis

muscle.[77,82] MR imaging or CT may demonstrate asymmetric enlargement or atrophy of the ipsilateral piriformis muscle (**Fig. 24**), although the significance of such findings is controversial.[83,84] Dedicated MR neurography may demonstrate enlargement and increased signal within the sciatic nerve on fluid-sensitive sequences.[83,85] Targeted ultrasonography may demonstrate asymmetry of the piriformis

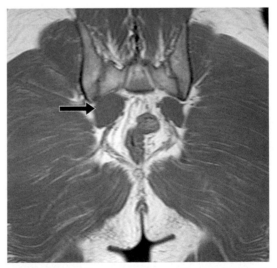

Fig. 24. Piriformis syndrome in a 25-year-old female softball player with right buttocks pain radiating down the right leg. Coronal T1 MR image demonstrates asymmetrically increased right piriformis muscle bulk (*arrow*), suggestive of piriformis syndrome. No additional abnormalities were identified in the right hip or pelvis by MR imaging. The patient experienced significant symptom relief following ultrasound-guided right piriformis injection of corticosteroid and anesthetic.

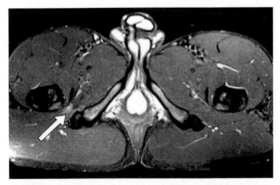

Fig. 23. Ischiofemoral impingement syndrome in a 19-year-old male track runner and football athlete with activity-induced right groin pain. Axial STIR MR image demonstrates asymmetric narrowing of the right ischiofemoral space and focal intramuscular edema in the quadratus femoris muscle belly (*arrow*), characteristic of ischiofemoral impingement syndrome.

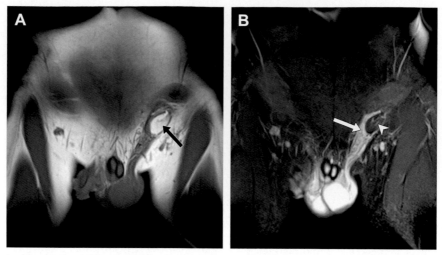

Fig. 25. Inguinal hernia in a 36-year-old ice hockey player with left groin pain and clinical concern for athletic pubalgia. (*A*) Coronal T1 and (*B*) coronal STIR MR images of the pelvis demonstrate a small fat-containing left indirect inguinal hernia (*arrow* [*A*]) with mild edema in the herniated omental fat (*arrowhead* [*B*]). The spermatic cord (*arrow* [*B*]) is intimate to the hernia within the inguinal canal.

muscle bulk and can be used to elicit tenderness by applying pressure with the ultrasound transducer at the greater sciatic notch. Other causes of sciatic nerve entrapment in the subgluteal space fall under the recently described spectrum of deep gluteal syndrome, which includes fibrous bands, hamstring tendon origin pathology, gluteus muscle abnormalities, and pathologies in the buttocks.[86] Potential interventions for piriformis syndrome include injection of corticosteroid and anesthetic, botulinum toxin injection, and even sciatic neurolysis in refractory cases.[87–89]

HERNIAS

True inguinal or other abdominal hernias may be encountered in individuals in whom a core injury is suspected and serve as a visceral source of pain. Strenuous activities leading to increased intra-abdominal pressure have been implicated in the development of inguinal hernias.[90] CT is the most commonly requested modality to evaluate for suspected hernia and potential associated complications, although small or subtle hernias may not always be detected on static imaging. In experienced hands, ultrasound is the most accurate modality to detect hernias, given its ability to perform dynamic assessment and lack of ionizing radiation.[91] The Valsalva maneuver increases intra-abdominal pressure and may allow otherwise occult hernias to become visible. Inguinal and other abdominal hernias may be evident on MR imaging obtained to evaluate for core injury (**Fig. 25**); thus, the visceral soft tissues should be carefully examined on such studies.

SUMMARY

Core injuries remote from the pubic symphysis are an important consideration in active individuals and athletes alike. The core is large in anatomic scope, including the musculoskeletal structures of the lower thorax, abdomen, pelvis, thoracolumbar spine, and proximal thighs. Numerous core injuries have been described, including many specific syndromes. MR imaging is the mainstay for imaging the core anatomy, although ultrasonography is particularly useful for dynamic imaging and image-guided therapeutic intervention. Using appropriate imaging studies and tailoring imaging protocols allow for more accurate diagnosis, improved treatment planning, and quicker patient recovery.

REFERENCES

1. Omar IM, Zoga AC, Kavanagh EC, et al. Athletic pubalgia and "sports hernia": optimal MR imaging technique and findings. Radiographics 2008;28(5):1415–38.
2. Zoga AC, Kavanagh EC, Omar IM, et al. Athletic pubalgia and the "sports hernia": MR imaging findings. Radiology 2008;247(3):797–807.
3. Stoller DW, Stoller DW. Magnetic resonance imaging in orthopaedics and sports medicine. 3rd edition. Philadelphia: Lippincott Williams & Wilkins; 2007.
4. Garrett WE Jr. Muscle strain injuries: clinical and basic aspects. Med Sci Sports Exerc 1990;22(4):436–43.
5. Mueller-Wohlfahrt HW, Haensel L, Mithoefer K, et al. Terminology and classification of muscle injuries in

sport: the Munich consensus statement. Br J Sports Med 2013;47(6):342–50.

6. Delos D, Maak TG, Rodeo SA. Muscle injuries in athletes: enhancing recovery through scientific understanding and novel therapies. Sports Health 2013;5(4):346–52.

7. Drakos M, Birmingham P, Delos D, et al. Corticosteroid and anesthetic injections for muscle strains and ligament sprains in the NFL. HSS J 2014; 10(2):136–42.

8. Nepple JJ, Matava MJ. Soft tissue injections in the athlete. Sports Health 2009;1(5):396–404.

9. Moraes VY, Lenza M, Tamaoki MJ, et al. Platelet-rich therapies for musculoskeletal soft tissue injuries. Cochrane Database Syst Rev 2014;(4):CD010071.

10. Cross KM, Saliba SA, Conaway M, et al. Days to return to participation after a hamstrings strain among American Collegiate Soccer Players. J Athl Train 2015;50(7):733–41.

11. Ekstrand J, Healy JC, Walden M, et al. Hamstring muscle injuries in professional football: the correlation of MRI findings with return to play. Br J Sports Med 2012;46(2):112–7.

12. Ahmad CS, Redler LH, Ciccotti MG, et al. Evaluation and management of hamstring injuries. Am J Sports Med 2013;41(12):2933–47.

13. Bowman KF Jr, Cohen SB, Bradley JP. Operative management of partial-thickness tears of the proximal hamstring muscles in athletes. Am J Sports Med 2013;41(6):1363–71.

14. Lempainen L, Sarimo J, Heikkila J, et al. Surgical treatment of partial tears of the proximal origin of the hamstring muscles. Br J Sports Med 2006; 40(8):688–91.

15. Hansford BG, Stacy GS. Musculoskeletal aspiration procedures. Semin Intervent Radiol 2012;29(4): 270–85.

16. Evans GF, Haller RG, Wyrick PS, et al. Submaximal delayed-onset muscle soreness: correlations between MR imaging findings and clinical measures. Radiology 1998;208(3):815–20.

17. Page P. Pathophysiology of acute exercise-induced muscular injury: clinical implications. J Athl Train 1995;30(1):29–34.

18. Cheung K, Hume P, Maxwell L. Delayed onset muscle soreness : treatment strategies and performance factors. Sports Med 2003;33(2):145–64.

19. Connell DA, Jhamb A, James T. Side strain: a tear of internal oblique musculature. AJR Am J Roentgenol 2003;181(6):1511–7.

20. Dragoni S, Giombini A, Di Cesare A, et al. Stress fractures of the ribs in elite competitive rowers: a report of nine cases. Skeletal Radiol 2007;36(10): 951–4.

21. Gerrie BJ, Harris JD, Lintner DM, et al. Lower thoracic rib stress fractures in baseball pitchers. Phys Sportsmed 2016;44(1):93–6.

22. Lord MJ, Ha KI, Song KS. Stress fractures of the ribs in golfers. Am J Sports Med 1996;24(1):118–22.

23. Miller TL, Harris JD, Kaeding CC. Stress fractures of the ribs and upper extremities: causation, evaluation, and management. Sports Med 2013;43(8): 665–74.

24. Udermann BE, Cavanaugh DG, Gibson MH, et al. Slipping rib syndrome in a collegiate swimmer: a case report. J Athl Train 2005;40(2):120–2.

25. Malghem J, Vande Berg B, Lecouvet F, et al. Costal cartilage fractures as revealed on CT and sonography. AJR Am J Roentgenol 2001;176(2):429–32.

26. Meuwly JY, Wicky S, Schnyder P, et al. Slipping rib syndrome: a place for sonography in the diagnosis of a frequently overlooked cause of abdominal or low thoracic pain. J Ultrasound Med 2002;21(3): 339–43.

27. Copeland GP, Machin DG, Shennan JM. Surgical treatment of the 'slipping rib syndrome'. Br J Surg 1984;71(7):522–3.

28. Meyers WC, Lanfranco A, Castellanos A. Surgical management of chronic lower abdominal and groin pain in high-performance athletes. Curr Sports Med Rep 2002;1(5):301–5.

29. Irshad K, Feldman LS, Lavoie C, et al. Operative management of "hockey groin syndrome": 12 years of experience in National Hockey League players. Surgery 2001;130(4):759–64 [discussion: 764–6].

30. Ziprin P, Williams P, Foster ME. External oblique aponeurosis nerve entrapment as a cause of groin pain in the athlete. Br J Surg 1999;86(4):566–8.

31. Bunker TD, Esler CN, Leach WJ. Rotator-cuff tear of the hip. J Bone Joint Surg Br 1997;79(4):618–20.

32. Kagan A 2nd. Rotator cuff tears of the hip. Clin Orthop Relat Res 1999;(368):135–40.

33. Grumet RC, Frank RM, Slabaugh MA, et al. Lateral hip pain in an athletic population: differential diagnosis and treatment options. Sports Health 2010; 2(3):191–6.

34. Dwek J, Pfirrmann C, Stanley A, et al. MR imaging of the hip abductors: normal anatomy and commonly encountered pathology at the greater trochanter. Magn Reson Imaging Clin N Am 2005; 13(4):691–704, vii.

35. Pfirrmann CW, Chung CB, Theumann NH, et al. Greater trochanter of the hip: attachment of the abductor mechanism and a complex of three bursae–MR imaging and MR bursography in cadavers and MR imaging in asymptomatic volunteers. Radiology 2001;221(2):469–77.

36. Chowdhury R, Naaseri S, Lee J, et al. Imaging and management of greater trochanteric pain syndrome. Postgrad Med J 2014;90(1068):576–81.

37. Kingzett-Taylor A, Tirman PF, Feller J, et al. Tendinosis and tears of gluteus medius and minimus muscles as a cause of hip pain: MR imaging findings. AJR Am J Roentgenol 1999;173(4):1123–6.

38. Mallow M, Nazarian LN. Greater trochanteric pain syndrome diagnosis and treatment. Phys Med Rehabil Clin N Am 2014;25(2):279–89.

39. Strauss EJ, Nho SJ, Kelly BT. Greater trochanteric pain syndrome. Sports Med Arthrosc 2010;18(2):113–9.

40. Williams BS, Cohen SP. Greater trochanteric pain syndrome: a review of anatomy, diagnosis and treatment. Anesth Analg 2009;108(5):1662–70.

41. Long SS, Surrey DE, Nazarian LN. Sonography of greater trochanteric pain syndrome and the rarity of primary bursitis. AJR Am J Roentgenol 2013;201(5):1083–6.

42. Wilson SA, Shanahan EM, Smith MD. Greater trochanteric pain syndrome: does imaging-identified pathology influence the outcome of interventions? Int J Rheum Dis 2014;17(6):621–7.

43. Arnaiz J, Piedra T, de Lucas EM, et al. Imaging findings of lower limb apophysitis. AJR Am J Roentgenol 2011;196(3):W316–25.

44. Sailly M, Whiteley R, Read JW, et al. Pubic apophysitis: a previously undescribed clinical entity of groin pain in athletes. Br J Sports Med 2015;49(12):828–34.

45. Jaimes C, Jimenez M, Shabshin N, et al. Taking the stress out of evaluating stress injuries in children. Radiographics 2012;32(2):537–55.

46. Roedl JB, Morrison WB, Ciccotti MG, et al. Acromial apophysiolysis: superior shoulder pain and acromial nonfusion in the young throwing athlete. Radiology 2015;274(1):201–9.

47. Roedl JB, Nevalainen M, Gonzalez FM, et al. Frequency, imaging findings, risk factors, and long-term sequelae of distal clavicular osteolysis in young patients. Skeletal Radiol 2015;44(5):659–66.

48. McKinney BI, Nelson C, Carrion W. Apophyseal avulsion fractures of the hip and pelvis. Orthopedics 2009;32(1):42.

49. Stevens MA, El-Khoury GY, Kathol MH, et al. Imaging features of avulsion injuries. Radiographics 1999;19(3):655–72.

50. Lazovic D, Wegner U, Peters G, et al. Ultrasound for diagnosis of apophyseal injuries. Knee Surg Sports Traumatol Arthrosc 1996;3(4):234–7.

51. Pisacano RM, Miller TT. Comparing sonography with MR imaging of apophyseal injuries of the pelvis in four boys. AJR Am J Roentgenol 2003;181(1):223–30.

52. Polster JM, Elgabaly M, Lee H, et al. MRI and gross anatomy of the iliopsoas tendon complex. Skeletal Radiol 2008;37(1):55–8.

53. Van Dyke JA, Holley HC, Anderson SD. Review of iliopsoas anatomy and pathology. Radiographics 1987;7(1):53–84.

54. Johnston CA, Wiley JP, Lindsay DM, et al. Iliopsoas bursitis and tendinitis. A review. Sports Med 1998;25(4):271–83.

55. Deslandes M, Guillin R, Cardinal E, et al. The snapping iliopsoas tendon: new mechanisms using dynamic sonography. AJR Am J Roentgenol 2008;190(3):576–81.

56. Pelsser V, Cardinal E, Hobden R, et al. Extraarticular snapping hip: sonographic findings. AJR Am J Roentgenol 2001;176(1):67–73.

57. Tatu L, Parratte B, Vuillier F, et al. Descriptive anatomy of the femoral portion of the iliopsoas muscle. Anatomical basis of anterior snapping of the hip. Surg Radiol Anat 2001;23(6):371–4.

58. Roedl JB, Gonzalez FM, Zoga AC, et al. Potential utility of a combined approach with US and MR arthrography to image medial elbow pain in baseball players. Radiology 2016;279(3):827–37.

59. Ilizaliturri VM Jr, Camacho-Galindo J. Endoscopic treatment of snapping hips, iliotibial band, and iliopsoas tendon. Sports Med Arthrosc 2010;18(2):120–7.

60. Yen YM, Lewis CL, Kim YJ. Understanding and Treating the Snapping Hip. Sports Med Arthrosc 2015;23(4):194–9.

61. Blankenbaker DG, Tuite MJ, Keene JS, et al. Labral injuries due to iliopsoas impingement: can they be diagnosed on MR arthrography? AJR Am J Roentgenol 2012;199(4):894–900.

62. Domb BG, Shindle MK, McArthur B, et al. Iliopsoas impingement: a newly identified cause of labral pathology in the hip. HSS J 2011;7(2):145–50.

63. Micheli LJ, Curtis C. Stress fractures in the spine and sacrum. Clin Sports Med 2006;25(1):75–88, ix.

64. Arendt EA, Griffiths HJ. The use of MR imaging in the assessment and clinical management of stress reactions of bone in high-performance athletes. Clin Sports Med 1997;16(2):291–306.

65. Romani WA, Gieck JH, Perrin DH, et al. Mechanisms and management of stress fractures in physically active persons. J Athl Train 2002;37(3):306–14.

66. Behrens SB, Deren ME, Matson A, et al. Stress fractures of the pelvis and legs in athletes: a review. Sports Health 2013;5(2):165–74.

67. Niva MH, Kiuru MJ, Haataja R, et al. Fatigue injuries of the femur. J Bone Joint Surg Br 2005;87(10):1385–90.

68. Wall J, Feller JF. Imaging of stress fractures in runners. Clin Sports Med 2006;25(4):781–802.

69. Daffner RH, Pavlov H. Stress fractures: current concepts. AJR Am J Roentgenol 1992;159(2):245–52.

70. Shin AY, Morin WD, Gorman JD, et al. The superiority of magnetic resonance imaging in differentiating the cause of hip pain in endurance athletes. Am J Sports Med 1996;24(2):168–76.

71. Sofka CM. Imaging of stress fractures. Clin Sports Med 2006;25(1):53–62, viii.

72. Lee JK, Yao L. Stress fractures: MR imaging. Radiology 1988;169(1):217–20.

73. Nguyen JT, Peterson JS, Biswal S, et al. Stress-related injuries around the lesser trochanter in long-distance runners. AJR Am J Roentgenol 2008; 190(6):1616–20.

74. Nattiv A, Kennedy G, Barrack MT, et al. Correlation of MRI grading of bone stress injuries with clinical risk factors and return to play: a 5-year prospective study in collegiate track and field athletes. Am J Sports Med 2013;41(8):1930–41.

75. Anderson MW, Kaplan PA, Dussault RG. Adductor Insertion avulsion syndrome (thigh splints): spectrum of MR imaging features. AJR Am J Roentgenol 2001;177(3):673–5.

76. Charkes ND, Siddhivarn N, Schneck CD. Bone scanning in the adductor insertion avulsion syndrome ("thigh splints"). J Nucl Med 1987;28(12): 1835–8.

77. Hopayian K, Song F, Riera R, et al. The clinical features of the piriformis syndrome: a systematic review. Eur Spine J 2010;19(12):2095–109.

78. Singer AD, Subhawong TK, Jose J, et al. Ischiofemoral impingement syndrome: a meta-analysis. Skeletal Radiol 2015;44(6):831–7.

79. Falotico GG, Torquato DF, Roim TC, et al. Gluteal pain in athletes: how should it be investigated and treated? Rev Bras Ortop 2015;50(4):462–8.

80. Torriani M, Souto SC, Thomas BJ, et al. Ischiofemoral impingement syndrome: an entity with hip pain and abnormalities of the quadratus femoris muscle. AJR Am J Roentgenol 2009;193(1):186–90.

81. Backer MW, Lee KS, Blankenbaker DG, et al. Correlation of ultrasound-guided corticosteroid injection of the quadratus femoris with MRI findings of ischiofemoral impingement. AJR Am J Roentgenol 2014; 203(3):589–93.

82. Miller TA, White KP, Ross DC. The diagnosis and management of Piriformis Syndrome: myths and facts. Can J Neurol Sci 2012;39(5):577–83.

83. Filler AG, Haynes J, Jordan SE, et al. Sciatica of non-disc origin and piriformis syndrome: diagnosis by magnetic resonance neurography and interventional magnetic resonance imaging with outcome study of resulting treatment. J Neurosurg Spine 2005;2(2): 99–115.

84. Russell JM, Kransdorf MJ, Bancroft LW, et al. Magnetic resonance imaging of the sacral plexus and piriformis muscles. Skeletal Radiol 2008;37(8): 709–13.

85. Petchprapa CN, Rosenberg ZS, Sconfienza LM, et al. MR imaging of entrapment neuropathies of the lower extremity. Part 1. The pelvis and hip. Radiographics 2010;30(4):983–1000.

86. Hernando MF, Cerezal L, Perez-Carro L, et al. Deep gluteal syndrome: anatomy, imaging, and management of sciatic nerve entrapments in the subgluteal space. Skeletal Radiol 2015;44(7): 919–34.

87. Jawish RM, Assoum HA, Khamis CF. Anatomical, clinical and electrical observations in piriformis syndrome. J Orthop Surg Res 2010;5:3.

88. Misirlioglu TO, Akgun K, Palamar D, et al. Piriformis syndrome: comparison of the effectiveness of local anesthetic and corticosteroid injections: a double-blinded, randomized controlled study. Pain Physician 2015;18(2):163–71.

89. Santamato A, Micello MF, Valeno G, et al. Ultrasound-guided injection of botulinum toxin type A for piriformis muscle syndrome: a case report and review of the literature. Toxins (Basel) 2015;7(8): 3045–56.

90. Sanjay P, Woodward A. Single strenuous event: does it predispose to inguinal herniation? Hernia 2007;11(6):493–6.

91. Arend CF. Static and dynamic sonography for diagnosis of abdominal wall hernias. J Ultrasound Med 2013;32(7):1251–9.

Algorithm for Imaging the Hip in Adolescents and Young Adults

Adam C. Zoga, MD[a],*, Tarek M. Hegazi, MD, MBBS, FRCPC[a,b], Johannes B. Roedl, MD, PhD[a]

KEYWORDS

- Algorithm • Imaging • Hip • Adolescents • Young adults • MRI

KEY POINTS

- Hip/groin pain in the prearthritic patient includes intra-articular, and/or extra-articular osseous, chondral or soft tissue lesions, with increasing role of the radiologist in the management algorithm of these patients.
- It is the role of imagers to facilitate and tailor the most appropriate imaging modalities and protocols to the clinical scenario of the patient.
- MR imaging should include large field of view imaging of the entire pelvis with dedicated high-resolution small field of view imaging of the involved hip to better assess both extra-articular and intra-articular causes of hip pain.
- Hallmark findings of cam-type femoroacetabular impingement is prominence at the anterosuperior femoral head/neck junction, as well as anterosuperior labral and cartilage tears.

INTRODUCTION

The hip is the last great frontier of untamed large joint injury in adolescents and young adults. Hip arthroscopy is still far less frequently performed than knee or shoulder arthroscopy, but it has become more mainstream in recent years. When the senior author (A.C.Z.) completed his musculoskeletal radiology fellowship in 2003, hip arthroscopy was exceedingly rare and our role as imagers was to identify periarticular lesions, developmental malalignments, or early arthritic conditions. This role has changed, as has radiology as a specialty. It is no longer an acceptable practice standard to ignore cartilage lesions and partial-thickness labrum tears at the femoroacetabular joint. Activity-related painful syndromes from internal derangements of the prearthritic hip are common, and, once accurately identified, often treatable. Simultaneously, extra-articular sources of pain mimicking internal derangements of the hip are also common, and amenable to both minimally invasive and noninvasive treatment regimens. Distinguishing intra-articular sources of pain from extra-articular or even referred sources can be clinically difficult, because many lesions can cause anterior symptoms radiating to the groin and are exacerbated by activity. In musculoskeletal radiology, hip imaging offers great opportunities to show the value of radiologists to the managing sports medicine clinicians and to the patients themselves. This article delineates an algorithm for imaging young patients with hip and groin pain and presents ideas on how imagers can contribute to treatment planning and return to play or to a pain-free life.

During the 2005 to 2006 academic year, the authors performed and interpreted 405 noncontrast MR imaging examinations of the hip and 145 direct or indirect MR arthrographic hip studies in our

[a] Division of Musculoskeletal Imaging and Interventions, Department of Radiology, Jefferson Medical College, Thomas Jefferson University Hospital, Thomas Jefferson University, 132 South 10th Street, Suite 1096, 1087 Main Building, Philadelphia, PA 19107, USA; [b] Department of Radiology, University of Dammam, PO Box 2114, Dammam 31451, Saudi Arabia, UAE
* Corresponding author.
E-mail address: adam.zoga@jefferson.edu

Radiol Clin N Am 54 (2016) 913–930
http://dx.doi.org/10.1016/j.rcl.2016.05.016

outpatient musculoskeletal radiology practice. In 2014 to 2015, we performed and interpreted 385 noncontrast MR imaging examinations of the hip, 636 direct MR arthrographic studies, and 78 indirect MR arthrograms. Our practice has changed over the years, but, during that same period, MR imaging examinations of the knee remained within the range of 3000 to 4000 each year. Imaging of the hip has increased significantly as part of our practice. At the same time, hip arthroscopy has increased in frequency in North America and throughout the industrialized world. In the United States, the annual number of billed arthroscopic hip procedures has increased precipitously, with more orthopaedic surgeons experienced in hip arthroscopy, more accepted arthroscopic techniques, and many more treatable prearthritic hip lesions. One series showed an increase of more than 600% in hip arthroscopic procedures performed by a cohort of newly trained surgeons taking the American Board of Orthopaedic Surgery Part II examination from 2006 to 2010.[1] Musculoskeletal imagers must embrace such operational changes in health management and work to help patients and managing clinicians arrive together at the optimal treatment plan. Establishing the value of advanced imaging in the setting of hip and groin pain in adolescents and young adults remains a major opportunity for musculoskeletal radiologists.

Not all intrinsic and periarticular lesions manifesting as hip and groin pain are surgical, and, of those that are, not all are best treated by an orthopaedic surgeon.[2] Referred sources of symptoms might respond well to directed physical therapy and strengthening programs. Periarticular maladies such as bursitis, tendinopathy, and nerve entrapment might be managed with image-guided percutaneous therapies. In addition, athletic pubalgia lesions or core muscle injuries might warrant evaluation and treatment by a subspecialized general surgeon. However, arthroscopic treatments have been proved effective for many internal derangements of the hip.[3] Physical examination is valuable, but accurately distinguishing intra-articular lesions from extra-articular sources of hip and groin pain can be daunting, even to experienced examiners. In this regard, musculoskeletal radiologists have a unique opportunity to not only effectively diagnose the underlying source of symptoms but also to guide patients toward the most appropriate subspecialist for treatment. The authors think that, in the setting of hip and groin pain in adolescents and the young adults, experienced musculoskeletal imagers are uniquely positioned to oversee treatment planning and therapeutic execution. Each case referred for imaging should be managed thoughtfully and systematically. When imaging is completed, the radiologist should almost always have a good idea of what treatment the patient needs next, and this decision should be conveyed in the imaging reports. For young, active patients with refractory deep hip and groin pain, musculoskeletal radiologists can therefore have great value in the management algorithm.

THE IMAGING PLAN

There are many options for imaging the hip, and no practitioner should be more familiar with the imaging options and indications for each of the various imaging protocols than musculoskeletal radiologists. The authors think that it would border on irresponsible to practice as if referrers, whether surgeons, primary care clinicians, or sports medicine experts, always know the most appropriate study to order. With this in mind, each order for imaging the hip or the musculoskeletal pelvis should be reviewed by the imager to ensure that an optimal examination and protocol is chosen. An 80-year-old emergency department patient with a suspected femoral neck fracture and equivocal radiographs should not endure imaging time or cost spent on high-resolution, small-field-of-view cartilage sequences dedicated to the ipsilateral hip when an inversion recovery sequence covering the entirety of the pelvis can diagnose the femoral neck fracture as well as other findings such as sacral insufficiency fractures or osseous metastases. Similarly, a teenaged girl with pincer impingement generally should not be exposed to the excessive ionizing radiation that accompanies high-resolution computed tomography (CT) of the pelvis using a bone algorithm when the needed anatomic information is available on high-quality radiographs. It is the job of imagers to facilitate appropriate imaging modalities and protocols.

Imaging of hip and groin pain should almost always begin with radiographs, but radiograph protocols can vary based on the clinical scenario. A hip fracture protocol can be as limited as a standing anteroposterior (AP) exposure of the pelvis and a frog lateral of the hip.[4] However, for young, active patients with activity-related hip or groin pain, a radiographic series should be built to identify developmental anatomic variations or syndromes, including developmental dysplasia of the hip, femoroacetabular impingement, slipped capital femoral epiphyses, and Legg-Calvé-Perthes. It should also allow the imager to identify lesions at the sacroiliac joints and the pubic symphysis. Our adolescent and young adult hip clinic radiograph protocol includes 5 views (**Fig. 1**):

1. Standing AP pelvis
2. Supine AP of hip only

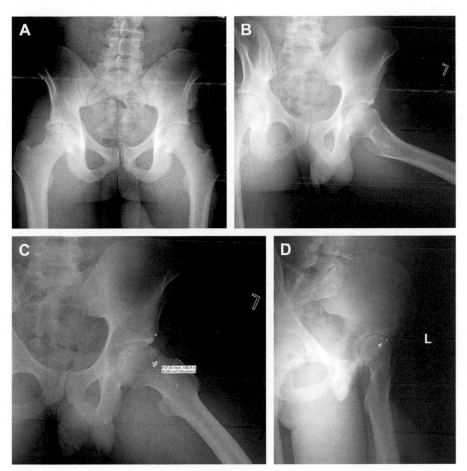

Fig. 1. Hip radiograph protocol. (*A*) Anteroposterior radiograph of the pelvis obtained with patient supine and both legs in 15° of internal rotation. The lateral center edge angle is measured from this view using 2 intersecting lines, one drawn vertically through the femoral head and the other from the femoral head isocenter to the lateral extent of the acetabular rim. Normal values range from 20° to 40°, with higher values indicating pincer-type impingement morphology and lower values indicating dysplasia. Acetabular retroversion can be evaluated on this view by showing lateral projection of the superior aspect of the anterior acetabulum relative to the posterior rim forming the figure-of-eight sign. (*B*) Frog-leg lateral radiograph is acquired with patient supine, the knee flexed, and the thigh abducted and externally rotated. (*C*) Elongated femoral neck view (Dunn view) obtained in 45° hip flexion. This view better visualizes the anterior femoral head-neck junction, evaluating for cam-type impingement morphology. The alpha angle quantifies the degree of femoral head asphericity and is best measured on the Dunn view using 2 intersecting lines, one along the central femoral neck and the other from the isocenter of the femoral head to a point where the sphericity of the femoral head is first lost, using 55° as the threshold of normal. (*D*) False profile view obtained in 65° of external rotation better visualizes anterior acetabular morphology. The anterior center edge angle is measured from this view using 2 intersecting lines, one drawn parallel to the femoral neck and the other from the central femoral head to the anterior acetabular rim. Normal values range from 20° to 40°.

3. Frog lateral of hip only
4. Dunn elongated femoral neck view of hip only
5. False profile of hip only

With these exposures, we routinely measure the femoral head extrusion index bilaterally to assess for dysplasia, the femoral head center edge angle, and the femoral head-neck alpha angle to assess for cam impingement and acetabular version as an indicator of pincer impingement. All of these calculations are then placed in the imaging report.

Skeletal maturity at the pelvis and at the proximal femora should also be reported, and particular attention should be given to symmetry of all osseous and physeal structures in skeletally immature patients. Other views can be performed for specific clinical indications.[5] In the setting of core muscle injury, if there is suspicion for instability at the pubic symphysis, the standing AP pelvis view can be compared with bilateral flamingo views, in which the patient sequentially bears full weight on a single extremity, then the other, during AP exposures of the pelvis. Inflammatory spondyloarthropathies may warrant bilateral oblique views angled to the sacroiliac joints, although asymmetry of the sacroiliitis may still be best assessed on the AP pelvis view, and inlet/outlet views are still useful in delineating the extent of pelvic ring fractures.

Observation and acknowledgement of sometimes subtle radiographic findings can often get the imager and the referrer into the correct spectrum of disorder, and govern the need for more tertiary imaging studies and particular imaging protocols.

NONCONTRAST MR IMAGING PROTOCOLS

Distinguishing intra-articular sources of symptoms from extra-articular sources can be particularly difficult with hip and groin pain, and this is a primary objective of MR imaging. The authors advocate using a multichannel phased array torso coil and a combination of lower-resolution, large-field-of-view survey imaging of the entire pelvis with dedicated high-resolution small-field-of-view imaging of the hip. All of our pelvis and hip protocols include 3 pelvis sequences: coronal short-tau inversion recovery (STIR), coronal T1, and axial T2 fast spin echo (FSE) with fat saturation. These lower-resolution sequences should identify any of the potential extra-articular sources of hip and groin pain, including bursitis, flexor and rotator tendinopathies, true hernias, athletic pubalgia lesions/core muscle injury, stress fractures, and masses or collections in the visceral pelvis.

For the high-resolution sequences, the authors use the same phased array torso coil, selecting elements in close proximity to the hip when feasible, and acquire true coronal and sagittal images prescribed along the acetabulum, and axial-oblique images prescribed along the femoral neck; all intermediate-weighted proton density FSE with fat saturation (Table 1). These sequences are optimized for assessment of the acetabular labrum,

articular cartilage, and subchondral bone at the femoroacetabular joint. Some investigators have shown the value of high-resolution, non–fat-suppressed, intermediate-weighted sequences, and planes prescribed along the acetabulum, as well as radial imaging dedicated to the ipsilateral hip (Swiss protocol). Valid points can be made on both sides of the argument over when to fat suppress and when to not fat suppress on high-resolution MR imaging of the hip (Fig. 2).[6]

Some hip arthroscopy subspecialists request radial imaging to further delineate osseous anatomy and labral tears, and this is easy to achieve when desired. Simply use an magnetic resonance cholangiopancreatography sequence from the biliary protocol, thin the slices to 4 to 5 mm, and place the center in the middle of the acetabular fossa en face along the acetabular rim. Another problem-solving imaging tool that can be useful is acquisition of an additional small-field-of-view coronal T2-weighted FSE fat-suppressed sequence with the patient positioned in femoral abduction and external rotation (FABER). Simply place the patient's ipsilateral foot behind the contralateral knee while the patient is supine on the scanner and allow the ipsilateral knee to fall to the side in external rotation. This technique can help identify nondisplaced anterosuperior labrum tears (Fig. 3).

INDIRECT MAGNETIC RESONANCE ARTHROGRAPHY

When direct MR arthrography is not feasible, an arthrographic MR imaging protocol after intravenous administration of a gadolinium-based contrast agent has been shown to be an accurate tool for identification and delineation of acetabular labrum tears and chondral lesions.[7] The authors use the same imaging planes and fields of view as in the noncontrast protocol, and the 3 survey sequences of the pelvis are identical,

Table 1 Routine hip MR imaging parameters								
Sequence	FOV (cm)	Matrix	Slice Thickness (mm)	Slice Gap (mm)	NEX	TR (ms)	TE (ms)	TI
Pelvis coronal T1	36–40	256 × 256	4	1	1	400–800	Minimum	—
Pelvis coronal STIR	36–40	256 × 192	4	1	2	>2000	20–40	150
Pelvis axial T2 FS	36–40	256 × 256	4	1	2	>2000	40–50	—
Hip axial-oblique PD FS	14–20	384 × 256	4	1	2	>2000	30–40	—
Hip coronal PD FS	14–20	384 × 256	4	1	2	>2000	40–50	—
Hip sagittal PD FS	14–20	384 × 256	4	1	2	>2000	40–50	—

Abbreviations: FOV, field of view; FS, fat suppressed; NEX, number of excitations; PD, proton density; TE, echo time; TI, inversion time; TR, repetition time.

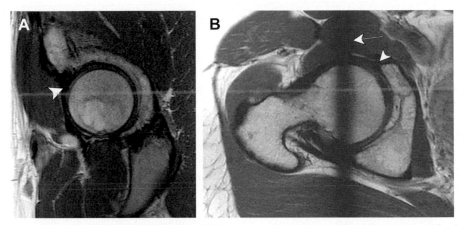

Fig. 2. High-resolution, noncontrast MR imaging (Swiss protocol). Sagittal oblique image prescribed along the acetabular rim (A) and radial (B) intermediate-weighted non–fat-suppressed MR image show a normal acetabular labrum (arrowheads). There is typical crosstalk artifact noted on the radial MR image (arrow).

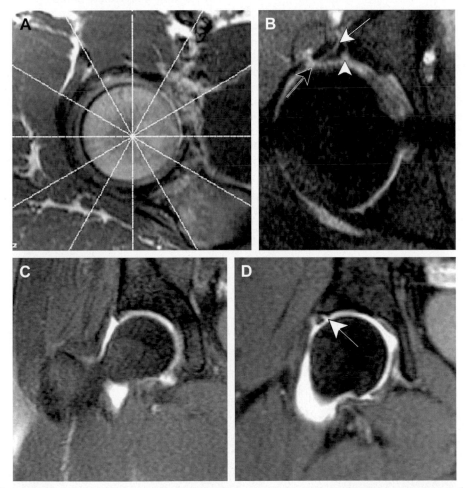

Fig. 3. Alternative imaging techniques. (A) MR image shows the prescription of radial sequencing at the acetabular opening. (B) Radial T2-weighted MR image shows a partial-thickness undersurface labral tear that was not clearly seen on conventional imaging planes (arrowhead). Also note partial-thickness cartilage thinning at the anterosuperior femoral head (black arrow). A potential pitfall when interpreting radial images is that the close proximity of the iliopsoas tendon to the anterior labrum can lead to misinterpretation of a labral tear (white arrow). Neutral (C) and FABER (D) MR arthrograms show an anterosuperior labral tear that was not seen on the neutral position but is clearly identified on the FABER position (arrow).

but the proton density–weighted small-field-of-view sequences are changed to arthrographic T1-weighted fat-saturated images, or, with some scanners, T1-weighted spoiled gradient echo sequences. Other factors being equal, the authors prefer the frequency-selective fat-saturated T1 images, because chondral and labral signal is robust and homogeneous, but an isotropic gradient echo sequence can be valuable for its thin slices and potential for multiplanar reconstructions. With indirect MR arthrography, there is generally little joint distension without a preexistent joint effusion, but contrast generally aggregates in regions of soft tissue and osseous injury.

DIRECT MAGNETIC RESONANCE ARTHROGRAPHY AND THE ANESTHETIC EXAMINATION

In our practice, direct MR arthrography is the workhorse imaging study for suspected internal derangements of the prearthritic hip. A dilute gadolinium-based contrast solution can be placed into the femoroacetabular joint with fluoroscopy, radiography, or sonographic guidance, but the authors advocate correlating MR findings with a radiographic series, and thus fluoroscopy guidance after scout radiographs can be the most efficient technique and also minimizes the ionizing

radiation dose (**Fig. 4**). We dilute the agent in normal saline and local anesthetic at approximately 1 mmol/L, with mild variation based on the particular agent and field strength. We find it necessary to use only 1 to 2 mL of nonionic, iodinated contrast to document an intra-articular position, and generally keep this distinct from the gadolinium-based contrast solution. We include 3 to 4 mL of anesthetic in the contrast solution, optimally a mixture of immediate-acting and longer-acting agents. Ultimately, although a palpable fullness and resistance to further infusion of fluid is a better gauge than any particular volume, most arthrographic hip injections should involve 12 to 18 mL of fluid in total.[8,9]

The anesthetic arthrogram plays a very important role in imaging hip and groin pain. The authors perform a physical examination with maneuvers directed to the hip before prepping the area for injection, and then repeat the same examination after intra-articular anesthetic administration. Our physical examination includes documentation of pain on a scale of 1 to 10 during passive hip flexion, flexion with external rotation and abduction, flexion with internal rotation and adduction, and active hip flexion (**Fig. 5**). Other maneuvers can be added based on activity and symptoms, but with these 4 basic examinations we have found a reproducible, algorithmic approach to the physical examination to be most useful to our subspecialty hip

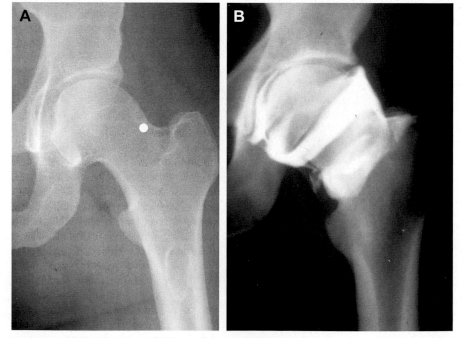

Fig. 4. Fluoroscopy-guided arthrogram. (*A*) Scout fluoroscopic image of the hip shows the typical location of needle placement at the superolateral aspect of the femoral head-neck junction. (*B*) Fluoroscopic image after administration of contrast for an MR arthrogram shows typical appearance of intra-articular contrast around the femoral neck.

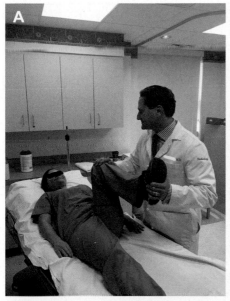
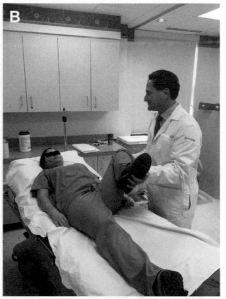
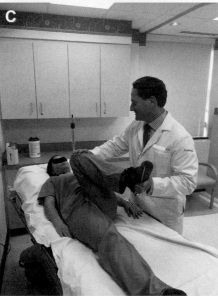

Fig. 5. Anesthetic examination maneuvers. (A) Passive hip flexion, (B) flexion with external rotation and abduction, (C) flexion with internal rotation and adduction. These maneuvers are performed before the injection and then repeated after the injection. Any change in symptoms is documented in the procedure report. Assessment of active hip flexion, abduction, and adduction can also be helpful, particularly for extra-articular sources of pain, but symptoms should not significantly change with intra-articular anesthetic.

arthroscopy referrers. The results of the anesthetic arthrogram are placed in our image-guided arthrogram report, but could also be placed in the MR imaging report. A distinct section of the report, Anesthetic Examination, details the reported pain score for each maneuver both before and after the injection. The longer-acting anesthetics can have more of an effect after the patient leaves for MR imaging, so we provide a printed pain score worksheet ranging out to 6 hours after the injection for completion and presentation to the referrer. This examination is not perfect, because the volume of injected fluid alone can exacerbate discomfort and some labral injuries may manifest with

exacerbation of pain during anesthetic injection, but, overall, the procedure has added value to our musculoskeletal practice. The anesthetic examination has generated reports of strong positive predictive value (89%) and specificity (83%) for acetabular labrum tear in a cohort of young adults, so these results are vital for optimization of the ultimate direct MR arthrogram interpretation.[10]

Our direct MR arthrographic protocol is essentially identical to the indirect MR arthrography protocol (Table 2). We again acquire 3 survey sequences of the pelvis followed by the 3 fat-suppressed T1-weighted sequences dedicated to the hip (Fig. 6). Technologists should be tutored

Table 2
Direct MR hip arthrogram imaging parameters

Sequence	FOV (cm)	Matrix	Slice Thickness (mm)	Slice Gap (mm)	NEX	TR (ms)	TE (ms)	TI
Pelvis coronal T1	36–40	256 × 256	4	1	1	400–800	Minimum	—
Pelvis coronal STIR	36–40	256 × 192	4	1	2	>2000	20–40	150
Pelvis axial T2 FS	36–40	256 × 256	4	1	2	>2000	40–50	—
Hip axial-oblique T1 FS	14–20	384 × 256	4	0.5	2	400–800	Minimum	—
Hip coronal T1 FS	14–20	384 × 256	4	0.5	2	400–800	Minimum	—
Hip sagittal T1 FS	14–16	384 × 256	4	0.5	2	400–800	Minimum	—

on the importance of prescribing the axial-oblique sequence along the femoral neck from a coronal localizer, because a suboptimal image plane can lead to inaccurate and nonreproducible alpha angle calculations. Radial imaging or FABER imaging can easily be acquired and added to this protocol when requested or warranted. Because there is already contrast within the joint, fat-suppressed T1-weighted imaging is generally the most appropriate for these additions.

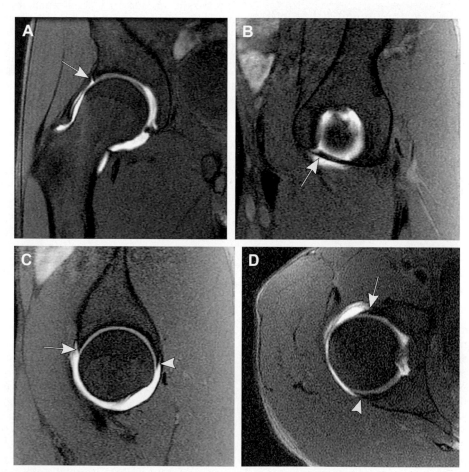

Fig. 6. Normal MR arthrogram. Coronal (*A*), sagittal (*B, C*), and axial (*D*) T1-weighted fat-suppressed MR arthrograms of a normal hip show the normal perilabral recess lateral to the superior labrum (*arrow in A*) and normal transverse ligament (*arrow in B*). Note the normal hypointense appearance of the anterior (*arrows in C and D*) and posterior (*arrowheads in C and D*) labrum.

COMPUTED TOMOGRAPHY APPLICATIONS

To experienced imagers, CT offers little more than quality radiographs in the setting of atraumatic hip and groin pain. However, three-dimensional (3D) models of the femoral head or the acetabulum with subtraction of the reciprocal joint surfaces can be useful to surgeons when mapping out a treatment plan. During image acquisition the entire pelvis is exposed to ionizing radiation, so we review 1 spiral acquisition of the pelvis to look for concomitant or incidental lesions, and then generate multiplanar two-dimensional (2D) reformats as well as 3D reformats of the femoral head and the acetabulum (**Fig. 7**).[11] As a protocol, we do not recommend CT of the prearthritic hip in the imaging algorithm, but, when requested, we try to use both its 2D and its 3D capabilities.

INTRINSIC FEMOROACETABULAR LESIONS

Many patients undergoing dedicated hip MR imaging have injury to intra-articular structures, including articular cartilage, subchondral bone, the acetabular labrum, and the ligamentum teres. With direct or indirect MR arthrography, contrast-enhanced joint fluid should outline soft tissue lesions on T1-weighted fat-suppressed images, whereas clinicians must rely on native joint fluid and T2-weighted fat-suppressed sequences to do the same with noncontrast protocols. With MR arthrography, it is critical to correlate arthrographic T1-weighted sequences with fluid-sensitive T2-weighted images for bone marrow edema, muscle edema, and preexisting fluid collections. Fractures and osseous lesions can be missed if an MR arthrographic protocol includes only T1 weighting. For intra-articular hips, a systematic approach to anatomy, pathology, and their relationship should be followed, using all imaging studies available.[12]

The Acetabulum

Many internal derangements of the hip reflect prominence (overcoverage) or deficiency (dysplasia) of the acetabulum. Acetabular version

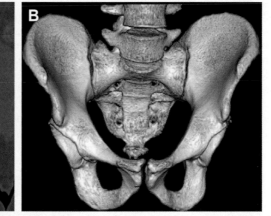
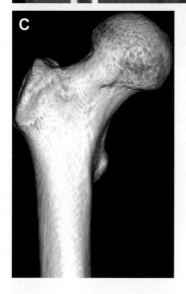

Fig. 7. (*A*) Coronal 2D reformat CT of the right hip showing prominence of the femoral head-neck junction, indicating cam-type femoroacetabular impingement morphology (*arrow*). 3D surface rendering CT of the pelvis with the femora subtracted (*B*) shows acetabular version and symmetry, and 3D image of the isolated femur (*C*) maps the osseous and articular surfaces.

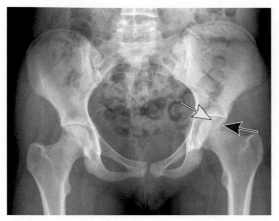

Fig. 8. Acetabular retroversion. AP radiograph of the pelvis in a skeletally immature teenaged girl shows bilateral crossover or figure-of-eight signs. The superior aspect of the anterior acetabular rim (*black arrow*) projects lateral to the posterior rim (*white arrow*), consistent with acetabular retroversion.

is best assessed on a standing AP radiograph of the pelvis (**Fig. 8**), but findings on that radiographic view can be reinforced at MR imaging and potential sequelae to anatomic aberrations detailed. A femoral head extrusion index can be measured at MR imaging on the coronal sequence at its anterior to posterior midline, and acetabular retroversion can be confirmed at the most superior margin of the acetabular rim, but these observations are best reported in support of subsequent labral and chondral injuries. With retroversion, during flexion

and internal rotation, the femoral head migrates too proximal into the region of acetabular deficiency, causing a transient overcoverage of the femoral head anteriorly. The result is often abruption of the anterior acetabular labrum at its base from the anterior acetabular rim, or a pincer-type anterior labrum tear.[13] With advanced developmental dysplasia of the hip, the superior acetabular rim is deficient and the superior acetabular labrum is enlarged or overgrown but also prone to tear (**Fig. 9**).

The Femoral Head-Neck Junction

Osseous prominence at the anterosuperior femoral head-neck junction has long been described as a developmental variation frequently associated with cam-type femoroacetabular impingement. This prominence can be measured on the elongated femoral neck radiographic view or on axial-oblique MR images with the femoral head-neck alpha angle (**Fig. 10**).[14] Frequently, there is a small cortical defect, or synovial herniation pit, at the exact site of the osseous prominence, likely reflecting repeated impaction on the anterosuperior acetabulum. This osseous morphology causes a grinding-type trauma leading to anterosuperior labrum tears and delaminating-type chondral lesions on the anterosuperior acetabulum and the anterosuperior femoral head-neck junction. These features are the hallmark MR imaging findings of cam-type femoroacetabular impingement.[15] As our experience with imaging and treating these

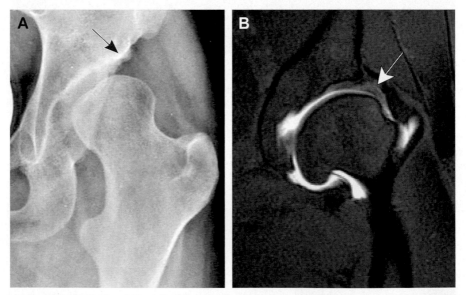

Fig. 9. Developmental dysplasia of the hip. (*A*) AP radiograph shows a deficient, hypoplastic, shallow superior acetabulum (*arrow*). (*B*) Coronal MR arthrogram shows acetabular undercoverage with hypertrophic superior labrum and intrasubstance labral degeneration (*arrow*).

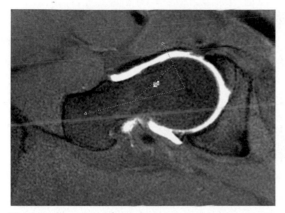

Fig. 10. Cam-type femoroacetabular impingement. Axial-oblique T1-weighted MR arthrogram of the right hip shows osseous protuberance at the anterior femoral head-neck junction, resulting in an increased alpha angle measuring 78°.

aberrations in osseous anatomy has grown, we have learned that the most common symptomatic scenario in young adults is a mixed cam-type and pincer-type impingement, which should be acknowledged by musculoskeletal imagers when detailing hip anatomy and injury.

The Acetabular Labrum

The fibrocartilaginous acetabular labrum, analogous to the glenoid labrum, is prone to degenerative tearing throughout life. However, most degenerative acetabular labrum tears are asymptomatic or minimally symptomatic. The hip is inherently more stable than the glenohumeral joint, and almost all hip labrum tears occur in reproducible locations with reproducible morphologies, most often related to the osseous variations discussed earlier. Several anatomic localization systems have been proposed for delineation of acetabular labrum tears, and the morphologic extent of labral injury can be described with many of the same terms as are routinely used for knee meniscus tears. Although a clock-face designation is popular in some regions, the authors use the zone classification system to reinforce the descriptive localization of acetabular labrum injury (Fig. 11).[16,17] The acetabular labrum can show regions of intrasubstance degeneration on MR sequences, but any incongruity at its undersurface can be considered a tear, whether symptomatic or not. Fluid signal extending from the joint into the labral substance is a reliable indicator of labral tear on noncontrast sequences, whereas contrast-enhanced fluid extending into the labrum indicates tear on arthrographic MR images. Further, the acetabular labrum should have neat margins and

hypointense signal on all MR images, and its free margin should show a sharp, acute angle. Aberrations in this morphology at MR imaging can be considered a labral tear.[18]

With cam-type impingement, labral tears are typically broad and complex, involving the undersurface of the anterosuperior labrum, or zone 2 (Fig. 12). The degree of complexity varies and tears can extend beyond zone 2 anteriorly to zone 1, or superiorly to zone 3. With pincer-type impingement, the labrum is more often abrupted from the acetabular rim at its base, anterior more common than posterior, and detachment from the osseous acetabulum is common (Fig. 13). A traumatic posterior subluxation injury can result in a detached posterior labrum tear, but these are uncommon, and degenerative-type tearing of the superior labrum (zone 3) is common with joint space narrowing and early osteoarthritis.

Paralabral cysts, analogous to parameniscal cysts at the knee, are a reliable indicator of acetabular labrum tear.[19] Cysts should be quantified in relative terms and location should be described with regard to proximity to surrounding structures. On noncontrast MR images, the neck from a paralabral cyst can often be tracked to the site of labrum tear (Fig. 14). A particular nuance of paralabral cysts at the hip is a tendency for cysts to extend from an anterosuperior labrum tear cephalad along the rectus femoris tendon to its origin at the anterior-inferior iliac spine. These paralabral cysts can cause pain with active hip flexion, particularly when they insinuate between the direct and indirect heads of the rectus femoris. In general, description of acetabular labrum tears in the prearthritic hip should include regions and/or zones involved, complexity, morphology, any detachment, paralabral cysts, and presence and degree of associated cartilage or subchondral injury.[20]

Articular Cartilage

As with other joints, including the knee and shoulder, articular cartilage lesions in the hip are most often associated with injury to the fibrocartilaginous stabilizing cuff, in this case the acetabular labrum. The paucity of hyaline cartilage on the femoral head and acetabulum (in contrast with the knee), the small amount of normal joint fluid, and the depth of the hip joint within the pelvis all contribute to challenges in imaging hip cartilage. Direct MR arthrographic protocols help with increased tissue contrast, but advanced cartilage imaging techniques, including T1 rho, T2 mapping, and delayed gadolinium enhanced MR imaging of cartilage (dGEMRIC), can be of great help when

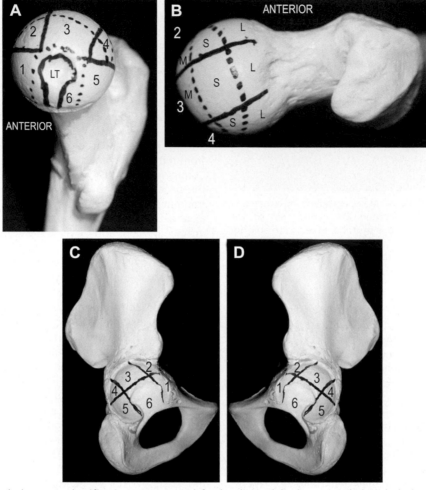

Fig. 11. Acetabular zone classification system used for localizing labral tears and chondral abnormalities. (*A*) Right hemipelvis model and (*B*) left hemipelvis model. (*C*) Front view of right proximal femur model. The head has been divided into 6 zones around the projection of the acetabular fossa (with a dotted line around the ligamentum transversum [LT]). Zone 1 is the anterior-inferior femoral head; zone 2, anterior-superior femoral head; zone 3, central superior femoral head; zone 4, posterior-superior femoral head; zone 5, posterior-inferior femoral head; and zone 6, area around ligamentum teres. (*D*) Superior view of right proximal femur model. The 3 subdivisions of zones 2, 3, and 4 are presented: medial (M), superior (S), and lateral (L). (*From* Ilizaliturri VM Jr, Byrd JW, Sampson TG, et al. A geographic zone method to describe intra-articular pathology in hip arthroscopy: cadaveric study and preliminary report. Arthroscopy 2008;24(5):534–9; with permission.)

assessing articular cartilage in the prearthritic hip.[21] When present, articular cartilage lesions should be localized using an adaptation of whatever system is used for localizing labral tears, and lesions should be graded based on size, depth, and morphology. Modified Outerbridge and Noyes classification systems (among others) can be applied to hip cartilage as they are at other joints, and particular attention should be given to delaminating-type chondral lesions that may be unstable with ranges of motion.[22] With cam impingement, chondral wearing and delaminating-type chondral lesions are prevalent

at the anterosuperior acetabulum (zone 2), but reciprocal lesions are also prevalent at the antero-superior femoral head-neck junction. Imagers should take care to assess for both traumatic and degenerative articular cartilage lesions after identification of an acetabular labrum tear, because these may factor into treatment planning and possibly arthroscopic technique.

The Ligamentum Teres

Ligamentum teres disruption is an uncommon finding at MR imaging, but, clinically, injury can

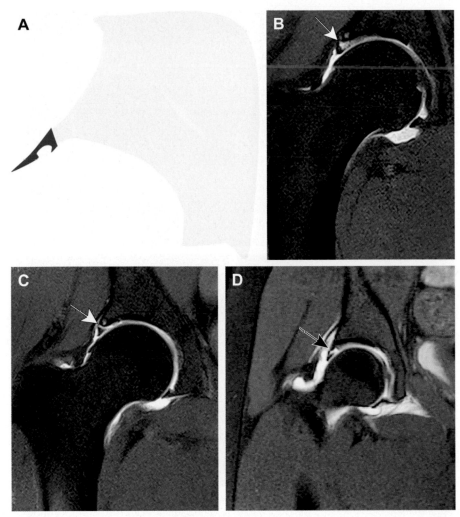

Fig. 12. Anterosuperior labral tears in cam-type impingement. (*A*) Typical undersurface tears at the anterosuperior labrum as well as chondrosis seen with cam-type impingement. (*B*) Coronal MR arthrogram showing partial-thickness undersurface anterosuperior labral tear (*arrow*). (*C*) Coronal MR arthrogram showing full-thickness, detached anterosuperior labral tear at the chondrolabral junction (*arrow*). (*D*) Coronal MR arthrogram showing a delaminating anterosuperior labral tear extending to the free edge of the labrum (*arrow*).

manifest as internal snapping, popping, or insta-bility.[23] The normal ligamentum teres has a broad origin from both the ischial and pubic sides of the acetabular notch, and tapers to its insertion on the fovea capitis femoris. The value of reporting partial or complete ligamentum teres tear at MR imaging is unclear, and numerous morphologic variants (bifid, trifid) have been reported.[21] It has been theorized that the ligamentum teres plays a stabilizing role because it is most taut in positions of femoroacetabular instability, but sometimes the ligamentum teres is deliberately transected or resected at arthroscopy, so its value in the adult hip is debatable. At MR imaging, an intact ligamentum teres should be easy to confirm with at least a small joint effusion or an MR arthrographic

protocol, but assessment can be difficult with a paucity of fluid in the joint (**Fig. 15**).[24]

Normal Variants

There is no widespread agreement in the imaging literature on the presence and prevalence of subla-bral sulci and sublabral recesses in the adult hip. Sublabral sulci have been reported with a prevalence of up to 25%, but the most commonly reported location for a sublabral sulcus is postero-superior on the acetabulum, a location where labral tear is very uncommon in the prearthritic hip. Anterior and anterosuperior sublabral sulci can also occur and are much more likely to be confounders for labral tears. The reported prevalence of anterior

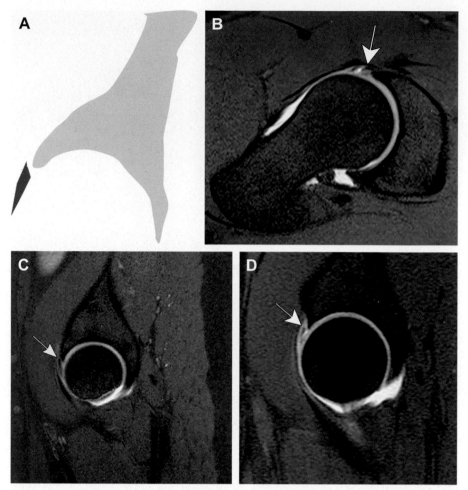

Fig. 13. Anterior labral tears in pincer-type impingement. (*A*) Typical detachment of the anterior labrum seen with pincer-type impingement. Axial-oblique MR arthrogram (*B*) and sagittal MR arthrogram (*C*) show full-thickness anterior labral tear with detachment from the osseous acetabular rim (*arrows*). (*D*) Sagittal MR arthrogram shows anterior labral tear with a delaminating component extending to the free edge of the labrum (*arrow*).

and anterosuperior sublabral sulci varies from less than 10% to 50%, and some investigators have suggested that all anterosuperior clefts are pathologic.[25,26] In our experience and with the guidance of our referring hip arthroscopy surgeons, normal-variant sublabral sulci or sublabral recesses anterior to the apex of the acetabular rim (zone 3) are uncommon, and should be considered at least suspicious for labral tear. Posterosuperior and posterior sublabral clefts or recesses are common, and often extend along the posterior acetabulum all the way to its posteroinferior region. At MR imaging or MR arthrography, a normal-variant sulcus or recess should have sharp, clean margins and simple geometric contours. If a cleft or defect extends into the labral substance, it should be considered a tear. If there is cartilage loss or subchondral edema subjacent to a cleft or defect, it should be considered a tear. If there is more than 1 mm of distraction

between the articular cartilage and the labrum, it should be considered a tear.

The supra-acetabular fossa, sometimes referred to as the pseudodefect of the acetabulum, is a focal defect in the subchondral bone of the acetabulum in a reproducible location, its apex (border of zones 3 and 6, or 12:00). It should be located at the apex of the acetabulum on both coronal and sagittal images. Traumatic osteochondral lesions are extremely uncommon in this location, so distinguishing the supra-acetabular fossa from a traumatic lesion is possible by location alone; however, with this normal structure, overlying hyaline cartilage should be intact, and subjacent bone marrow signal should be normal. The stellate crease is another normal variant; a focal area of hyaline cartilage deficiency in the acetabular roof, medial to the supracetabular fossa (**Fig. 16**). At MR imaging, chondral margins of the stellate

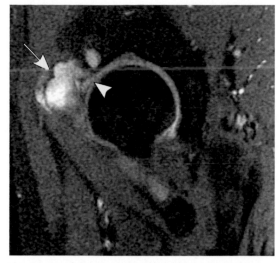

Fig. 14. Paralabral cyst. Sagittal T1-weighted fat-suppressed image from an indirect MR arthrogram shows a lobulated, enhancing paralabral cyst (*arrow*) related to an underlying anterosuperior full-thickness, detached labral tear (*arrowhead*).

crease should be neat, in contrast with traumatic lesions, but again the location far medial on the acetabular roof is atypical for trauma.[27]

POSTOPERATIVE IMAGING CONSIDERATIONS

Guidance on imaging the postoperative hip is available from several recent articles. The noncontrast and arthrographic protocols discussed earlier can be used for most postoperative indications, including acetabular labrum retear, progressive chondrosis, and repair failure.

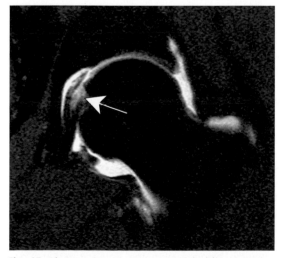

Fig. 15. Ligamentum teres tear. Axial-oblique proton density fat-suppressed MR image shows partial-thickness tear of the proximal ligamentum teres at its insertion on the fovea capitis with underlying bone marrow edema (*arrow*).

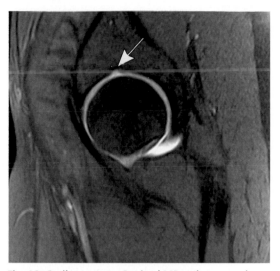

Fig. 16. Stellate crease. Sagittal MR arthrogram shows shallow articular cartilage deficiency at the acetabular roof with neat chondral margins (*arrow*).

A high-resolution, intermediate-weighted, non–fat-suppressed sequence can be added for optimal assessment of sutures or suture anchors in the acetabular rim if there has been a labral repair. For postoperative infection or fluid collection, a before and after intravenous contrast mass or infection protocol can be considered.

When evaluating the postoperative labrum, it is important to gather information on the arthroscopic technique and the surgical objective. After debridement, the labrum often shows blunting or truncation of its free edge and hyperintense signal at its undersurface, similar to the debrided meniscus in the knee. Direct MR arthrographic images are helpful in this setting, distinguishing enhanced fluid signal from the less T2-hyperintense signal at the labral undersurface with evolving granulation tissue. It is a good sign of healing when the site of labral tear shows granulation tissue but does not allow joint fluid, enhanced or nonenhanced, to extend into the labral substance. With labral repair, the labrum can be primarily sutured to the acetabular rim, or the acetabular rim can be taken down, debrided, and then reattached along with the labrum (rim takedown repair). Both types of repair should be tight, not allowing joint fluid to pass through the repair, but granulation tissue at the site of the repair is expected. Femoral osteotomy defects can be identified at the anterosuperior femoral head-neck junction, ideally at the site of previous impingement.[28]

EXTRA-ARTICULAR HIP LESIONS

Hip and groin pain in young adults can result from both intra-articular and extra-articular lesions. Although MR arthrographic protocols are tailored to optimal contrast within the joint, identification of periarticular disorder is equally important. Radiographs and CT are sensitive for soft tissue calcification/ossification, but offer little else in the setting of periarticular sources of hip pain. Sonography has become a primary imaging tool for tendinopathies and fluid collections about the hip, but it fails in the assessment of osseous and chondral lesions. MR imaging allows the reliable identification of both intra-articular and extra-articular sources of pain in the prearthritic hip. Thus, a systematic approach should be taken to assess periarticular structures about the hip, and throughout the pelvis.

Gluteus Minimus and Medius

The gluteus medius and gluteus minimus have been called the rotator cuff of the hip, and are commonly involved in disorders ranging from peritendinitis to degenerative tendinopathies and tears.[26] These lesions, along with fluid collections near gluteal insertions on the femur, are an exceedingly common extra-articular source of hip pain (**Fig. 17**). Anatomic considerations and a spectrum of lesions about the gluteus minimus and medius are covered by Belair and colleagues (See Belair JA, Hegazi TM, Roedl JB, et al: Core Injuries Remote from the Pubic Symphysis, in this issue), so the discussion here is limited, but these lesions are best assessed on fluid-sensitive, fat-suppressed images in all planes available.[29]

Rectus Femoris, Iliopsoas, and Hip Flexors

Hip flexors and accessory hip flexors are also commonly involved in both degenerative and inflammatory conditions manifesting as anterior or anterolateral hip pain.[27] At the physical examination performed as a part of the anesthetic arthrogram, hip flexors can be assessed with active maneuvers: leg flexion and flexion with abduction and adduction. Lesions ranging from origin to insertion and involving the rectus femoris, sartorius, and iliopsoas

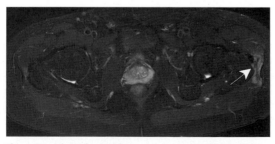

Fig. 17. Gluteal tendon tear. Large-field-of-view, T2-weighted, fat-suppressed MR image shows partial-thickness tear of the gluteus medius tendon at its insertion on the lateral facet of the greater trochanter with surrounding soft tissue edema and peritendinitis (*arrow*).

are covered by Belair and colleagues (See Belair JA, Hegazi TM, Roedl JB, et al: Core Injuries Remote from the Pubic Symphysis, in this issue).

Bursitis and Ischiofemoral Impingement

These lesions are also covered by Belair and colleagues (See Belair JA, Hegazi TM, Roedl JB, et al: Core Injuries Remote from the Pubic Symphysis, in this issue), but are an important consideration when interrogating potential extra-articular sources of hip and groin pain, and warrant mention in the algorithmic imaging evaluation. With arthrographic protocols, imagers must distinguish extension of joint fluid into the iliopsoas bursa from preexisting iliopsoas bursitis by comparing T1-weighted and T2-weighted sequences. With indirect MR arthrography, even low-grade impingement lesions enhance, so ischiofemoral impingement is best diagnosed on the T2-weighted fat-suppressed images.

REFERRED SOURCES OF HIP AND GROIN PAIN

Stress fractures, core muscle injuries, and piriformis syndromes are all potential sources of referred pain to the hip and groin. The anesthetic arthrogram examination can be very helpful in leading imagers to one of these diagnoses, because intra-articular anesthetic should not make a significant impact on pain, and pain should not be elicited with typical passive maneuvers directed to intrinsic hip structures. Sacroiliitis and even lower lumbar spondylopathy are other potential sources of referred pain, and visceral lesions, including inguinal hernia, inflammatory bowel disease, and endometriosis can play a role in musculoskeletal pain generation. The prevalence of these lesions is the primary impetus for including large-field-of-view, fluid-sensitive, fat-suppressed, and anatomy-specific sequences in hip imaging radiographic, CT, and MR imaging protocols.

CONCOMITANT LESIONS

As discussed earlier, hip and groin pain in prearthritic patients can reflect both intra-articular and/or extra-articular osseous, chondral, or soft tissue lesions. Symptoms therefore do not necessarily reflect only a single disorder. An association between core muscle injury and ipsilateral intrinsic hip disorder has been established.[28] This scenario can render results of the anesthetic arthrogram confusing, and imagers must be diligent in following through with the entire imaging algorithm, even after an injury is identified. Finding a soft tissue injury such as gluteus medius tear and a simultaneous ipsilateral intrinsic chondral-labral lesion is a common event when imaging the hip, and either or both can be pain generators. Similarly, potential referred sources of pain, including inguinal hernia and lumbar spondylopathy, can be present along with an acetabular labrum tear. Identifying concomitant lesions as possible sources of hip and groin pain is easier with MR imaging using the protocols detailed in this article than with ultrasonography or conventional radiographs.[30]

Another helpful tool in the imaging armamentarium is image-guided (generally ultrasonography-guided) selective diagnostic injections for extra-articular structures. Focused musculoskeletal ultrasonography and ultrasonography-guided anesthetic and/or steroid injections have become a significant part of our practice in the work-up of young patients with hip and groin pain. This practice is detailed by Roedl and colleagues (See McCarthy E, Hegazi T, Zoga AC, et al: Ultrasound-Guided Interventions for Core and Hip Injuries in Athletes, in this issue).

SUMMARY

Accurate diagnosis of musculoskeletal sources of hip and groin pain is often clinically difficult, because a myriad of intra-articular and extra-articular lesions can contribute to symptoms. The imaging work-up should begin with a dedicated radiographic series, including a standing AP view of the pelvis and views tailored to femoroacetabular anatomy. MR imaging and MR arthrography remain workhorse imaging tools in young adult and prearthritic patients, and MR imaging protocols combining sequences dedicated to the hip as well as sequences covering the musculoskeletal pelvis offer the best chance of identifying all potential sources of symptoms. With MR arthrography, the anesthetic arthrogram can be an extremely useful tool, but imagers must be wary of potential concomitant lesions.

REFERENCES

1. Bozic KJ, Chan V, Valone FH 3rd, et al. Trends in hip arthroscopy utilization in the United States. J Arthroplasty 2013;28(8 Suppl):140–3.
2. Philippon MJ, Faucet SC, Briggs KK. Arthroscopic hip labral repair. Arthrosc Tech 2013;2(2):e73–6.
3. McCarthy JC, Lee JA. Hip arthroscopy: indications, outcomes, and complications. Instr Course Lect 2006;55:301–8.
4. Campbell SE. Radiography of the hip: lines, signs, and patterns of disease. Semin Roentgenol 2005; 40(3):290–319.
5. Clohisy JC, Carlisle JC, Beaule PE, et al. A systematic approach to the plain radiographic evaluation of the young adult hip. J Bone Joint Surg Am 2008;90(Suppl 4):47–66.
6. Potter HG, Schachar J. High resolution noncontrast MRI of the hip. J Magn Reson Imaging 2010;31(2): 268–78.
7. Zlatkin MB, Pevsner D, Sanders TG, et al. Acetabular labral tears and cartilage lesions of the hip: indirect MR arthrographic correlation with arthroscopy–a preliminary study. AJR Am J Roentgenol 2010;194(3):709–14.
8. Fitzgerald RH Jr. Acetabular labrum tears. Diagnosis and treatment. Clin Orthop Relat Res 1995;(311):60–8.
9. Conway WF, Totty WG, McEnery KW. CT and MR imaging of the hip. Radiology 1996;198(2):297–307.
10. Zoga AC, Shortt CP, Morrison WB, et al. SSC12–08. MRI of athletic pubalgia: incidence and imaging of concomitant pubic symphysis and ipsilateral hip pathology. SSC12-08, musculoskeletal (hip and groin disorders). Proceedings of the Radiologic Society of North America. Chicago, IL, November 30-December 4, 2008.
11. Tannast M, Siebenrock KA, Anderson SE. Femoroacetabular impingement: radiographic diagnosis–what the radiologist should know. AJR Am J Roentgenol 2007;188(6):1540–52.
12. Petersilge CA. From the RSNA refresher courses. Radiological Society of North America. Chronic adult hip pain: MR arthrography of the hip. Radiographics 2000;20:S43–52.
13. Carballido-Gamio J, Link TM, Li X, et al. Feasibility and reproducibility of relaxometry, morphometric, and geometrical measurements of the hip joint with magnetic resonance imaging at 3T. J Magn Reson Imaging 2008;28(1):227–35.
14. Barton C, Salineros MJ, Rakhra KS, et al. Validity of the alpha angle measurement on plain radiographs in the evaluation of cam-type femoroacetabular impingement. Clin Orthop Relat Res 2011;469(2):464–9.
15. Kassarjian A, Yoon LS, Belzile E, et al. Triad of MR arthrographic findings in patients with cam-type femoroacetabular impingement. Radiology 2005; 236(2):588–92.
16. Blankenbaker DG, De Smet AA, Keene JS, et al. Classification and localization of acetabular labral tears. Skeletal Radiol 2007;36(5):391–7.
17. Ilizaliturri VM Jr, Byrd JW, Sampson TG, et al. A geographic zone method to describe intra-articular pathology in hip arthroscopy: cadaveric study and preliminary report. Arthroscopy 2008;24(5):534–9.
18. Groh MM, Herrera J. A comprehensive review of hip labral tears. Curr Rev Musculoskelet Med 2009;2(2): 105–17.
19. Armfield DR, Towers JD, Robertson DD. Radiographic and MR imaging of the athletic hip. Clin Sports Med 2006;25(2):211–39, viii.
20. Hodler J, Trudell D, Pathria MN, et al. Width of the articular cartilage of the hip: quantification by using fat-suppression spin-echo MR imaging in cadavers. AJR Am J Roentgenol 1992;159(2):351–5.

21. Sutter R, Zanetti M, Pfirrmann CW. New developments in hip imaging. Radiology 2012;264(3):651–67.

22. Gold GE, Chen CA, Koo S, et al. Recent advances in MRI of articular cartilage. AJR Am J Roentgenol 2009;193(3):628–38.

23. Bardakos NV, Villar RN. The ligamentum teres of the adult hip. J Bone Joint Surg Br 2009;91(1):8–15.

24. Cerezal L, Kassarjian A, Canga A, et al. Anatomy, biomechanics, imaging, and management of ligamentum teres injuries. Radiographics 2010;30(6):1637–51.

25. Nguyen MS, Kheyfits V, Giordano BD, et al. Hip anatomic variants that may mimic abnormalities at MRI: labral variants. AJR Am J Roentgenol 2013;201(3):W394–400.

26. Saddik D, Troupis J, Tirman P, et al. Prevalence and location of acetabular sublabral sulci at hip arthroscopy with retrospective MRI review. AJR Am J Roentgenol 2006;187(5):W507–11.

27. Stoller D. Magnetic resonance imaging in orthopedics and sports medicine. 3rd edition. Philadelphia: Wolters Kluwer/Lippincott; 2007.

28. Blankenbaker DG, De Smet AA, Keene JS. MR arthrographic appearance of the postoperative acetabular labrum in patients with suspected recurrent labral tears. AJR Am J Roentgenol 2011;197(6):W1118–22.

29. Chi AS, Long SS, Zoga AC, et al. Prevalence and pattern of gluteus medius and minimus tendon pathology and muscle atrophy in older individuals using MRI. Skeletal Radiol 2015;44(12):1727–33.

30. Meyers WC, McKechnie A, Philippon MJ, et al. Experience with "sports hernia" spanning two decades. Ann Surg 2008;248(4):656–65.

Section III - New Ideas for Imaging Sports Injuries in the Lower Extremity

Postoperative Imaging of the Knee
Meniscus, Cartilage, and Ligaments

Daniel M. Walz, MD

KEYWORDS

- MR imaging • Meniscus repair • Anterior cruciate ligament reconstruction • Postoperative

KEY POINTS

- MR imaging is able to depict the normal and abnormal postoperative appearance of patients who have undergone meniscus surgery, ligament reconstruction, and cartilage repair.
- Understanding the options of repair, resect, or replace for meniscal surgery is key to the interpretation of postoperative knee MR imaging.
- A practical approach to the evaluation of MR images in patients who have undergone cartilage grafting includes a description of defect fill, integration, subchondral bone, repair tissue character, and non–repair site complications.
- MR imaging can be used to evaluate graft placement and integrity in patients following ligament reconstruction, aiding in the diagnosis of graft complications such as tear, impingement, instability and perigraft fibrosis.

INTRODUCTION

Orthopedic surgical interventions in the knee, including ligament reconstruction, meniscus repair and resection, as well as cartilage repair, transplant, and augmentation, occur with increasing frequency. Specifically, arthroscopic (partial) meniscectomy is the most commonly performed orthopedic procedure in the United States.[1] Although often successful, these procedures can result in short-term and long-term morbidity requiring postoperative imaging and subsequent further intervention. In a typical musculoskeletal imaging practice, postoperative examinations of the knee are performed on a daily basis with magnetic resonance (MR) imaging being one of the most commonly performed and most useful modalities in diagnosing recurrent disorders and directing further treatment.

This article reviews the normal and abnormal postoperative imaging appearance of frequently performed surgical procedures of the meniscus, articular cartilage, and ligaments. Imaging algorithms and protocols are discussed with particular attention to MR imaging techniques. Attention is paid to understanding the surgical procedure performed and the expected postsurgical appearance as well as commonly identified recurrent and residual disorders and surgical complications.

MENISCUS

The meniscus is a C-shaped fibrocartilaginous structure that functions to maintain joint congruity and stability while converting and distributing force applied to the knee to avoid injury. Thick, circumferentially oriented collagen fibers are interwoven with radial fibers to provide tensile strength and the ability to distribute force. Compared with hyaline cartilage, the meniscus has a higher collagen, lower proteoglycan, and lower water content.[2] However, zonal variations are present

Disclosure: The author has nothing to disclose.
Division of Musculoskeletal Imaging, Department of Radiology, Hofstra Northwell School of Medicine, Northwell Health, 611 Northern Boulevard, Suite 250, Great Neck, NY 11020, USA
E-mail address: dwalz@northwell.edu

Radiol Clin N Am 54 (2016) 931–950
http://dx.doi.org/10.1016/j.rcl.2016.04.011

depending on the function of different parts of the meniscus; the thicker periphery of the meniscus functions to absorb tensile load and has low proteoglycan content, whereas the free edge absorbs compressive forces and has high proteoglycan content.[2,3]

The vascular supply of the meniscus is directly related to its ability to heal. With respect to vascularity, the meniscus is divided into a red or vascular peripheral zone and a white or inner avascular zone. The red zone tears can be expected to heal with a significantly higher rate compared with white zone tears.[4] White zone tears rarely heal and are more often treated with partial resection as opposed to repair. Tears between these two zones are termed red-white tears and do not heal at nearly the same rate as red zone tears.[5]

Meniscus injury is one of the most common causes for knee pain and tears of the meniscus are a leading reason for patients to undergo arthroscopy. Post–meniscus surgery pain, whether new or residual, can have several causes and often leads to referral for repeat MR imaging. Before attempting to interpret the postoperative meniscus on knee MR imaging, clinicians need to have a thorough understanding of the different meniscus surgical interventions; namely the concept of repair, resect, or replace. Knowledge of which of these three was performed as part of the pre–MR imaging clinical information is very important. Availability of the surgical report detailing the type of surgery performed, although not always available, along with the preoperative MR imaging, allows an ideal evaluation of the postoperative MR imaging.

POSTOPERATIVE MR IMAGING PROTOCOL FOR EVALUATION OF THE MENISCUS

There remains some debate in the literature as to the ideal techniques and protocols to evaluate the postoperative knee.[6–11] The techniques include conventional MR imaging, indirect MR arthrography, direct MR arthrography, as well as computed tomography (CT) arthrography. Although some research shows an overall increase in accuracy of MR arthrography compared with other techniques, a prospective study by White and colleagues[12] showed no statistical significance in these differences. For this and other reasons, in our practice, and anecdotally in most other practices, conventional MR imaging is used with 3 planes of intermediate-weighted fast spin-echo sequences along with 2 planes of fat-suppressed T2-weighted or short tau inversion recovery (STIR) sequences. However, MR arthrography is used for troubleshooting in difficult or confusing cases, or on specific request. CT arthrography is used for patients who cannot undergo MR imaging.

MR IMAGING APPEARANCE AFTER MENISCUS REPAIR

Meniscus repair is typically indicated for peripheral or red zone tears that are longitudinal in orientation and in younger patients, typically 40 to 50 years old and younger. These tears are often larger than 1 cm as tears smaller than this have been shown to heal spontaneously.[4,13,14] Three major techniques are used to repair the meniscus: inside out, outside in, and all inside. Various alterations of these techniques, with or without the use of biologic augmentation, are used in modern clinical practice with the specifics of these operations beyond the scope of this article.

- The criteria for a meniscus tear (abnormal signal and/or morphology) are the same for evaluation of the repaired meniscus but are less accurate compared with preoperative knee MR imaging.[15]
- The MR appearance of a successfully repaired meniscus should ideally show resolution of the previously identified bright signal abnormality as well as maintenance of the normal meniscus size and morphology (**Fig. 1**). The degree of healing can be classified as partial if there is bright signal extending into less than 50% of the tear site (**Fig. 2**).[2]

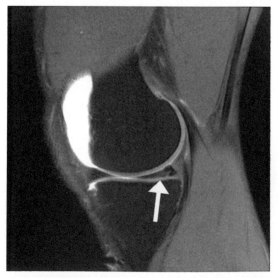

Fig. 1. Sagittal T1 fat-suppressed MR arthrogram after repair of a posterior horn tear shows minimal patchy intermediate signal abnormality (*white arrow*) with a normal size and shape of the meniscus and no bright signal gadolinium entering the meniscus, confirming a healed tear.

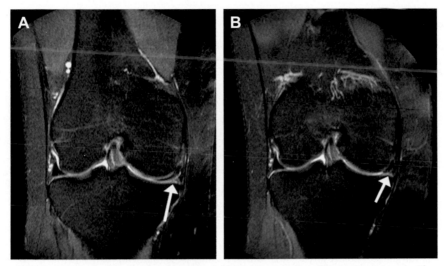

Fig. 2. Coronal T2 fat-suppressed image of the knee before (*A*) and after (*B*) meniscus repair. The preoperative MR imaging (*A*) shows obliquely oriented bright signal within the body segment of the medial meniscus consistent with a tear (*white arrow*). The postoperative MR imaging (*B*) shows minimal bright signal at the undersurface of the tear site (*white arrow*) but near-complete resolution of the abnormal signal consistent with an almost completely healed meniscus tear or a completely healed tear with minimal bright signal granulation tissue at the undersurface of the meniscus.

- However, complete resolution of signal at the tear site is rare. Particularly within the first 1 to 2 years following surgery, persistent intermediate to bright signal abnormality in a healed meniscus can be related to fibrovascular granulation tissue and/or fibrocartilaginous scar tissue.[10,16,17] In these cases, if no other cause for knee pain is present (eg, tear at another site, displaced meniscus, cartilage injury), MR arthrography may be useful to look for extension of gadolinium into the tear (**Fig. 3**).

- Persistent and definitive fluid bright signal at the repair site as well as the presence of a new parameniscal cyst significantly heightens the suspicion of a recurrent tear (**Fig. 4**).[18–23]

- Meniscal sutures do not typically create artifact but metallic darts, arrows, and anchors can create artifact, requiring specific artifact-reducing sequences or MR/CT arthrography.

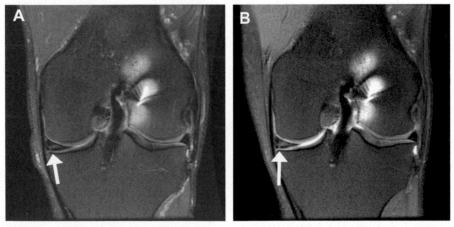

Fig. 3. Coronal T2 fat-suppressed MR image (*A*) and T1-weighted fat-suppressed MR arthrogram (*B*) after meniscus repair. Mildly complex intermediate signal (*white arrow*) is seen at the tear repair site on T2-weighted imaging but does not fill with gadolinium on T1-weighted fat-suppressed imaging (*white arrow* in *B*). Arthroscopy confirmed no residual or recurrent tear. This signal is likely secondary to granulation and scar tissue.

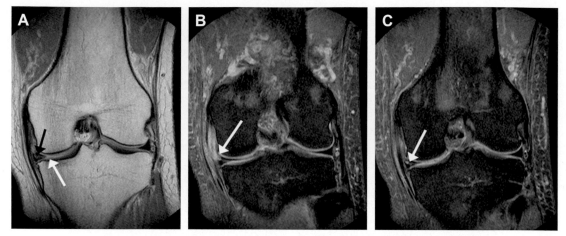

Fig. 4. Coronal intermediate-weighted image (*A*) shows blunting of the free edge of the medial meniscus (*white arrow* in *A*) with faint intermediate linear signal within the meniscus (*black arrow* in *A*). Coronal T2-weighted fat-suppressed images (*B* and *C*) more clearly show the linear bright signal (*white arrow* in *C*) as well as parameniscal cyst formation (*white arrow* in *B*) indicating a recurrent meniscus tears.

MR IMAGING AFTER PARTIAL MENISCUS RESECTION

Partial meniscectomy is the most commonly performed meniscus procedure and is used for treatment of all white zone tears as well as radial, parrot beak, horizontal cleavage, complex, and displaced flap tears. The end point is to resect as little meniscus as possible while still removing all unstable or displaced meniscal tissue. There is significant debate in the recent literature as to the success of partial meniscectomy, with several studies indicating that meniscectomy does not benefit most patients with or without osteoarthritis (OA). However, there is strong criticism of the validity and clinical application of these investigations.[24–30]

- The expected appearance after partial meniscectomy includes a more diminutive appearance of the meniscus with blunted rather than sharp edges (**Fig. 5**). This appearance is more pronounced when greater than 25% of the meniscus is resected. For smaller resections, the meniscus often maintains a nearly normal shape and size.
- When less than 25% of the meniscus is resected, the same criteria for tears can be applied for the postoperative meniscus as for the preoperative meniscus, with accuracy reported as high as 90%.[6]
- When greater than 25% of the meniscus is resected, there is reduction in accuracy in diagnosing meniscus tears.[15] In these cases, intermediate signal at the free edge of the remaining meniscus can be from a tear, scar

tissue, or residual grade 2 degenerative-type signal. The brighter the signal at these sites on T2-weighed imaging the higher the specificity for tear at the cost of lower sensitivity.[2]

- A postoperative phenomenon in which grade 2 signal converts to grade 3 signal (linear signal extending to articular surface and indicating meniscal tear) at the free edge adjacent to meniscus resection can also limit

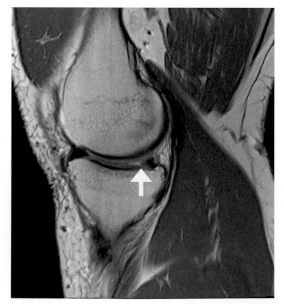

Fig. 5. Sagittal intermediate-weighted image shows mild free edge blunting (*white arrow*) of the posterior horn of the medial meniscus with mild decrease in the expected size of the meniscus.

evaluation of recurrent tear and lead to false-positive interpretations.[31]

- When greater than 25% of the meniscus is resected, Applegate and colleagues[6] reported that direct MR arthrography has an accuracy of 87% versus 65% for conventional MR imaging. Significant advances in MR imaging since 1993 are likely to result in an improvement in the accuracy of conventional MR but this has not been specifically reported and compared.

MR IMAGING AFTER MENISCAL REPLACEMENT

Meniscal resection and replacement is the least commonly performed meniscus surgery. This surgery is reserved for a smaller group of patients: nonobese adults younger than 55 years of age with significant unicompartmental meniscal disorder but intact cartilage, a stable and normally aligned joint, and the ability to undergo the necessary rehabilitation.[2] Allograft or synthetic transplant are the 2 major options for meniscal replacement. Allograft is frequently harvested with attached bone, which is then used for fixation. Biologic augmentation can be used to promote fixation and stable incorporation. Correct sizing of the graft is essential and can be better achieved with synthetic material.

- Conventional MR imaging is routinely used for evaluation of patients after meniscal transplant.
- Displaced meniscal tissue, discrete fluid-filled clefts, and gross morphologic change are indications of tears of the transplanted meniscus. During the first postoperative year, meniscus extrusion, shrinkage, and degenerative signal

are common findings that are not definitively related to clinical outcome (**Fig. 6**).[32,33]

- A meniscal allograft that extrudes early tends to remain extruded. When it does not extrude, it tends to remain in place. Meniscus extrusion has been linked to progression of osteoarthrosis but not definitively leading to a worsened clinical outcome.[34,35]

HYALINE CARTILAGE

Articular cartilage lesions, both partial and full thickness, are a significant cause of knee pain across all age groups. In a review of athletic injuries in professional and amateur athletes, Flanigan and colleagues[36] showed that 36% of these patients had a chondral injury as part of their disorder. In addition to causing acute and subacute pain, chondral lesions can predispose patients to the development of premature osteoarthrosis. Mature cartilage has little or no ability to heal because of poor vascularity, an inability to recruit undifferentiated cells, and limitations of cell replication and migration.[37,38] For these reasons, surgical interventions for chondral injuries are becoming common in many orthopedic practices, as is imaging of such in radiology practices.

Essential to the understanding of the postoperative imaging appearance of cartilage repair procedures is knowledge of the types of surgical interventions. The commonly used procedures include bone marrow stimulation/microfracture, osteochondral allograft, osteochondral autograft (osteochondral autograft transfer system [OATS]), cartilage autograft implantation system (CAIS), and autologous chondrocyte implantation (ACI). ACI is now most commonly used with associated scaffolding systems to increase stability and

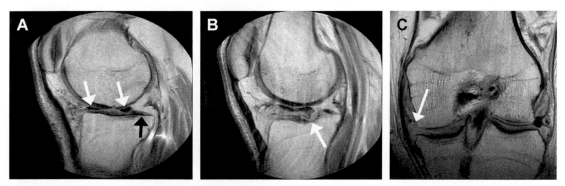

Fig. 6. Sagittal intermediate-weighted MR image (*A*) after meniscus transplant with attached bone block, showing intact meniscus tissue (*white arrows*) that does not cover the posterior articular cartilage (*black arrow*). Sagittal intermediate-weighted MR image (*B*) near the central attachments of the meniscus transplant shows no incorporation of the bone-meniscus allograft (*white arrow*) with the underlying tibial plateau. Coronal intermediate-weighted MR image (*C*) in a different patient after meniscus transplant shows diffuse degenerative signal throughout the extruded meniscus transplant (*white arrow*). (*Courtesy of* Michael S. Brown, MD, Hofstra Northwell Health, Great Neck, New York.)

incorporation. As with the meniscus, availability of the surgical report as well as detailed information from the surgeon can greatly aid the interpretation of such studies.

BONE MARROW STIMULATION/ MICROFRACTURE

Marrow stimulation is the most common surgical procedure for chondral lesions, with microfracture being the most often used. Before treating a lesion with microfracture, the chondral lesion is debrided to perpendicular shoulders at the periphery, and 1-mm to 2-mm holes are drilled 3 to 5 mm apart throughout the lesion about 2 to 4 mm deep, reaching and exposing subchondral bone. The purpose of these procedures is to expose the sub-chondral marrow, therefore filling pluripotent cells into the chondral defect, releasing cytokines to stimulate the growth of fibrocartilage. Bleeding from the procedure helps to form a fibrin clot, which provides stability for the repair tissue within the defect. More recent advances in microfracture involve the use of various scaffolds to improve stability and promote higher quality repair tissue.

- Greater success is achieved in patients younger than 40 years of age with lesions smaller than 2 cm^2, but can be performed for lesions measuring up to 4 cm^2.[38]
- The goal of microfracture is congruent fill of the defect with intact borders and normal sub-chondral signal. The fibrocartilage when imaged in the first year shows brighter signal than the adjacent hyaline cartilage secondary to highly water permeable fibrocartilage. This signal decreases with time to match the normal signal of fibrocartilage, which is hypo-intense to normal hyaline cartilage (**Fig. 7**).
- Worse outcomes are associated with persistent subchondral cystic change and edema signal, loss of congruity, incomplete fill, and cortical flattening.[39,40]
- Subchondral osseous productive change can be seen and is of uncertain clinical significance,[39] whereas frank osteophyte formation can be a marker of microfracture failure (**Fig. 8**).[41]

OSTEOCHONDRAL ALLOGRAFT AND AUTOGRAFT

Osteochondral allograft involves the grafting of cadaver tissue (bone and cartilage) after preservation of chondrocyte viability. Chondrocytes are thought to be immunoprivileged and the marrow elements are removed, minimizing the risk of immunologic complications. This procedure is

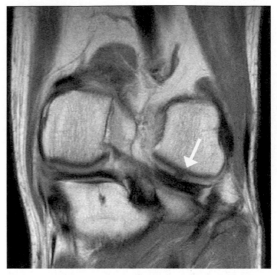

Fig. 7. Coronal intermediate-weighted MR image after prior microfracture with low-signal fibrocartilage (*white arrow*) filling a prior chondral defect with smooth borders and complete fill. (*Courtesy of Michael S. Brown, MD, Hofstra Northwell Health, Great Neck, New York.*)

reserved for larger lesions (>2.5 cm^2), which are debrided to smooth margins peripherally and deep to the level of bone. The subchondral bone is then abraded to promote ingrowth. The allograft

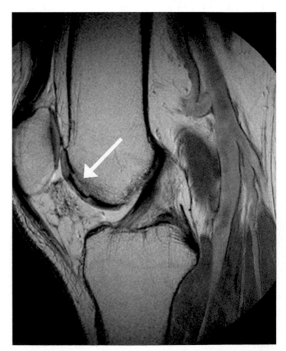

Fig. 8. Sagittal intermediate-weighted MR image after microfracture of a trochlear sulcus chondral lesion shows protuberant osseous overgrowth (*white arrow*) with thin intermediate signal overlying hyaline cartilage.

sometimes requires pin fixation. Advantages of the use of allograft include the ability to match the size of the lesion with a single graft without donor site morbidity. Disadvantages include graft availability, cost, disease transmission, and technical challenges of matching size and shape.

Osteochondral autograft (OATS) uses a donor site within the patient's ipsilateral knee, often from the lateral trochlea. This technique uses plugs from the donor site to fill defects typically between 1 and 4 cm². The donor plugs can vary in size, often between 4 and 5 mm. For this reason, multiple osteochondral plugs can be used for 1 lesion; a process termed mosaicplasty. The donor sites can be left alone, undergo microfracture, or be repaired with allograft. Advantages of the use of autograft include the ability to use the patient's own tissue at the expense of donor site morbidity and size limitations. The osteochondral graft can also function to repair subchondral bone loss up to 10 mm.[42]

- As with all cartilage repair procedures, MR imaging should show congruity with adjacent cartilage (**Fig. 9**). Malpositioning or development of subsidence or protuberance often leads to failure.

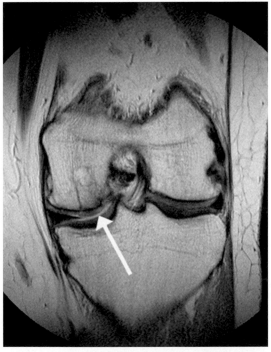

Fig. 9. Coronal intermediate-weighted MR image after osteochondral autograft transplant of the medial femoral condyle (*white arrow*) shows an intact graft with osseous incorporation and normal signal hyaline cartilage. Very thin shallow fissures are seen at the borders without full-thickness fissuring or subchondral signal abnormality.

- With mosaicplasty, lower signal fibrocartilage often fills the gaps between the plugs.
- Marrow edema-type signal is often seen below the graft but should resolve by 1 to 2 years (**Fig. 10**). Marrow edema or cystic change after this time is abnormal and a sign of poor incorporation.
- Donor site disorder should be identified, including cartilage delamination at the borders of the donor site. At the graft site, progression of adjacent cartilage loss or persistent subsidence or protuberance of the graft and progressive subchondral signal abnormality should be noted (**Fig. 11**).

CARTILAGE AUTOGRAFT IMPLANTATION SYSTEM/PARTICULATE CARTILAGE ALLOGRAFT

CAIS is a single surgical procedure in which cartilage is harvested at a remote site from the chondral lesion to be treated; typically from the margin of the intercondylar notch. This cartilage is minced and placed into a biodegradable scaffold with fibrin glue, and is then placed into the defect using bioabsorbable anchors. The basis for this type of repair is that the chondrocytes are freed from their typical dense matrix via the mincing process, thus allowing proliferation and ingrowth into adjacent cartilage.[43] Lu and colleagues[43] propose that this process allows adult chondrocytes to behave more like juvenile chondrocytes in producing extracellular matrix and achieving a hyaline-type cartilage repair.

Particulate cartilage allograft is obtained from donors younger than 13 years of age and cut into small pieces (1-mm cubes). Similar to CAIS, the underlying concept is allowing the cells to migrate and multiply, forming an incorporated hyaline cartilage matrix. This allograft is implanted into the recipient chondral lesion in a single surgery and secured with fibrin glue.

AUTOLOGOUS CHONDROCYTE IMPLANTATION

ACI is a 2-surgery procedure in which cartilage is initially harvested from a non–weight-bearing portion of the knee and then cultured for 4 weeks to allow for an increase in the number of chondrocytes. At this time, the cartilage is implanted into the chondral lesion using a periosteal or synthetic collagen cover. Graft hypertrophy can be seen and is thought to most often result from the periosteal cover. This condition can be treated with arthroscopic debridement. Matrix ACI (MACI) is a

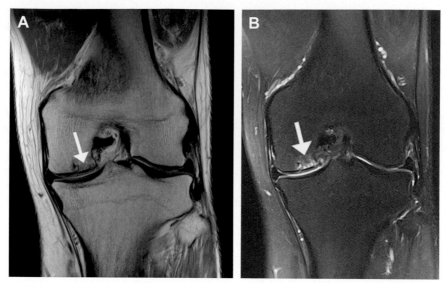

Fig. 10. Coronal intermediate-weighted (*A*) and T2 fat-suppressed images (*B*) in a patient who had undergone osteochondral autograft transplant 8 months earlier with edema signal and cystic change in the subchondral bone (*white arrows*). There is a thin full-thickness chondral fissure at the medial margin of the graft with associated cystic change. The remainder of the imaging findings show solid incorporation of the graft without complication. This cystic change and edema signal can be a normal finding in the first 1 to 2 years after surgery. The fissure may fill in or persist with stable or worsening subchondral cystic change.

technique in which scaffolds are used to hold the implanted chondrocytes, leading to a more stable repair. This technique shows reduced graft hypertrophy and incidence of delamination relative to conventional ACI.[44,45]

- The signal of the cartilage should match that of the adjacent hyaline cartilage by 12 to 18 months. As with the previously described cartilage procedures, marrow signal abnormality at the procedure site is common early and should slowly resolve over 12 to 18 months. Persistent edema signal intensity or increasing edema signal, with or without cysts, is considered pathologic and a sign of impending or active failure.

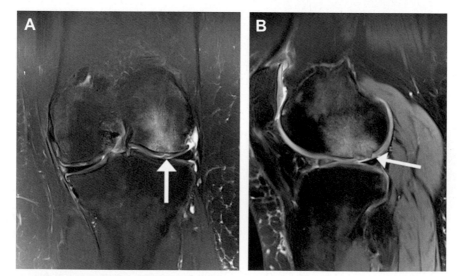

Fig. 11. Coronal (*A*) and sagittal (*B*) T2 fat-suppressed images in a patient with a failed osteochondral implant, showing chondral delamination and fissuring (*white arrow* in *A*) with extensive subchondral marrow edema. The graft is rotated with osseous protrusion at the joint line; a change from its original location (*white arrow* in *B*).

- The repair site initially shows brighter signal intensity but decreases during the first 12 to 18 months to match that of adjacent hyaline cartilage.[44]
- Incomplete integration into adjacent cartilage is often initially seen but should resolve with smooth, imperceptible margins by 1 to 2 years.[45]
- For ACI, complete fill or slight overfill is expected. With MACI, defect underfill can be seen initially as a normal finding.[45]

POSTOPERATIVE MR IMAGING PROTOCOL FOR EVALUATION OF HYALINE CARTILAGE

Similar to postoperative imaging of the meniscus, there is no definitive imaging technique or protocol that has been consistently proved to be superior to another. Postoperative protocols in these patients should be built based on optimizing the visualization of findings relevant to published MR-based scoring systems for cartilage repair. In our practice, we use high-resolution intermediate-weighted fast spin-echo imaging in 3 planes along with T2 fat-suppressed or STIR sequences, also in 3 planes. With more frequency, an isotropic three-dimensional (3D) TSE (Turbo Spin Echo) sequence with slice thickness of 0.6 mm (acquired in the sagittal or coronal plane and reconstructed into each of the 3 classic planes or into a custom plane based on the radiologist's needs) is added to the protocol. This method allows improved definition of fissures at the margins and within the chondral repair sites. Some investigators propose the use of 3D gradient recalled echo (GRE) sequences with fat suppression as a way to better depict the surface and overall thickness of cartilage. As with all GRE sequences, these sequences are prone to susceptibility artifact at the operated sites. Quantitative compositional biochemical cartilage imaging, such as T2 mapping, dGEMRIC (Delayed gadolinium enhanced Magnetic Resonance Imaging of cartilage), and T1rho is sometimes used in these patients. These techniques have been more vigorously studied in the nonoperated knee but can be applied when evaluating incorporation of cartilage grafts into adjacent cartilage and assessment of return of normal biochemical makeup of hyaline cartilage. MR arthrography, as with meniscus surgery, is reserved for trouble shooting or when specifically requested.

MR IMAGING AFTER CARTILAGE SURGERY

Several research-based systems have been proposed and developed, often for specific cartilage procedures. In clinical practice it is probably best to combine information from each of these systems to develop a concise and conclusive report while avoiding reporting information that may not have clinical relevance.

In 2003, Henderson and colleagues[46] reported on a scoring system to evaluate cartilage repair after ACI. This system evaluated chondral fill, repaired cartilage signal intensity, bone marrow edema, and the presence of a joint effusion. A similar system was described by Roberts and colleagues[47] in 2003 with evaluation categories including surface integrity and contour, signal intensity of the repaired cartilage, cartilage thickness, and subchondral bone signal. The following year, Marlovits and colleagues[48] described the MOCART (magnetic resonance observation of cartilage repair tissue) MR-based scoring system for patients who had undergone microfracture, ACI, or autologous osteochondral transplant. This system evaluated 9 parameters: defect filling, repair tissue integration, repair tissue surface, repair tissue structure, repair tissue signal intensity, subchondral lamina status, subchondral bone status, the presence of adhesions, and the presence of synovitis. This system was further modified by Welsch and colleagues[49] in 2009 as the 3D-MOCART system using isotropic 3D acquisitions and further defining some of the original 9 parameters based on information gained through these sequences. The MOCART systems are the most commonly applied systems both in clinical practice and research but are limited to solely evaluating the cartilage repair sites. The cartilage repair OA knee score (CROAKS) combines MOCART with the MR OA Knee Score to provide a system that can evaluate the site of cartilage repair as well as the remainder of the knee articulation and provide longitudinal postoperative assessment.[45]

In 2013, 2 reviews and meta-analyses of MR imaging and clinical outcomes after cartilage repair surgery were published evaluating the systems discussed earlier for various cartilage procedures.[50,51] Blackman and colleagues,[50] in their meta-analysis, revealed that MR imaging findings correlate with clinical outcomes after cartilage repair surgery. However, the specific parameters that correlate best differ based on the procedure performed. They also showed that no MR-based system correlated with clinical outcomes after all types of surgery. De Windt and colleagues[51] similarly determined that morphologic MR is unreliable in predicting clinical outcome. These studies indicate that a single system may not be applicable to all cartilage repair procedures. Chang and colleagues[52] proposed a comprehensive Osteochondral Allograft MR Imaging Scoring System (OCAMRISS) with parameters grading 5 cartilage parameters, 4 bone parameters, and 4 additional joint findings. The investigators validated this system with histopathologic and micro-CT reference standards as well as biomechanics indentation testing in goats.

The number of systems and the parameters as well as their subdivisions can be overwhelming in a typical busy clinical imaging practice and can yield confusing results to orthopedists. For this reason and more, simplification of these systems into a descriptive report detailing what are thought to be the most relevant findings is essential. Forney and colleagues[38] proposed a practical reporting system that includes descriptions of defect fill (volume, thickness, and surface contour), integration (underlying bone and adjacent cartilage), subchondral bone status (edemalike marrow signal, cysts, osteophytes), repair tissue character (signal intensity), and non–repair site complications (cartilage defects, adhesions, donor site appearance, meniscus and ligament disorder). Although not completely applicable in research settings, this is likely more appropriate and useful for referring orthopedic surgeons, as has been reported anecdotally in our practice.

CRUCIATE AND COLLATERAL LIGAMENTS

Injuries to the cruciate and collateral ligaments of the knee are common, particularly in the athletic population, leading to an increase in the frequency of surgical intervention to treat instability created by these ligament tears. The anterior cruciate ligament (ACL) and medial collateral ligament (MCL) are the two most commonly injured ligaments, with the ACL being the most commonly reconstructed knee ligament. The purpose of reconstructing knee ligaments in high-performance athletes and in the general population is to return them to previous ability levels as well as to prevent joint instability and subsequent premature arthrosis.

POSTOPERATIVE IMAGING OF LIGAMENT RECONSTRUCTION/REPAIR

Standard preoperative MR imaging protocols are typically used for evaluation of postoperative imaging of repaired knee ligaments. In cases in which metallic fixation is used, metal artifact–reducing sequences are advocated as well as the use of STIR or Dixon-type fat-suppression techniques. 3D-FSE sequences can also be used, with the advantage of being able to reconstruct these thinly acquired, signal-rich sequences into planes relative to the postsurgical anatomy. The MR imaging findings of graft tear are similar to those of primary ligament tear, including discontinuity, abnormal bowing or position of the graft, and internal signal abnormality (**Fig. 12**). For the ACL, several studies have shown mixed results in evaluating for graft tears. Horton and colleagues[53] reported a sensitivity and specificity of 36% and 80% for detection of partial-thickness and full-thickness tears, whereas Rak and colleagues[54] reported a 100% accuracy in diagnosing graft tears. In one study, MR arthrography was shown to yield higher specificity and sensitivity compared with conventional MR imaging.[55] Partial graft tears present a greater diagnostic challenge, with the most important finding being change in caliber of the graft.[53]

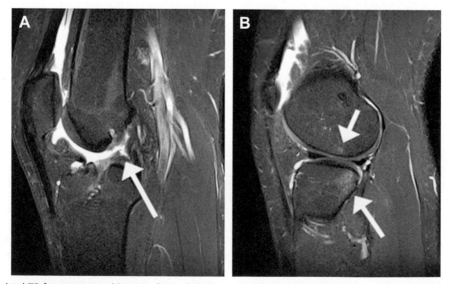

Fig. 12. Sagittal T2 fat-suppressed images (*A* and *B*) show complete disruption of the midportion of the patient's ACL graft (*white arrow* in *A*) with typical osseous contusions in the posterior lateral tibial plateau and midportion of the lateral femoral condyle (*white arrows* in *B*).

Osseous contusion patterns typical of an ACL injury can be used as secondary signs of tear but can also be seen in the setting of graft laxity, poorly placed graft, and graft stretching.[56]

ANTERIOR CRUCIATE LIGAMENT

Ligament reconstruction is the mainstay of surgical treatment of ACL tears, with primary repair rarely, if ever, performed. The most common choice for reconstruction is the use of autografts rather than allografts. Bone-patella tendon-bone (BTB) and hamstring tendon are the most commonly used autografts and each has its own appearance. There has not been shown to be a significant difference in outcome between the two autografts.[56] Although uncommon, complications related to the harvest site have been reported with greater frequency with BTB graft and include tendon tear/tendinosis, patella fracture (**Fig. 13**), and patella chondrosis.[57] The tendon nearly always shows thickening, a central defect, and signal abnormality for the first year after harvesting. This condition eventually resolves with only mild tendon thickening after the first year, which is not typically symptomatic or pathologic (**Fig. 14**). In addition there is a higher rate of arthrofibrosis with BTB grafts.[58] Hamstring grafts are obtained from the distal semitendinosus and gracilis tendons, which are folded over and sutured together, resulting in a distinctive layered appearance compared with other graft sources.[44] Graft site complications with hamstring grafts are uncommon and it is reported that the donor site tendons regain 80% to 90% of their original strength within 6 months.[59] Single-bundle reconstruction is more commonly performed compared with double-bundle reconstruction. However, some clinicians advocate the use of double-bundle reconstruction to more closely replicate the function of the native ACL.[60,61]

- ACL grafts typically show low signal from the immediate postoperative period through the first 4 months, followed by a period of revascularization and resynovialization in which intermediate signal can be seen on all imaging sequences.[44,62–65]
- Typically by 1 year, the graft undergoes ligamentization, returning to low signal (**Fig. 15**). However, some intermediate signal has been reported to persist for a much longer time, sometimes with enhancement on postcontrast imaging, indicating persistent vascularization.[66]

ANTERIOR CRUCIATE LIGAMENT GRAFT POSITIONING

Correct ACL graft placement is key in preventing many of the postoperative complications that are

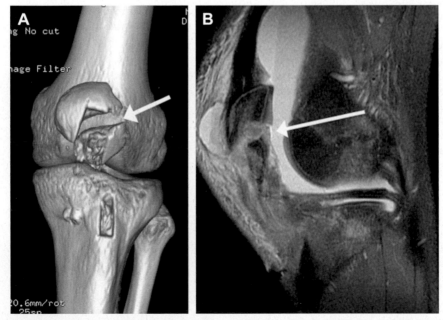

Fig. 13. 3D reconstructed CT image (*A*) 3 weeks after BTB grafting for ACL reconstruction with an atraumatic fracture (*white arrow*) likely secondary to excessive bone resection. T2 fat-suppressed sagittal image (*B*) performed on the same date shows the fracture (*white arrow*) with a large lipohemarthrosis and extravasation of joint fluid through the patella defect.

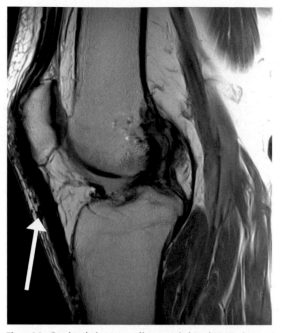

Fig. 14. Sagittal intermediate-weighted MR image 4 years after BTB grafting for ACL reconstruction with mild patellar tendon thickening (*white arrow*) without signal abnormality. The patient did not report anterior knee pain or symptoms related to the patella tendon.

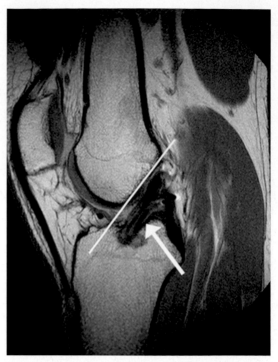

Fig. 15. Sagittal intermediate-weighted MR image shows a properly placed ACL graft with the tibial tunnel positioned just posterior to the Blumensaat line (*white line*). The graft shows minimal linear intermediate signal between the folds of the graft as is normal for a hamstring autograft (*white arrow*).

encountered, including graft tear, graft impingement, knee laxity, and generalized knee pain. Correct femoral tunnel position is essential in creating isometry with correct tibial tunnel position and important in preventing graft impingement and instability.[67] The location of the tibial and femoral tunnels created for graft fixation can be evaluated on radiographs, CT, and MR imaging, with CT recently shown to be most consistently reliable in depicting exact tunnel location.[68] In modern clinical practice, MR is often preferred given its superiority in evaluating the soft tissue, cartilage, and marrow, whereas CT is less commonly used secondary to radiation exposure.

- The tibial tunnel should be placed such that on sagittal MR imaging a line drawn along the course of the Blumensaat line is anterior to the graft and tunnel position (see **Fig. 20**). If the graft and tunnel position is anterior to this line, graft impingement is likely. Graft impingement can also occur from osteophytes from within the intercondylar notch, which may require a notchplasty for treatment.
- If the tibial tunnel is too far posteriorly (posterior to the midpoint of the tibia), a vertically oriented graft can result in instability and graft laxity (**Fig. 16**).

- On coronal images, the graft should ideally be oriented 60° to 65° and definitively less than 75° relative to the joint line.[56,65,67] Excessive vertical orientation can lead to instability and impingement (**Fig. 17**).

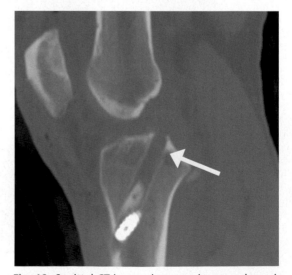

Fig. 16. Sagittal CT image shows an improperly positioned ACL graft tibial tunnel, posterior to the midpoint of the tibia (*white arrow*).

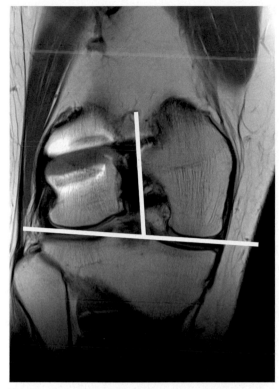

Fig. 17. Coronal intermediate-weighted MR image after ACL reconstruction shows a vertically oriented graft that forms an approximately 80° angle (*white lines*) relative to the joint line with the tunnel positioned between 11 and 12 o'clock.

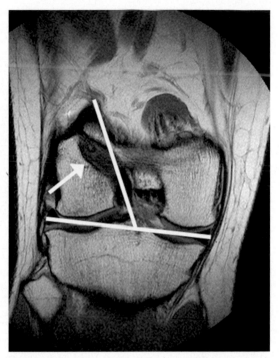

Fig. 18. Coronal intermediate-weighted MR image after ACL reconstruction with a properly positioned graft forming a 65° angle (*white lines*) with the joint line and the femoral tunnel positioned at 10 o'clock (*white arrow*).

- Femoral tunnel positioning should be at the junction of the roof of the intercondylar notch and the posterior femoral cortex, as seen on sagittal imaging.[56]
- The femoral tunnel should be between 10 and 11 o'clock and 1 to 2 o'clock for the right and left knee respectively on coronal imaging (**Fig. 18**). With double-bundle reconstruction, the posterolateral bundle should be between 9 and 10 o'clock or 2 and 3 o'clock for the right and left knee, with the anteromedial bundle being the same as a single-bundle reconstruction.

ANTERIOR CRUCIATE LIGAMENT COMPLICATIONS

The common complications following ACL graft reconstruction include reinjury, graft impingement, arthrofibrosis, donor site morbidity, ganglion cyst formation, tunnel widening and resorption, hardware failure, and foreign body reaction, as well as long-term progressive arthrosis.

- Partial-thickness (**Fig. 19**) or full-thickness ACL graft tear is the most common cause of failure and can occur with a properly or improperly placed graft.[69]
- As described earlier, graft impingement is a result of poor tunnel placement or osteophytes within the intercondylar notch. These findings, along with graft thickening and increased signal intensity, particularly within the distal graft, are typical of graft impingement (**Fig. 20**).
- Arthrofibrosis can be a cause of stiffness and restricted motion with loss of terminal extension. It can be focal with nodular scarring anterior to the graft (the so-called cyclops lesion) (**Fig. 21**) or more diffuse, surrounding the graft. Arthrofibrosis is more commonly seen in cases of early postinjury reconstruction and in patients who do not follow presurgical and postsurgical rehabilitation and motion recommendations.
- Donor site morbidity, although not common, more often is secondary to BTB grafts and includes tendon tear/tendinosis, patella fracture, and patella chondrosis.
- A small amount of bright or intermediate signal can be seen within the tunnels after

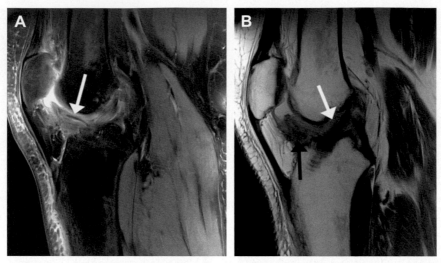

Fig. 19. Sagittal T2 fat-suppressed (*A*) and intermediate-weighted (*B*) MR images show a small partial-thickness tear of the distal graft with a displaced flap from the graft (*white arrow* in *A*) with surrounding scarring/arthrofibrosis (*black arrow* in *B*). Subtle change in caliber of the graft can be identified secondary to the tear (*white arrow* in *B*).

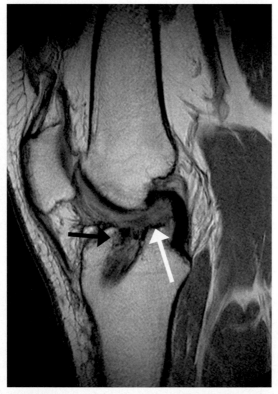

Fig. 20. Sagittal intermediate-weighted MR image shows a tibial tunnel (*black arrow*) that is slightly too far anterior relative to the Blumensaat line with subsequent graft impingement manifested by abnormal signal, thickening, and altered contour of the mid and distal aspects of the graft (*white arrow*).

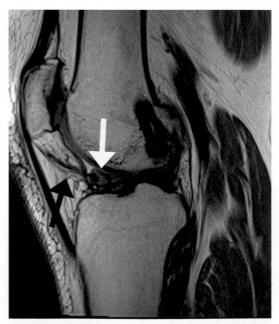

Fig. 21. Sagittal intermediate-weighted MR image shows lobulated scarring (*white arrow*) anterior to the graft, consistent with focal arthrofibrosis (cyclops lesion). Linear scarring (*black arrow*) is seen in the Hoffa fat, as is expected after arthroscopy.

surg
treat
thes
beca
cult
in th
opel
eral
com
with
con:
stru
opel
edge

PEA

•

•

hamstring reconstruction given the folding of the graft fibers (see **Fig. 15**). However, large or progressively growing fluid collections within the graft or within the tunnels are considered to be abnormal and signs of instability and potential graft failure (**Fig. 22**).

- Tunnel widening can be secondary to ganglion cyst formation, from repetitive graft cycling and motion within a tunnel, or from foreign body and immunologic reaction (**Fig. 23**).[70] The latter is more often seen with synthetic grafts or secondary to fixation devices. Revision surgery in the setting of tunnel widening and osteolysis often requires a 2-stage procedure; the first involving bone grafting within the tunnel.
- Hardware complications can lead to loss of graft fixation if they occur before solid graft incorporation and can result in intra-articular bodies and foreign body reaction at any time.

In children, the physes and bones at the knee are often more vulnerable to injury than the ligaments. This condition is also seen elsewhere in the pediatric musculoskeletal system.[71,72] Avulsion ACL tears are therefore common in children. Surgical management of ACL tears in children is complex because of the potential risk of injury to the physis and growth disturbance. Delaying ACL reconstruction until maturity is possible but risks

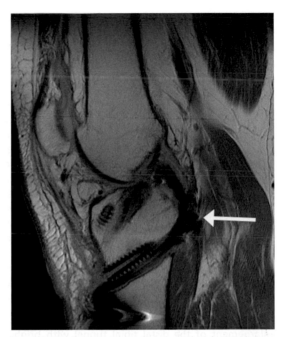

Fig. 23. Sagittal intermediate-weighted MR image shows that the patient has had ACL and PCL reconstruction. The so-called killer turn is shown as the graft enters into the tibial tunnel (*white arrow*). This turn presents a surgical challenge and can result in graft complications from excessive stress.

instability episodes and intra-articular damage. Surgical options include physeal sparing, partial transphyseal procedures, and complete transphyseal procedures.

POSTERIOR CRUCIATE LIGAMENT

The posterior cruciate ligament (PCL) is injured with much less frequency than the ACL. Injuries to the PCL can be isolated or part of a multiligamentous injury; the latter more often leading to PCL reconstruction (**Fig. 24**). Isolated PCL injuries are typically only reconstructed if they are full-thickness tears with persistent instability following nonoperative treatment. Autograft choices are similar to the ACL with options for single-bundle or double-bundle reconstruction. As with the ACL, tunnel positioning is essential. However, there is a greater degree of variability in tunnel positioning depending on the surgeon's preferred technique. The femoral tunnel is typically situated at the anterior aspect of the PCL footprint at the anterior portion of the intercondylar notch.[56] The tibial side of the graft can be tunneled or fixated using an inlay technique with BTB graft. Tibial tunnel techniques present a challenge, particularly because of the so-called killer turn; the sharp

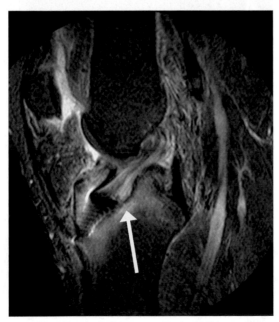

Fig.
a pa
reco
fibul
later

Fig. 22. Sagittal T2 fat-suppressed MR image shows enlargement of the tibial tunnel (*white arrow*) with abnormal graft signal and extensive surrounding bone marrow edema signal.

REFERENCES

1. Mather RC 3rd, Garrett WE, Cole BJ, et al. Cost-effectiveness analysis of the diagnosis of meniscus tears. Am J Sports Med 2015;43(1):128–37.
2. Boutin RD, Fritz RC, Marder RA. Magnetic resonance imaging of the postoperative meniscus: resection, repair, and replacement. Magn Reson Imaging Clin N Am 2014;22(4):517–55.
3. Sanchez R, Strouse PJ. The knee: MR imaging of uniquely pediatric disorders. Radiol Clin North Am 2009;47(6):1009–25.
4. Kijowski R, Rosas HG, Lee KS, et al. MRI characteristics of healed and unhealed peripheral vertical meniscal tears. AJR Am J Roentgenol 2014;202(3):585–92.
5. Barber-Westin SD, Noyes FR. Clinical healing rates of meniscus repairs of tears in the central-third (red-white) zone. Arthroscopy 2014;30(1):134–46.
6. Applegate GR, Flannigan BD, Tolin BS, et al. MR diagnosis of recurrent tears in the knee: value of intraarticular contrast material. AJR Am J Roentgenol 1993;161(4):821–5.
7. Lim PS, Schweitzer ME, Bhatia M, et al. Repeat tear of postoperative meniscus: potential MR imaging signs. Radiology 1999;210(1):183–8.
8. Magee T, Shapiro M, Rodriguez J, et al. MR arthrography of postoperative knee: for which patients is it useful? Radiology 2003;229(1):159–63.
9. Hantes ME, Zachos VC, Zibis AH, et al. Evaluation of meniscal repair with serial magnetic resonance imaging: a comparative study between conventional MRI and indirect MR arthrography. Eur J Radiol 2004;50(3):231–7.
10. Pujol N, Panarella L, Selmi TA, et al. Meniscal healing after meniscal repair: a CT arthrography assessment. Am J Sports Med 2008;36(8):1489–95.
11. Cardello P, Gigli C, Ricci A, et al. Retears of postoperative knee meniscus: findings on magnetic resonance imaging (MRI) and magnetic resonance arthrography (MRA) by using low and high field magnets. Skeletal Radiol 2009;38(2):149–56.
12. White LM, Schweitzer ME, Weishaupt D, et al. Diagnosis of recurrent meniscal tears: prospective evaluation of conventional MR imaging, indirect MR arthrography, and direct MR arthrography. Radiology 2002;222(2):421–9.
13. Weiss CB, Lundberg M, Hamberg P, et al. Non-operative treatment of meniscal tears. J Bone Joint Surg Am 1989;71(6):811–22.
14. DeHaven KE. Decision-making factors in the treatment of meniscus lesions. Clin Orthop Relat Res 1990;(252):49–54.
15. Recht MP, Kramer J. MR imaging of the postoperative knee: a pictorial essay. Radiographics 2002;22(4):765–74.
16. Hoffelner T, Resch H, Forstner R, et al. Arthroscopic all-inside meniscal repair–Does the meniscus heal? A clinical and radiological follow-up examination to verify meniscal healing using a 3-T MRI. Skeletal Radiol 2011;40(2):181–7.
17. Miao Y, Yu JK, Ao YF, et al. Diagnostic values of 3 methods for evaluating meniscal healing status after meniscal repair: comparison among second-look arthroscopy, clinical assessment, and magnetic resonance imaging. Am J Sports Med 2011;39(4):735–42.
18. Deutsch AL, Mink JH, Fox JM, et al. Peripheral meniscal tears: MR findings after conservative treatment or arthroscopic repair. Radiology 1990;176(2):485–8.
19. Farley TE, Howell SM, Love KF, et al. Meniscal tears: MR and arthrographic findings after arthroscopic repair. Radiology 1991;180(2):517–22.
20. Kent RH, Pope CF, Lynch JK, et al. Magnetic resonance imaging of the surgically repaired meniscus: six-month follow-up. Magn Reson Imaging 1991;9(3):335–41.
21. Eggli S, Wegmuller H, Kosina J, et al. Long-term results of arthroscopic meniscal repair. An analysis of isolated tears. Am J Sports Med 1995;23(6):715–20.
22. Muellner T, Egkher A, Nikolic A, et al. Open meniscal repair: clinical and magnetic resonance imaging findings after twelve years. Am J Sports Med 1999;27(1):16–20.
23. Barber BR, McNally EG. Meniscal injuries and imaging the postoperative meniscus. Radiol Clin North Am 2013;51(3):371–91.
24. Herrlin SV, Wange PO, Lapidus G, et al. Is arthroscopic surgery beneficial in treating non-traumatic, degenerative medial meniscal tears? A five year follow-up. Knee Surg Sports Traumatol Arthrosc 2013;21(2):358–64.
25. Katz JN, Brophy RH, Chaisson CE, et al. Surgery versus physical therapy for a meniscal tear and osteoarthritis. N Engl J Med 2013;368(18):1675–84.
26. Sihvonen R, Paavola M, Malmivaara A, et al. Arthroscopic partial meniscectomy versus sham surgery for a degenerative meniscal tear. N Engl J Med 2013;369(26):2515–24.
27. Vermesan D, Prejbeanu R, Laitin S, et al. Arthroscopic debridement compared to intra-articular steroids in treating degenerative medial meniscal tears. Eur Rev Med Pharmacol Sci 2013;17(23):3192–6.
28. Yim JH, Seon JK, Song EK, et al. A comparative study of meniscectomy and nonoperative treatment for degenerative horizontal tears of the medial meniscus. Am J Sports Med 2013;41(7):1565–70.
29. Elattrache N, Lattermann C, Hannon M, et al. New England Journal of Medicine article evaluating the usefulness of meniscectomy is flawed. Arthroscopy 2014;30(5):542–3.
30. Krych AJ, Carey JL, Marx RG, et al. Does arthroscopic knee surgery work? Arthroscopy 2014;30(5):544–5.

31. Vance K, Meredick R, Schweitzer ME, et al. Magnetic resonance imaging of the postoperative meniscus. Arthroscopy 2009;25(5):522–30.

32. Lee DH, Lee BS, Chung JW, et al. Changes in magnetic resonance imaging signal intensity of transplanted meniscus allografts are not associated with clinical outcomes. Arthroscopy 2011;27(9): 1211–8.

33. Lee BS, Chung JW, Kim JM, et al. Morphologic changes in fresh-frozen meniscus allografts over 1 year: a prospective magnetic resonance imaging study on the width and thickness of transplants. Am J Sports Med 2012;40(6):1384–91.

34. Potter HG, Rodeo SA, Wickiewicz TL, et al. MR imaging of meniscal allografts: correlation with clinical and arthroscopic outcomes. Radiology 1996;198(2): 509–14.

35. Ha JK, Jang HW, Jung JE, et al. Clinical and radiologic outcomes after meniscus allograft transplantation at 1-year and 4-year follow-up. Arthroscopy 2014;30(11):1424–9.

36. Flanigan DC, Harris JD, Trinh TQ, et al. Prevalence of chondral defects in athletes' knees: a systematic review. Med Sci Sports Exerc 2010; 42(10):1795–801.

37. Buckwalter JA, Mankin HJ. Articular cartilage: degeneration and osteoarthritis, repair, regeneration, and transplantation. Instr Course Lect 1998; 47:487–504.

38. Forney MC, Gupta A, Minas T, et al. Magnetic resonance imaging of cartilage repair procedures. Magn Reson Imaging Clin N Am 2014;22(4):671–701.

39. Mithoefer K, Williams RJ 3rd, Warren RF, et al. The microfracture technique for the treatment of articular cartilage lesions in the knee. A prospective cohort study. J Bone Joint Surg Am 2005;87(9):1911–20.

40. Ramappa AJ, Gill TJ, Bradford CH, et al. Magnetic resonance imaging to assess knee cartilage repair tissue after microfracture of chondral defects. J Knee Surg 2007;20(3):228–34.

41. Gomoll AH, Madry H, Knutsen G, et al. The subchondral bone in articular cartilage repair: current problems in the surgical management. Knee Surg Sports Traumatol Arthrosc 2010;18(4):434–47.

42. Chang G, Horng A, Glaser C. A practical guide to imaging of cartilage repair with emphasis on bone marrow changes. Semin Musculoskelet Radiol 2011;15(3):221–37.

43. Lu Y, Dhanaraj S, Wang Z, et al. Minced cartilage without cell culture serves as an effective intraoperative cell source for cartilage repair. J Orthop Res 2006;24(6):1261–70.

44. Sanders TG. Imaging of the postoperative knee. Semin Musculoskelet Radiol 2011;15(4):383–407.

45. Guermazi A, Roemer FW, Alizai H, et al. State of the art: MR imaging after knee cartilage repair surgery. Radiology 2015;277(1):23–43.

46. Henderson IJ, Tuy B, Connell D, et al. Prospective clinical study of autologous chondrocyte implantation and correlation with MRI at three and 12 months. J Bone Joint Surg Br 2003;85(7):1060–6.

47. Roberts S, McCall IW, Darby AJ, et al. Autologous chondrocyte implantation for cartilage repair: monitoring its success by magnetic resonance imaging and histology. Arthritis Res Ther 2003;5(1):R60–73.

48. Marlovits S, Striessnig G, Resinger CT, et al. Definition of pertinent parameters for the evaluation of articular cartilage repair tissue with high-resolution magnetic resonance imaging. Eur J Radiol 2004; 52(3):310–9.

49. Welsch GH, Zak L, Mamisch TC, et al. Three-dimensional magnetic resonance observation of cartilage repair tissue (MOCART) score assessed with an isotropic three-dimensional true fast imaging with steady-state precession sequence at 3.0 Tesla. Invest Radiol 2009;44(9):603–12.

50. Blackman AJ, Smith MV, Flanigan DC, et al. Correlation between magnetic resonance imaging and clinical outcomes after cartilage repair surgery in the knee: a systematic review and meta-analysis. Am J Sports Med 2013;41(6):1426–34.

51. de Windt TS, Welsch GH, Brittberg M, et al. Is magnetic resonance imaging reliable in predicting clinical outcome after articular cartilage repair of the knee? A systematic review and meta-analysis. Am J Sports Med 2013;41(7):1695–702.

52. Chang EY, Pallante-Kichura AL, Bae WC, et al. Development of a Comprehensive Osteochondral Allograft MRI Scoring System (OCAMRISS) with histopathologic, micro-computed tomography, and biomechanical validation. Cartilage 2014; 5(1):16–27.

53. Horton LK, Jacobson JA, Lin J, et al. MR imaging of anterior cruciate ligament reconstruction graft. AJR Am J Roentgenol 2000;175(4):1091–7.

54. Rak KM, Gillogly SD, Schaefer RA, et al. Anterior cruciate ligament reconstruction: evaluation with MR imaging. Radiology 1991;178(2):553–6.

55. McCauley TR, Elfar A, Moore A, et al. MR arthrography of anterior cruciate ligament reconstruction grafts. AJR Am J Roentgenol 2003;181(5):1217–23.

56. Naraghi A, White LM. MR imaging of cruciate ligaments. Magn Reson Imaging Clin N Am 2014; 22(4):557–80.

57. Papakonstantinou O, Chung CB, Chanchairujira K, et al. Complications of anterior cruciate ligament reconstruction: MR imaging. Eur Radiol 2003;13(5): 1106–17.

58. Marrale J, Morrissey MC, Haddad FS. A literature review of autograft and allograft anterior cruciate ligament reconstruction. Knee Surg Sports Traumatol Arthrosc 2007;15(6):690–704.

59. Rispoli DM, Sanders TG, Miller MD, et al. Magnetic resonance imaging at different time periods

following hamstring harvest for anterior cruciate ligament reconstruction. Arthroscopy 2001;17(1): 2–8.

60. Hofbauer M, Muller B, Murawski CD, et al. Strategies for revision surgery after primary double-bundle anterior cruciate ligament (ACL) reconstruction. Knee Surg Sports Traumatol Arthrosc 2013;21(9): 2072–80.

61. Muller B, Hofbauer M, Wongcharoenwatana J, et al. Indications and contraindications for double-bundle ACL reconstruction. Int Orthop 2013;37(2):239–46.

62. Arnoczky SP, Tarvin GB, Marshall JL. Anterior cruciate ligament replacement using patellar tendon. An evaluation of graft revascularization in the dog. J Bone Joint Surg Am 1982;64(2):217–24.

63. Boynton MD, Fadale PD. The basic science of anterior cruciate ligament surgery. Orthop Rev 1993; 22(6):673–9.

64. Murakami Y, Sumen Y, Ochi M, et al. MR evaluation of human anterior cruciate ligament autograft on oblique axial imaging. J Comput Assist Tomogr 1998; 22(2):270–5.

65. Saupe N, White LM, Chiavaras MM, et al. Anterior cruciate ligament reconstruction grafts: MR imaging features at long-term follow-up–correlation with functional and clinical evaluation. Radiology 2008; 249(2):581–90.

66. Muramatsu K, Hachiya Y, Izawa H. Serial evaluation of human anterior cruciate ligament grafts by contrast-enhanced magnetic resonance imaging: comparison of allografts and autografts. Arthroscopy 2008;24(9):1038–44.

67. Gnannt R, Chhabra A, Theodoropoulos JS, et al. MR imaging of the postoperative knee. J Magn Reson Imaging 2011;34(5):1007–21.

68. Parkar AP, Adriaensen ME, Fischer-Bredenbeck C, et al. Measurements of tunnel placements after anterior cruciate ligament reconstruction - A comparison between CT, radiographs and MRI. Knee 2015; 22(6):574–9.

69. Carson EW, Anisko EM, Restrepo C, et al. Revision anterior cruciate ligament reconstruction: etiology of failures and clinical results. J Knee Surg 2004; 17(3):127–32.

70. Wilson TC, Kantaras A, Atay A, et al. Tunnel enlargement after anterior cruciate ligament surgery. Am J Sports Med 2004;32(2):543–9.

71. Roedl JB, Morrison WB, Ciccotti MG, et al. Acromial apophysiolysis: superior shoulder pain and acromial nonfusion in the young throwing athlete. Radiology 2015;274(1):201–9.

72. Roedl JB, Nevalainen M, Gonzalez FM, et al. Frequency, imaging findings, risk factors, and long-term sequelae of distal clavicular osteolysis in young patients. Skeletal Radiol 2015;44(5):659–66.

73. Roedl JB, Gonzalez FM, Zoga AC, et al. Potential utility of a combined approach with US and MR arthrography to image medial elbow pain in baseball players. Radiology 2016;279(3):827–37.

74. Corten K, Hoser C, Fink C, et al. Case reports: a Stener-like lesion of the medial collateral ligament of the knee. Clin Orthop Relat Res 2010;468(1): 289–93.

75. Harish S, O'Donnell P, Connell D, et al. Imaging of the posterolateral corner of the knee. Clin Radiol 2006;61(6):457–66.

76. Schechinger SJ, Levy BA, Dajani KA, et al. Achilles tendon allograft reconstruction of the fibular collateral ligament and posterolateral corner. Arthroscopy 2009;25(3):232–42.

The Hindfoot Arch
What Role Does the Imager Play?

Yu-Ching Lin, MD[a], John Y. Kwon, MD[b], Mohammad Ghorbanhoseini, MD[b],
Jim S. Wu, MD[c],*

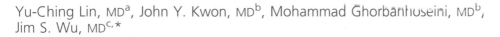

KEYWORDS

- Flatfoot • Pes planus • Radiography • MR imaging • Medial longitudinal arch
- Posterior tibial tendon • Spring ligament • Deltoid ligament

KEY POINTS

- Collapse of the hindfoot arch leads to a flatfoot deformity, which can be classified into flexible and fixed subtypes.
- Flatfoot deformity can be caused by both osseous deformities and injury to the soft tissue supporting structures, particularly the posterior tibial tendon and spring ligament.
- Imaging plays an important role in the assessment of flatfoot deformity, with radiographs and computed tomography useful in characterizing the degree of osseous deformity and magnetic resonance imaging and ultrasonography most useful in the evaluation of the supporting soft tissue structures.
- The role of the imager is to identify the structural causes of the flatfoot deformity and delineate the anatomy for treatment.
- Effective treatment of flatfoot deformity depends on attempting to restore normal foot biomechanics and alignment through strengthening exercises, orthotics, and surgery.

INTRODUCTION

Flatfoot deformity is a common disorder of the foot and ankle that occurs with loss of the hindfoot arch.[1] Although the condition can be asymptomatic, certain subtypes can lead to pain and debilitating loss of function.[1–3] Understanding the various conditions that affect the hindfoot arch leading to flatfeet can be a daunting process for radiologists and clinicians if they are not familiar with the anatomy and the various imaging criteria used to assess injury to the supporting structures. The longitudinal arch of the foot has medial and lateral components that provide structural support to the body. Abnormalities of mainly the medial longitudinal arch (MLA) lead to flatfeet; however, both arches have important bony and soft tissue components that maintain the hindfoot arch, and injury or congenital deformities of these structures can lead to a painful flatfoot.[4–7] This article discusses the anatomy of the hindfoot longitudinal arch and the biomechanical consequences of injury to the medial hindfoot supporting structures. Next, it discusses the various imaging modalities used to evaluate injury of these structures. In addition, the surgical and nonsurgical treatments available for the treatment of flatfoot deformity are discussed.

Disclosure: The authors have nothing to disclose.
[a] Department of Medical Imaging and Intervention, Chang Gung Memorial Hospital, Keelung and Chang Gung University, 5 Fu-Shin Street, Kueishan, Taoyuan, Taiwan 333, China; [b] Division of Foot and Ankle Surgery, Department of Orthopedic Surgery, Beth Israel Deaconess Medical Center, Harvard Medical School, 330 Brookline Avenue, Boston, MA 02215, USA; [c] Department of Radiology, Beth Israel Deaconess Medical Center, Harvard Medical School, 330 Brookline Avenue, Boston, MA 02215, USA
* Corresponding author.
E-mail address: jswu@bidmc.harvard.edu

Radiol Clin N Am 54 (2016) 951–968
http://dx.doi.org/10.1016/j.rcl.2016.04.012

CLASSIFICATION OF FLATFEET

Flatfoot deformity, or pes planus, can be classified as flexible versus fixed, or congenital versus acquired.[1–3,8] In flexible flatfeet, there is loss of the MLA with weight bearing, which corrects with heel rise. Flexible flatfeet is a normal finding in infants and children and is caused by a normal prominence of fat underneath the midfoot (Fig. 1).[3] With growth and progressive weight bearing, a normal arch should form by 8 years of age.[3] Flexible flatfeet can persist into adulthood, with most cases being asymptomatic and requiring no treatment.[1] However, symptomatic flexible flatfeet can require treatment with orthotics, strengthening and stretching exercises, and surgery.[2,3,9,10] Fixed flatfeet can have a variety of causes (Box 1),[3] with the most common cause being tarsal coalitions (Fig. 2).[11] In these cases, normal joint alignment and motion are altered because of congenital bridging between bones.

Both pediatric flexible flatfoot and tarsal coalitions can be classified as congenital flatfoot disorders. In acquired flatfoot, the MLA is initially normal but subsequently fails because of injury of the supporting structures of the MLA.[2,4] The most common cause of acquired flatfoot is progressive tendinopathy of the posterior tibialis tendon (PTT).[2,4,12–14] This failure can lead to a cascade of additional injuries caused by imbalance of the biomechanical forces that maintain the hindfoot arch.[4,9,15] Deformities secondary to trauma, arthritic processes, and neuropathic arthropathy (Fig. 3) are other causes of acquired flatfoot deformity.

ANATOMIC CONSIDERATIONS IN FLATFEET

The longitudinal arch of the foot has medial and lateral components. The higher and more important MLA is formed by the calcaneus, talus, cuneiforms, and first and second metatarsals. The most superior aspect of the MLA is the talar head, whereas the calcaneus and first and second metatarsal heads form the proximal and distal aspects of the arch, respectively.[6,7] Elasticity of the MLA is important in order to provide cushioning and support of the body during motion and is a result of several supporting tendinous and ligamentous structures.[6,7,16–18] These include the PTT, spring ligament, deltoid ligament complex, and other midfoot capsular structures.[4,9,19–21] The lateral longitudinal arch is formed by the calcaneus, cuboid, and fourth and fifth metatarsals; its main supporting soft tissue structures are the peroneus brevis (which opposes the effects of the posterior tibialis), the long plantar ligament, plantar calcaneocuboid ligament, extensor tendons, and intrinsic muscles to the fifth toe.[6,7] Integrity and stabilization of the hindfoot rely on an interaction between these bones, muscles, tendons, ligaments, and fascia.

The PTT is arguably the most important dynamic stabilizer of MLA and hindfoot.[22,23] With PTT tear or tendinopathy, the unopposed peroneus brevis abducts the forefoot into pronation, the calcaneus into valgus (eversion), and the talus into plantarflexion.[2,24] As the hindfoot arch collapse progresses, increasing stress shifts to secondary supporting structures, which include the spring ligament, deltoid ligament complex, plantar fascia,

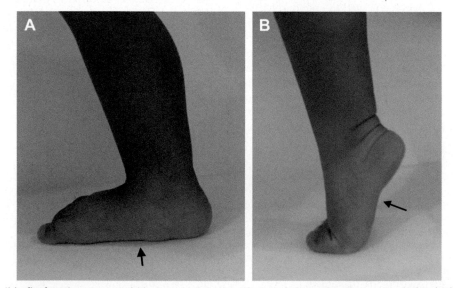

Fig. 1. Flexible flatfoot in a 2-year-old boy. Loss of the hindfoot arch (*arrow*) with standing (*A*), which returns to normal with heel rise (*B*).

Box 1
Causes of flatfeet

Flexible

Normal physiologic variant

Posterior tibial tendon injury

Accessory navicular

Obesity

Neurologic disorders

　Cerebral palsy

　Hypotonia

Muscular dystrophy

Osteogenesis imperfecta

Marfan syndrome

Down syndrome

Ehlers-Danlos

Fixed

Tarsal coalition

Posterior tibial tendon tear

Congenital vertical talus

Trauma

Inflammatory arthritides

Neuropathic arthropathy (Charcot)

Peroneal spastic flatfoot

and Achilles tendon (**Box 2**), in order to prevent further arch collapse.[2,22,23,25] Injury to these additional supporting structures leads to worsening of the flatfoot deformity (**Fig. 4**).[21] It is crucial to evaluate carefully the bony and soft tissue components of the MLA in order to determine the appropriate treatment options.

Posterior Tibial Tendon

PTT injury or tendinopathy is the most common cause of acquired adult flatfeet.[4,12,14,26] The PTT lies anterior to the flexor digitorum longus and the flexor hallucis longus tendons (**Fig. 5**) and courses behind the medial malleolus in a fibro-osseous groove. It travels anteriorly to insert primarily on the navicular bone. Secondary insertion sites are present on the cuneiforms, second to fourth metatarsal bases, sustentaculum tali, and cuboid.[24,27] The primary static function of the PTT is to invert the foot and flex the ankle to maintain the longitudinal arch of the foot.[21,24,27] During normal gait, the PTT pulls the hindfoot into varus and locks the transverse tarsal joints (calcaneocuboid, talonavicular, and transverse tarsal joints) to provide a rigid foot for push-off/heel-off.[16,24,27] Injury of the PTT leads to collapse of the MLA, subtalar joint eversion, foot abduction at the talonavicular joint, and hindfoot valgus.[16,28] Moreover, if the PTT becomes injured, abnormal stress is exerted on the additional supporting structures. Studies report a high association of PTT tears with abnormalities of the spring ligament (82%–92%)[19,25,27] and sinus tarsi (72%).[27]

Although PTT injury is often caused by tendon degeneration from repetitive microtrauma, acute traumatic injury to the tendon leading to a tear has been reported, and is often related to sports activity.[9] Sports create higher loading forces on the hindfoot arch and PTT, compared with typical activities of daily living.[9] Moreover, repetitive injury from sports activity can also lead to an inflamed PTT or tenosynovitis, leading to tendon tear and rupture.[29] In addition, the PTT can be predisposed to injury from impingement of the tendon at the fibro-osseous groove, inflammatory arthropathies, hypovascularity of tendon at the level of medial malleolus, and the presence of an accessory navicular.[27,29–31]

The accessory navicular, or os naviculare, deserves special discussion because it has a high association with painful flatfeet because of its alteration of the normal anatomy and distribution of forces related to the PTT.[30–32] The accessory navicular has 3 subtypes.[33,34] Type 1, os tibiale

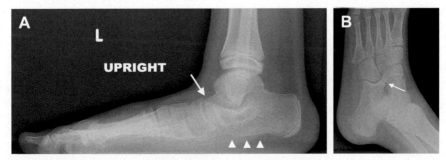

Fig. 2. Fixed (rigid) flatfeet in a 14-year-old boy with tarsal coalition. (*A*) Lateral standing radiograph shows pes planus with inferior tilting of the talar head (*arrow*) and flattening of the MLA (*arrowheads*). (*B*) Oblique radiograph shows a calcaneonavicular (nonosseous) coalition (*arrow*).

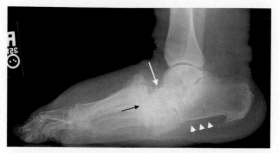

Fig. 3. Flatfoot deformity in a 59-year-old woman with severe foot pain and diabetes. Lateral standing radiograph shows pes planus with inferior tilting of the talar head (*white arrow*), severe proliferative neuropathic bony changes of the midfoot (*black arrow*), and flattening of the MLA (*arrowheads*).

externum, is a sesamoid in the distal tendon of the posterior tibialis and is typically asymptomatic. The type II accessory navicular is a heart-shaped ossicle that represents an unfused secondary ossification of the navicular bone (**Fig. 6**). The PTT attaches onto the accessory navicular, which is attached to the main navicular bone by a fibro-cartilaginous complex.[34] Type II is the most common symptomatic subtype because there can be pain at the fibrocartilaginous attachment from abnormal motion or injury.[34] Moreover, the action of the PTT is displaced upward and inward, altering the normal biomechanics of the PTT, so that it no longer functions effectively as an invertor

of the foot.[30,31] The cornuate navicular is the third subtype and is an especially prominent medial navicular tuberosity with symptoms related to bunion formation from the bony prominence.[34]

Spring Ligament

The spring ligament (also known as the plantar cal-caneonavicular ligament) is a thick triangular structure that originates from the undersurface of the sustentaculum tali and inserts onto the inferior and medial surfaces of the navicular bone.[35] It is supported medially by anterior fibers of the deltoid ligament and is superficially covered by the PTT.[35] The spring ligament has 3 components. The superomedial component originates from the medial aspect of sustentaculum tali, attaches to the superomedial aspect of navicular bone, and is a main contributor to hindfoot stability.[23,36] The medioplantar oblique component originates from the coronoid fossa of the calcaneus and attaches to the navicular tuberosity. The inferoplantar longi-tudinal component originates from the coronoid fossa of the calcaneus and attaches to the navic-ular beak. The spring ligament forms a fibrocartila-ginous sling or hammock that supports the medial and plantar portions of the talar head and holds the talus in a correct position, ensuring stability of the hindfoot (**Fig. 7**). If the spring ligament is torn (especially the superomedial component), the talar head rotates inferiorly (plantarflex) and medially (adduction). Moreover, the calcaneus progres-sively tilts into valgus malalignment and static sta-bility of MLA is lost.[19,21–23]

Deltoid Ligament Complex

The deltoid ligament complex (as known as the medial collateral ligament) is composed of superfi-cial and deep layers (**Fig. 8**). The superficial layer is composed of the tibionavicular ligament (TNL), tibiospring ligament (TSL), and tibiocalcaneal liga-ments (TCL).[37–39] They form a fan-shaped struc-ture originating from the anterior colliculus of the medial malleolus and inserting onto the navicular, spring ligament, and calcaneus, respectively. The deep layer is composed of the anterior and poste-rior tibiotalar ligaments, which originate from the posterior colliculus and insert onto the talus ante-riorly and posteriorly.[37–39] The deltoid ligament provides restraint against valgus tilt and external rotation of the talus, with the deep layer playing a major role in restraining pronation and hindfoot valgus.[24,37,38]

Tarsal Sinus

The tarsal sinus (**Fig. 9**) is a cone-shaped region between the posterior subtalar joint and the

---

Box 2
Soft tissue supporting structures of the medial longitudinal arch

Posterior tibial tendon

Spring ligament

  Superomedial

  Medioplantar oblique

  Inferoplantar longitudinal

Deltoid ligament complex

  Superficial layer

    Tibionavicular

    Tibiospring

    Tibiocalcaneal

  Deep layer

    Anterior tibiotalar

    Posterior tibiotalar

Plantar fascia

Achilles tendon

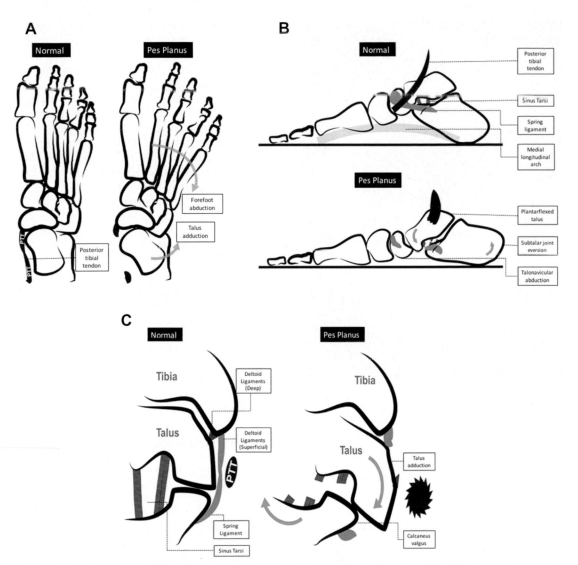

Fig. 4. Normal and abnormal foot alignment with pes planus when there is injury of the PTT and other supporting structures depicted in the (*A*) axial, (*B*) sagittal, and (*C*) coronal planes.

talocalcaneonavicular joint. It contains fat, blood vessels, nerves, and several ligaments (cervical, interosseous, talocalcaneal, and anterior capsular ligaments and inferior extensor retinaculum).[40–42] The main function of the tarsal sinus ligaments is to maintain the alignment between the talus and calcaneus by limiting talar tilting and calcaneus inversion.[41,43] Tarsal sinus ligamentous injury may lead to subtalar joint instability and is a major cause of sinus tarsi syndrome.[42]

Achilles Tendon and Plantar Fascia

The Achilles tendon and plantar fascia play important roles in the support of the hindfoot arch. When the PTT is torn, there is unopposed action by the

peroneus brevis and calf muscles through the Achilles tendon. The pull of these muscles leads to shortening of the lateral hindfoot and brings the calcaneus into valgus alignment. Contracture of the Achilles tendon and tightness of the gastrocnemius/soleus complex can develop.[44,45] Thus, exercises to decrease calf muscle tightness can be helpful in these patients.[2]

The plantar fascia attaches to the posterior inferior aspect of the calcaneus and the base of the metatarsal heads anteriorly. With flatfoot deformity, the MLA collapses and there is increased stress and elongation of the plantar fascia as it tries to maintain the hindfoot arch (**Fig. 10**). Cadaveric studies have shown that sectioning the plantar fascia can lead to 25%

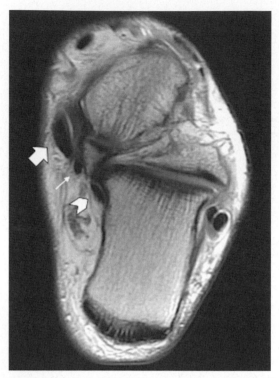

Fig. 5. Axial T1-weighted MR image shows the normal posterior tibial (*thick arrow*), flexor digitorum longus (*thin arrow*), and flexor hallucis longus tendons (*arrowhead*).

loss of stiffness of the MLA and there is a higher association of plantar fasciitis in patients with flatfeet.[46,47]

Tarsal Coalitions

Fixed flatfeet are most commonly caused by tarsal coalition, which is present in 1% of the population and bilateral in 50% to 80% of cases.[11,48] The most common tarsal coalitions occur between the anterior calcaneus and navicular (calcaneonavicular) and between the talus and sustentaculum tali (talocalcaneal); these account for 90% of tarsal coalitions.[11] Coalitions can be osseous, cartilaginous, or fibrous and all 3 types can be associated with a rigid flatfoot deformity.[11] The rigidity of the affected joint can lead to pain and abnormal stresses on adjacent tendons and ligaments about the foot and ankle. On radiographs, a talar beak may form secondary to restricted motion, leading to enthesopathic changes at the talonavicular ligament.[11] A C sign can be seen with talocalcaneal coalition and is formed by the medial margin of the talar dome and the posteroinferior margin of the sustentaculum tali (**Fig. 11**).[49] Many coalitions can be diagnosed on radiographs alone and an oblique view of the foot is especially helpful when evaluating for calcaneonavicular coalitions. In difficult cases, cross-sectional imaging with computed tomography (CT) or magnetic resonance (MR) imaging can be helpful, with several studies favoring CT rather than MR imaging because of its ability to optimally assess the osseous anatomy and assist in presurgical planning.[11,50,51]

IMAGING CONSIDERATIONS

Imaging studies play an important role in the evaluation of the hindfoot arch. The role of the imager is to identify the structural cause of the flatfoot deformity and delineate the anatomy for treatment. Radiography, ultrasonography (US), CT, and MR imaging are the best radiologic tests to use when evaluating flatfoot deformity.[16]

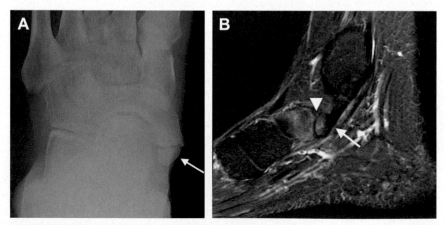

Fig. 6. Accessory navicular (type II) in a 45-year-old woman with medial foot pain. (*A*) AP radiograph shows a heart shaped ossicle (*arrow*) posterior to the navicular tuberosity. (*B*) Sagittal T2-weighted fat-saturated MR image shows the distal posterior tibial tendon (*arrow*) attaching onto a type II nonosseous accessory navicular with edema at the fibrocartilaginous attachment (*arrowhead*).

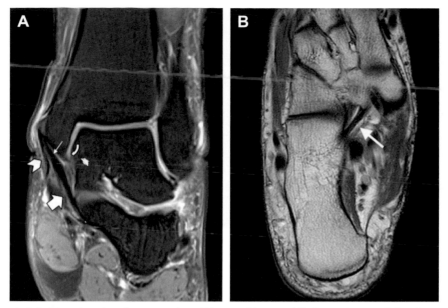

Fig. 7. Normal deltoid and spring ligaments in a 34-year-old man. (*A*) Coronal proton density–weighted fat-saturated MR image shows the anterior tibiotalar ligament (*curved arrow*), a component of the deltoid ligament complex deep layer; tibiospring ligament (*thin arrow*), a component of the deltoid ligament complex superficial layer; flexor retinaculum (*arrowhead*); and superomedial component of spring ligament (*thick arrow*). (*B*) Axial T1-weighted MR image shows the normal medioplantar oblique component of the spring ligament (*arrow*) extending from the posterior navicular to the anterior medial calcaneus.

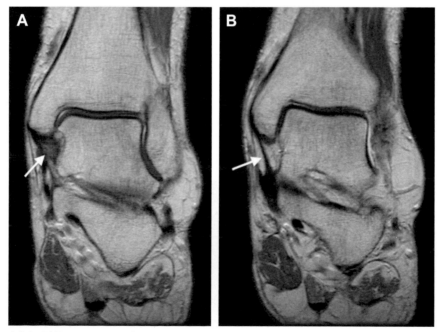

Fig. 8. Normal deltoid ligament complex in 28-year-old woman. Coronal proton-weighted MR images show (*A*) a normal posterior tibiotalar ligament with faint striations (*arrow*), a component of the deep layer; and (*B*) normal tibiospring ligament (*arrow*), a component of the superficial layer. These two components should be visible on nearly all normal MR imaging examinations.

Table 2
Johnson and Strom classification of PTT disorder in flatfoot deformity

Stage	Description	Treatment
Stage 1	1. Inflamed PTT with pain located medially 2. No deformity 3. Able to do single heel rise	1. Conservative treatment 2. Debridement of PTT
Stage 2	1. PTT elongation and degeneration with both medial and lateral foot pain 2. Flexible flatfoot deformity with hindfoot valgus, forefoot abduction, and forefoot varus 3. Difficult to do single heel rise	1. Conservative treatment 2. Debridement and augmentation of PTT 3. Surgical Correction

Stage 3	1. PTT ruptured with pain located laterally
	2. Fixed hindfoot valgus and often fixed forefoot varus deformity
	3. Unable to do single heel rise
		1. Surgical reconstruction
		  a. Soft tissue
		  b. Bone

Stage 4	1. Talus tilts into valgus within the ankle mortise secondary to deltoid ligament insufficiency
	  a. Flexible ankle valgus without substantial tibiotalar arthritis
	  b. Rigid ankle valgus or flexible ankle valgus with significant tibiotalar arthritis
		1. Surgical reconstruction
		  a. Soft tissue
		  b. Bone

help with hindfoot eversion.[8,86] In addition to exercises, orthotics to maintain the MLA can be helpful in symptomatic patients.[8,86] Over-the-counter nonindividualized orthotics can be used initially; however, orthotics molded to the patients foot can provided more personalized support. Initially orthotics should be accommodative; however, with worsening flatfoot deformity, more rigid foot and ankle orthotics can be considered.[1,3,8,86] The efficacy of these nonsurgical management options is unclear because there is a lack of randomized controlled clinical trials.[88]

When nonoperative treatment fails, surgery can be performed in an attempt to restore the normal biomechanics of the hindfoot arch. Soft tissue surgical procedures include debridement of the PTT in cases of tendinosis without foot deformity (stage 1).[89,90] Augmentation of the PTT can be performed when the PTT is elongated (stage II) or has a severe tear (stages III–IV). In certain cases, PTT can be strengthened by imbrication or by reattachment to the navicular bone. However, in severe cases of PTT tear with associated malalignment, tendon transfer with the flexor digitorum longus or, less commonly, the flexor hallucis longus tendon can be performed in addition to other bony procedures.[89,90] Achilles tendon/gastrocnemius complex lengthening can be performed in cases in which the patient has an equinus deformity, and is often an adjuvant procedure to flatfoot correction.[91] In addition, surgical repair of the spring ligament is becoming more common as surgeons realize the importance of this ligament in maintaining the hindfoot arch. Correcting only the PTT when both the PTT and spring ligament are abnormal can lead to persistent symptoms.

There are several osseous surgical procedures that can be performed to correct flatfoot deformity. The calcaneal slide osteotomy is a common procedure in which an osteotomy is performed at the midbody of the calcaneus and the posterior tuber is shifted 1 to 2 cm medially and fixed in relation the anterior calcaneus (**Fig. 22**). This procedure corrects the hindfoot valgus that occurs with flatfeet. The dorsal opening wedge osteotomy of the medial cuneiform, Cotton procedure, is another common procedure designed to lengthen the medial column, which becomes narrowed with flatfoot deformity. A transverse osteotomy line is created in the medial cuneiform and bone allograft, often iliac crest, is place in the osteotomy site (**Fig. 23**). Lateral column lengthening of the distal calcaneus (Evans procedure) or calcaneocuboid distraction arthrodesis can also correct adduction of the midfoot, especially in cases with significant adduction. Arthrodesis of the first tarsometatarsal joint and/or navicular-cuneiform are additional procedures used to correct pes planus deformities of the foot. In the presence of a painful accessory navicular (type II), simple resection of the os naviculare is the treatment of choice,[92] which has also been the established treatment of other symptomatic accessory ossa

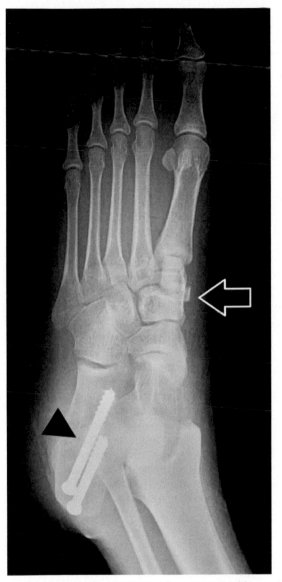

Fig. 22. Oblique foot radiograph in 37-year-old man after surgery for pes planus deformity. Calcaneal slide osteotomy (*arrowhead*) and medial cuneiform wedge osteotomy (*white arrow*) were performed.

in the musculoskeletal system; for example, an os trigonum or at the acromioclavicular joint (os acromiale).[93,94]

When patients present with stage IV deformity, additional procedures are warranted. If significant tibiotalar arthritis exists, ankle arthrodesis or ankle replacement is performed in additional to procedures to correct alignment. If arthritis is not present, deltoid ligament reconstruction and/or corrective supramalleolar tibial osteotomy can be performed in additional to the other procedures listed earlier.

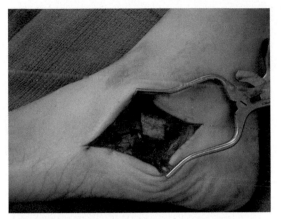

Fig. 23. Intraoperative view of a 28-year-old woman with pes planus, showing a medial cuneiform opening wedge osteotomy and bone graft placement (*arrow*).

SUMMARY

Flatfoot deformity can be flexible or fixed and can be caused by both osseous deformities and injuries to the soft tissue supporting structures, particularly the PTT and spring ligament. Knowledge of the relevant anatomic structures and their importance in maintaining the hindfoot arch is important in the diagnosis and treatment of these patients. The imager plays an important role by identifying the structural causes of the flatfoot deformity and delineating the anatomy for treatment. Radiographs and CT are most useful in characterizing the degree of osseous deformity, and US and MR imaging are most useful in the evaluation of the supporting soft tissue structures. Overall, MR imaging is likely the most useful imaging study. Treatment depends on the clinical symptoms and involves restoring the normal biomechanics of the hindfoot arch through strengthening exercises, foot/ankle orthotics, and surgery.

ACKNOWLEDGMENTS

The authors thank Kuo-Feng Weng and Benjamin Chen Fulop for assistance in creating the figures.

REFERENCES

1. Sheikh Taha AM, Feldman DS. Painful flexible flatfoot. Foot Ankle Clin 2015;20(4):693–704.
2. Van Gestel L, Van Bouwel S, Somville J. Surgical treatment of the adult acquired flexible flatfoot. Acta Orthop Belg 2015;81(2):172–83.
3. Halabchi F, Mazaheri R, Mirshahi M, et al. Pediatric flexible flatfoot; clinical aspects and algorithmic approach. Iran J Pediatr 2013;23(3):247–60.

4. Lin YC, Mhuircheartaigh JN, Lamb J, et al. Imaging of adult flatfoot: correlation of radiographic measurements with MRI. AJR Am J Roentgenol 2015;204(2): 354–9.

5. Williams DS 3rd, Tierney RN, Butler RJ. Increased medial longitudinal arch mobility, lower extremity kinematics, and ground reaction forces in high-arched runners. J Athletic Train 2014;49(3):290–6.

6. Yalcin N, Esen E, Kanatli U, et al. Evaluation of the medial longitudinal arch: a comparison between the dynamic plantar pressure measurement system and radiographic analysis. Acta Orthop Traumatol Turc 2010;44(3):241–5.

7. Fukano M, Fukubayashi T. Motion characteristics of the medial and lateral longitudinal arch during landing. Eur J Appl Physiol 2009;105(3):387–92.

8. Frances JM, Feldman DS. Management of idiopathic and nonidiopathic flatfoot. Instr Course Lect 2015; 64:429–40.

9. Ribbans WJ, Garde A. Tibialis posterior tendon and deltoid and spring ligament injuries in the elite athlete. Foot Ankle Clin 2013;18(2):255–91.

10. Bourdet C, Seringe R, Adamsbaum C, et al. Flatfoot in children and adolescents. Analysis of imaging findings and therapeutic implications. Orthop Traumatol Surg Res 2013;99(1):80–7.

11. Cass AD, Camasta CA. A review of tarsal coalition and pes planovalgus: clinical examination, diagnostic imaging, and surgical planning. J Foot Ankle Surg 2010;49(3):274–93.

12. Karasick D, Schweitzer ME. Tear of the posterior tibial tendon causing asymmetric flatfoot: radiologic findings. AJR Am J Roentgenol 1993; 161(6):1237–40.

13. Narvaez J, Narvaez JA, Sanchez-Marquez A, et al. Posterior tibial tendon dysfunction as a cause of acquired flatfoot in the adult: value of magnetic resonance imaging. Br J Rheumatol 1997;36(1):136–9.

14. Deland JT. The adult acquired flatfoot and spring ligament complex. Pathology and implications for treatment. Foot Ankle Clin 2001;6(1):129–35, vii.

15. Lee KM, Chung CY, Kwon SS, et al. Relationship between stress ankle radiographs and injured ligaments on MRI. Skeletal Radiol 2013;42(11):1537–42.

16. Imhauser CW, Siegler S, Abidi NA, et al. The effect of posterior tibialis tendon dysfunction on the plantar pressure characteristics and the kinematics of the arch and the hindfoot. Clin Biomech 2004;19(2): 161–9.

17. Tome J, Nawoczenski DA, Flemister A, et al. Comparison of foot kinematics between subjects with posterior tibialis tendon dysfunction and healthy controls. J Orthop Sports Phys Ther 2006;36(9): 635–44.

18. Richie DH Jr. Biomechanics and clinical analysis of the adult acquired flatfoot. Clin Podiatr Med Surg 2007;24(4):617–44, vii.

19. Deland JT, de Asla RJ, Sung IH, et al. Posterior tibial tendon insufficiency: which ligaments are involved? Foot Ankle Int 2005;26(6):427–35.

20. Mengiardi B, Zanetti M, Schottle PB, et al. Spring ligament complex: MR imaging-anatomic correlation and findings in asymptomatic subjects. Radiology 2005;237(1):242–9.

21. Jennings MM, Christensen JC. The effects of sectioning the spring ligament on rearfoot stability and posterior tibial tendon efficiency. J Foot Ankle Surg 2008;47(3):219–24.

22. Orr JD, Nunley JA 2nd. Isolated spring ligament failure as a cause of adult-acquired flatfoot deformity. Foot Ankle Int 2013;34(6):818–23.

23. Toye LR, Helms CA, Hoffman BD, et al. MRI of spring ligament tears. AJR Am J Roentgenol 2005;184(5): 1475–80.

24. Smith JT, Bluman EM. Update on stage IV acquired adult flatfoot disorder: when the deltoid ligament becomes dysfunctional. Foot Ankle Clin 2012;17(2): 351–60.

25. Gazdag AR, Cracchiolo A 3rd. Rupture of the posterior tibial tendon. Evaluation of injury of the spring ligament and clinical assessment of tendon transfer and ligament repair. J Bone Jt Surg Am 1997;79(5): 675–81.

26. Pomeroy GC, Pike RH, Beals TC, et al. Acquired flatfoot in adults due to dysfunction of the posterior tibial tendon. J Bone Jt Surg Am 1999;81(8): 1173–82.

27. Balen PF, Helms CA. Association of posterior tibial tendon injury with spring ligament injury, sinus tarsi abnormality, and plantar fasciitis on MR imaging. AJR Am J Roentgenol 2001;176(5):1137–43.

28. Younger AS, Sawatzky B, Dryden P. Radiographic assessment of adult flatfoot. Foot Ankle Int 2005; 26(10):820–5.

29. Arai K, Ringleb SI, Zhao KD, et al. The effect of flatfoot deformity and tendon loading on the work of friction measured in the posterior tibial tendon. Clin Biomech 2007;22(5):592–8.

30. Kiter E, Gunal I, Karatosun V, et al. The relationship between the tibialis posterior tendon and the accessory navicular. Ann Anat 2000;182(1):65–8.

31. Kiter E, Erdag N, Karatosun V, et al. Tibialis posterior tendon abnormalities in feet with accessory navicular bone and flatfoot. Acta Orthop Scand 1999; 70(6):618–21.

32. Wong MW, Griffith JF. Magnetic resonance imaging in adolescent painful flexible flatfoot. Foot Ankle Int 2009;30(4):303–8.

33. Lawson JP, Ogden JA, Sella E, et al. The painful accessory navicular. Skeletal Radiol 1984;12(4): 250–62.

34. Miller TT, Staron RB, Feldman F, et al. The symptomatic accessory tarsal navicular bone: assessment with MR imaging. Radiology 1995;195(3):849–53.

35. Williams G, Widnall J, Evans P, et al. MRI features most often associated with surgically proven tears of the spring ligament complex. Skeletal Radiol 2013;42(7):969-73.

36. Yao L, Gentili A, Cracchiolo A. MR imaging findings in spring ligament insufficiency. Skeletal Radiol 1999;28(5):245-50.

37. Mengiardi B, Pfirrmann CW, Vienne P, et al. Medial collateral ligament complex of the ankle: MR appearance in asymptomatic subjects. Radiology 2007;242(3):817-24.

38. Ellis SJ, Williams BR, Wagshul AD, et al. Deltoid ligament reconstruction with peroneus longus autograft in flatfoot deformity. Foot Ankle Int 2010;31(9):781-9.

39. Jeng CL, Bluman EM, Myerson MS. Minimally invasive deltoid ligament reconstruction for stage IV flatfoot deformity. Foot Ankle Int 2011;32(1):21-30.

40. Klein MA, Spreitzer AM. MR imaging of the tarsal sinus and canal: normal anatomy, pathologic findings, and features of the sinus tarsi syndrome. Radiology 1993;186(1):233-40.

41. Li SY, Hou ZD, Zhang P, et al. Ligament structures in the tarsal sinus and canal. Foot Ankle Int 2013;34(12):1729-36.

42. Thacker P, Mardis N. Ligaments of the tarsal sinus: improved detection, characterisation and significance in the paediatric ankle with 3-D proton density MR imaging. Pediatr Radiol 2013;43(2):196-201.

43. Cahill DR. The anatomy and function of the contents of the human tarsal sinus and canal. Anat Rec 1965;153(1):1-17.

44. Arangio G, Rogman A, Reed JF 3rd. Hindfoot alignment valgus moment arm increases in adult flatfoot with Achilles tendon contracture. Foot Ankle Int 2009;30(11):1078-82.

45. DiGiovanni CW, Langer P. The role of isolated gastrocnemius and combined Achilles contractures in the flatfoot. Foot Ankle Clin 2007;12(2):363-79, viii.

46. Huang CK, Kitaoka HB, An KN, et al. Biomechanical evaluation of longitudinal arch stability. Foot Ankle 1993;14(6):353-7.

47. Wearing SC, Smeathers JE, Urry SR, et al. The pathomechanics of plantar fasciitis. Sports Med 2006;36(7):585-611.

48. Stormont DM, Peterson HA. The relative incidence of tarsal coalition. Clin Orthop Relat Res 1983;(181):28-36.

49. Moraleda L, Gantsoudes GD, Mubarak SJ. C sign: talocalcaneal coalition or flatfoot deformity? J Pediatr Orthop 2014;34(8):814-9.

50. Emery KH, Bisset GS 3rd, Johnson ND, et al. Tarsal coalition: a blinded comparison of MRI and CT. Pediatr Radiol 1998;28(8):612-6.

51. Crim J. Imaging of tarsal coalition. Radiol Clin North Am 2008;46(6):1017-26, vi.

52. Toullec E. Adult flatfoot. Orthop Traumatol Surg Res 2015;101(1 Suppl):S11-7.

53. Kong A, Van Der Vliet A. Imaging of tibialis posterior dysfunction. Br J Radiol 2008;81(970):826-36.

54. Vanderwilde R, Staheli LT, Chew DE, et al. Measurements on radiographs of the foot in normal infants and children. J Bone Jt Surg Am 1988;70(3):407-15.

55. Levy JC, Mizel MS, Clifford PD, et al. Value of radiographs in the initial evaluation of nontraumatic adult heel pain. Foot Ankle Int 2006;27(6):427-30.

56. Ellis SJ, Yu JC, Williams BR, et al. New radiographic parameters assessing forefoot abduction in the adult acquired flatfoot deformity. Foot Ankle Int 2009;30(12):1168-76.

57. Pehlivan O, Cilli F, Mahirogullari M, et al. Radiographic correlation of symptomatic and asymptomatic flexible flatfoot in young male adults. Int Orthop 2009;33(2):447-50.

58. Lo HC, Chu WC, Wu WK, et al. Comparison of radiological measures for diagnosing flatfoot. Acta Radiol 2012;53(2):192-6.

59. Ippolito E, Fraracci L, Farsetti P, et al. Validity of the anteroposterior talocalcaneal angle to assess congenital clubfoot correction. AJR Am J Roentgenol 2004;182(5):1279-82.

60. Coughlin MJ, Kaz A. Correlation of Harris mats, physical exam, pictures, and radiographic measurements in adult flatfoot deformity. Foot Ankle Int 2009;30(7):604-12.

61. Sensiba PR, Coffey MJ, Williams NE, et al. Inter- and intraobserver reliability in the radiographic evaluation of adult flatfoot deformity. Foot Ankle Int 2010;31(2):141-5.

62. Bryant A, Tinley P, Singer K. A comparison of radiographic measurements in normal, hallux valgus, and hallux limitus feet. J Foot Ankle Surg 2000;39(1):39-43.

63. Metcalfe SA, Bowling FL, Baltzopoulos V, et al. The reliability of measurements taken from radiographs in the assessment of paediatric flat foot deformity. Foot 2012;22(3):156-62.

64. Hoffman D, Bianchi S. Sonographic evaluation of plantar hindfoot and midfoot pain. J Ultrasound Med 2013;32(7):1271-84.

65. Hoffman DF, Grothe HL, Bianchi S. Sonographic evaluation of hindfoot disorders. J Ultrasound 2014;17(2):141-50.

66. Arnoldner MA, Gruber M, Syre S, et al. Imaging of posterior tibial tendon dysfunction–Comparison of high-resolution ultrasound and 3T MRI. Eur J Radiol 2015;84(9):1777-81.

67. Harish S, Jan E, Finlay K, et al. Sonography of the superomedial part of the spring ligament complex of the foot: a study of cadavers and asymptomatic volunteers. Skeletal Radiol 2007;36(3):221-8.

68. Harish S, Kumbhare D, O'Neill J, et al. Comparison of sonography and magnetic resonance imaging

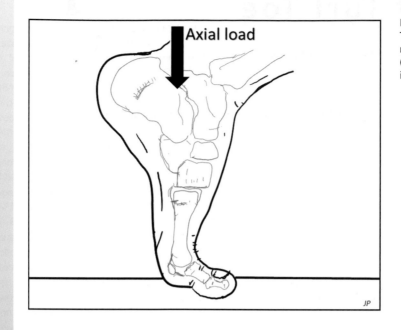

Fig. 1. Mechanism of turf toe injury. The planted forefoot with the heel raised is subjected to an axial load (*arrow*) forcing the 1st MTP joint into extreme dorsiflexion.

NORMAL ANATOMY

The 1st MTP joint is a modified hinge joint. The shallow groove of the 1st proximal phalangeal base contributes to the joint's inherent instability. The 1st MTP joint derives stability from the hallux sesamoids and its surrounding, supporting capsuloligamentous structures. The medial and lateral sesamoids add a layer of complexity to the 1st MTP joint relative to the lesser MTP joints. The sesamoids serve as a fulcrum for push-off power during gait and athletic endeavors. The 1st MTP joint bears up to 60% of body weight during normal gait and up to 3 to 8 times body weight during push-off activities.[5,7,8]

The 1st MTP joint range of motion is greatest in the sagittal plane, approximately 15° of plantar flexion and approximately 80° of dorsiflexion when standing.[9]

The 1st MTP joint anatomy can be challenging. It is important that referring teams and radiologists are familiar with and share the same anatomic nomenclature because variations in terminology exist.

To approach the 1st MTP joint anatomy, it helps to focus on its central structures and then extend to its periphery. At its core, the 1st MTP joint consists of the articulation of the 1st metarsal head and 1st proximal phalangeal base as well as the paired articulations of the 1st metatarsal head-medial sesamoid and 1st metatarsal head-lateral sesamoid.

The plantar plate of the 1st MTP joint is used as a broad encompassing term of the plantar capsule. It may be visualized as a hammock extending from the 1st metatarsal neck, encasing the sesamoids and inserting onto the base of the 1st proximal phalanx. The proximal thinner portion of the hammock, the paired confluent metatarso-sesamoid (MT-S) ligaments, originates from the metatarsal neck and inserts on the respective sesamoid (**Fig. 2**A). The distal thicker aspect of the hammock, the paired sesamoid phalangeal (SP) ligaments, originates from the respective sesamoid and inserts on the proximal phalangeal base (see **Fig. 2**A; **Fig. 3**A). There is thinner plantar plate capsular tissue between these 2 ligaments. The SP ligament has a taut appearance on MR imaging in neutral position. The SP ligaments are key stabilizers of the 1st MTP joint.

The intersesamoid (IS) ligament is an additional thick structure bridging the medial and lateral sesamoids (**Fig. 4**A). The literature varies in terms of the histologic nature of the IS ligament and other portions of the plantar plate reporting both fibrous and fibrocartilaginous tissue at this location.[5,10,11] The IS ligament is designated as the plantar plate by Netter[12] in his illustrations.

The plantar capsuloligamentous complex is composed of all the aforementioned structures of the plantar plate in addition to the collateral ligaments, the overlying tendinous confluences, and remaining nondesignated capsular tissue.

At the periphery of the 1st MTP joint lie the medial and lateral collateral ligaments. Medial

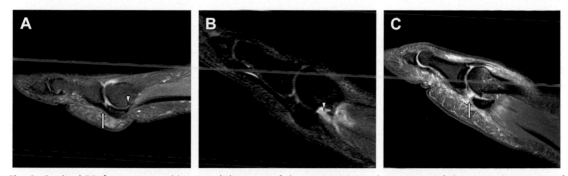

Fig. 2. Sagittal PD fat-suppressed images. (A) Image of the 1st MTP joint shows some of the normal anatomy of the plantar plate, including the SP ligament (arrow) and MT-S ligament (arrowhead) deep to the flexor hallucis tendon. (B) Image shows full-thickness tearing of the medial MT-S ligament (arrowhead) off its sesamoid insertion with associated edema in the flexor hallucis brevis muscle belly. (C) Image demonstrates a full-thickness tear of the medial SP ligament (arrow) off the sesamoid. There is associated proximal retraction of the sesamoid. The 1st MTP joint line serves as a good reference point to assess sesamoid retraction in the setting of turf toe.

and lateral collateral ligaments respectively add valgus and varus stability to the 1st MTP joint. Each fan-shaped collateral ligament originates at the metatarsal condyle tubercle and travels obliquely in a plantar direction (see **Fig. 4**A). On MR imaging, the lateral collateral ligament is typically thinner than the medial collateral ligament. The collateral ligaments consist of a collateral ligament proper and a confluent accessory collateral ligament. The collateral ligament proper inserts on the 1st proximal phalangeal base. Each accessory collateral ligament blends with its respective medial and lateral joint capsule and attaches to its respective sesamoid (see **Fig. 4**A).[5]

In the literature, there are multiple variations of the nomenclature of the medial and lateral plantar capsular attachments to the respective medial and lateral sesamoids. These include MT-S ligaments,[5,8,13] MT-S suspensory ligaments,[14] sesamoid suspensory ligaments,[8,15] MT-S slips,[16] sesamoid collateral ligaments,[17] accessory sesamoid ligaments,[18] and sesamoid ligaments[19] to name several. The aforementioned nomenclatures should not be confused with the proximal capsular tissue designated in this article as the MT-S ligaments. Subsequently, accessory collateral ligament is the terminology used in this descriptive effort of the complex 1st MTP joint anatomy to maintain consistency with the anatomy of the remaining hinge joints of the hands and feet. The 1st MTP joint anatomy is similar to the 1st metacarpophangeal joint.[20] Ultimately, this emphasizes the importance of good communication among the treating team.

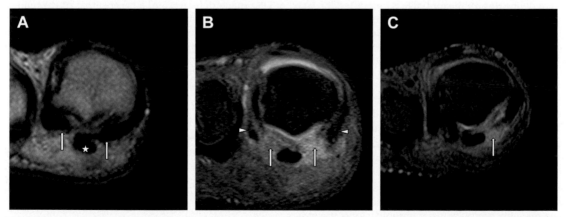

Fig. 3. Coronal images obtained distal to the sesamoids. (A) PD image demonstrates normal medial and lateral SP ligaments (arrows) confluent with the thinner central plantar plate capsular tissue deep to the flexor hallucis longus tendon (star). (B) PD fat-suppressed image demonstrates disruption of both medial and lateral SP ligaments (arrows) in a football player. Peripheral to these tear defects, the abductor and adductor hallucis tendons are intact (arrowheads). (C) PD fat-suppressed image of a basketball player shows a medial SP ligament fluid-filled tear (arrow).

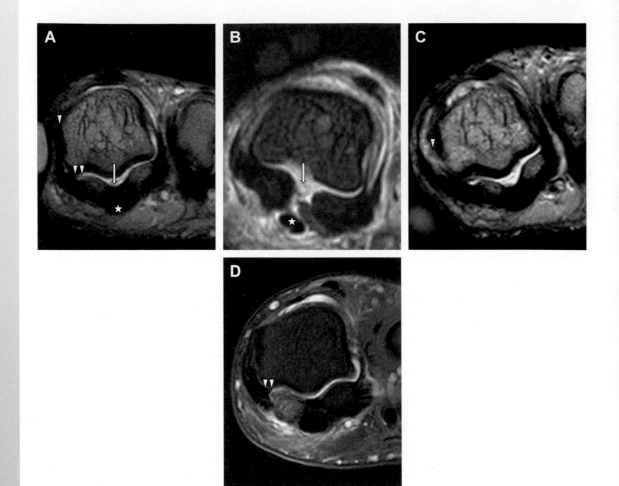

Fig. 4. Coronal images obtained at the level of the sesamoids. (*A*) PD image shows the intact IS, medial and lateral collateral ligaments. The IS ligament (*arrow*) abuts the underlying flexor hallucis longus tendon (*star*). Deep to the skin surface marker, the medial collateral ligament components, medial collateral ligament proper (*arrowhead*) and accessory medial collateral ligament (*double arrowheads*), are outlined on the image. (*B*) PD fat-suppressed image highlights an acute rupture of the IS ligament (*arrow*) in a defensive lineman. Associated fluid delineates the flexor hallucis longus tendon (*star*). (*C*) PD image demonstrates a chronic tear of the medial collateral ligament characterized by a large gap (*arrowhead*) in an amateur wrestler. (*D*) PD fat-suppressed image shows stripping of the accessory medial collateral ligament off its medial sesamoid insertion (*double arrowheads*). The injury occurred in a baseball player as he was sliding into base. Note the associated edema superficial to and in the medial sesamoid.

The tendinous confluences of the plantar capsuloligamentous complex include the flexor hallucis brevis, abductor hallucis, and adductor hallucis. The flexor hallucis brevis medial and lateral heads attach to the proximal and peripheral margins of the respective sesamoid, superficial to the MT-S ligaments. They merge with fibrous capsular tissue at the plantar surface of the medial and lateral sesamoids. Abductor and adductor hallucis tendons merge with capsular attachments along the periphery of the respective medial and lateral sesamoids (**Fig. 5**A). These tendinous confluences contribute to the plantar capsuloligamentous complex with distal insertions at the base of the 1st proximal phalanx.

IMAGING PROTOCOL

Advances in MR imaging and coil technology have made a more detailed diagnosis of turf toe possible. It remains paramount that the proper parameters are applied during the examination to obtain the best images possible.

In the setting of turf toe, standard coverage of the entire foot or forefoot should be avoided. The 1st MTP joint should be imaged using a dedicated extremity coil with the joint of interest in its isocenter. Knee and ankle coils are both good options for moderate to large feet. A knee coil is typically favored over an ankle coil because it does not suffer from signal drop-off at the

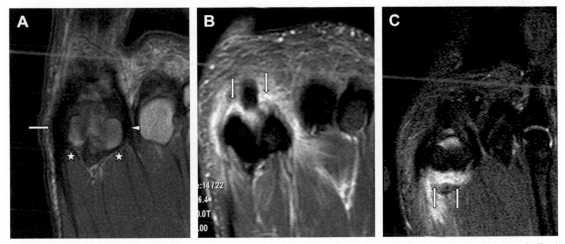

Fig. 5. Axial images. (*A*) PD image shows the confluence of the flexor hallucis brevis (*stars*), abductor hallucis (*arrow*), and adductor hallucis (*arrowhead*) tendons to the intact 1st MTP joint capsule. (*B*) PD fat-suppressed image illustrates bilateral SP ligament tears (*arrows*). The proximal, medial, and lateral capsular attachments are all intact. (*C*) PD fat-suppressed image shows broad proximal capsular defect from bilateral MT-S ligament tears (*arrows*). Distal, medial, and lateral capsular attachments are intact.

level of the 1st MTP joint. For smaller feet, an 8-channel wrist coil provides focused 1st MTP joint imaging with superior resolution; however, most turf toes do not come in small sizes. Optimal protocol parameters vary depending on multiple factors, including the scanner strength, inherent vendor sequences, type of extremity coil used, and the foot size. Isocenter placement in the coil and immobilization of the painful mobile great toe are critical to optimal images. Immobilization should be achieved by taping, sandbagging, and positioning foam.

Proton density (PD) sequence in all 3 planes is recommended for evaluation of the anatomy and chronic pathology. PD has soft tissue detail superior to T1 images for depicting the capsuloligamentous complex and cartilage of the 1st MTP joint. If time permits or if a high index of suspicion exists for an occult fracture, a T1 sequence can be done as a substitute or in addition to sagittal PD images. In addition to these anatomy-focused sequences, fat-suppressed fluid-weighted sequences in all 3 planes are recommended for optimal evaluation of acute pathology. Fat-suppressed PD images (echo time [TE] of 45–55 milliseconds) offer better resolution than short tau inversion recovery (STIR) and heavily weighted T2 images. STIR imaging is warranted if homogeneous fat suppression cannot be obtained.

It is ideal to keep the field of view, slice thickness, and slice spacing as low as signal-to-noise ratio allows for evaluation of the 1st MTP joint.

Since the SP ligament is on average of 2 mm in depth and 3 mm in width, it is important to set adequate parameters to obtain optimal diagnostic images. The parameters provided are vendor independent (**Table 1**).

Lower matrix, larger field of view, and slightly thicker sections should be used with low-field scanners. Vendor-dependent parameters in acquiring turf toe images are beyond the scope of this article.

PATHOLOGY

Turf toe is synonymous with a plantar plate sprain of the 1st MTP joint. Variations of turf toe include injury to any portion of the plantar capsuloligamentous complex. Several classifications have been devised to grade turf toe (**Table 2**). In a clinical setting, 3 grades of turf toe injury have generally been described.[15,21] MR imaging of turf toe is an adjunct tool to turf toe classification because it details the injured portion of the plantar capsuloligamentous complex and grades severity of the injury.

MR grading of ligamentous injury is consistent throughout the body and is intended to match clinical evaluation. A grade 1 ligament sprain presents on MR imaging as contiguous ligament fibers with adjacent soft tissue edema; a grade 2 ligament injury presents with partial disruption of fibers and edema; finally, a grade 3 ligament injury presents with full-thickness disruption of fibers.

Table 1
Turf toe magnetic resonance protocol for high-field scanner, 4–8 channel coil

Sequence	Repetition Time/ Echo Time (milliseconds)	Field of View	Matrix	Slice Thickness (mm)	Slice Spacing (mm); No More than 10% Gap	Number of Excitations
Coronal PD FSE	2–4K/35–45	10–12	384/224	3	0.3	2–3
Coronal PD FSE FS	3–4K/45–55	10–12	320/224	3	0.3	2–3
Axial PD FSE	2–4K/35–45	10–12	384/224	2.5–3	0.25–0.3	2–3
Axial PD FSE FS	3–4K/45–55	10–12	320/224	2.5–3	0.25–0.3	2–3
Sagittal PD FSE	2–4K/35–45	10–12	320/224	2.5–3	0.25–0.3	2–3
Sagittal PD FSE FS	3–4K/45–55	10–12	320/224	2.5–3	0.25–0.3	2–3

Abbreviations: FS, fat-suppressed; FSE, fast spin-echo.

In turf toe, SP ligament is a commonly injured structure and is used interchangeably with the term plantar plate. SP ligament injury may be unilateral or bilateral (**Fig. 3**B). Although best seen on sagittal and coronal images, a large SP ligament tear defect may also be well depicted on axial images (**Fig. 5**B). As always, it emphasizes the importance of visualizing any anatomic structure in 3 planes. In cases of unilateral SP ligament injury, the medial SP ligament is more commonly injured (**Figs. 2**C and **3**C). Lack of excursion of the sesamoid on plain film or fluoroscopy with stress (dorsiflexion) lateral view indicates SP ligament tear (**Fig. 6**). Ultrasound has been shown of great value in diagnosing ligament tears by measuring increased joint laxity with stress, for example, with ulnar collateral ligament tears in baseball pitchers.[22] Similarly, ultrasound has been useful to show increased gapping of the SP interval and lack of sesamoid excursion with stress (dorsiflexion).[23] It is clinically relevant for radiologists to note the presence and amount of sesamoid retraction that can occur with SP ligament injury on plain film and MR imaging. The 1st MTP joint line and the contralateral sesamoid serve as good reference points to assess for retraction.

In cases of loading of force proximal on the dorsiflexed 1st MTP joint, the resulting injury involves the proximal capsule termed, in this article, the MT-S ligaments (**Fig. 2**B). The tear is often

Table 2
Classification of acute turf toe

Grade	Clinical	Radiograph	MR Imaging	Pathology
1	Mild swelling, point tenderness, no ecchymosis	Normal	Edema of any portion of the PLC, no tear	No fiber disruption
2	Diffuse tenderness, mild to moderate swelling, ecchymosis, decreased ROM	Normal	Partial tear of any portion of the PLC, edema if acute	Partial tear of any portion of the PLC
3	Severe diffuse tenderness, marked swelling and ecchymosis, marked decreased ROM	Possible fracture, sesamoid retraction, or diastasis of bipartite sesamoid. Lack of sesamoid excursion with stress view	Full thickness tear of any portion of the PLC, edema if acute. Possible fracture, sesamoid retraction, or diastasis of bipartite sesamoid	Full-thickness tear of any portion of the PLC

Summation of classifications by Clanton, Rodeo, and Anderson.
Abbreviations: PLC, plantar capsuloligamentous complex; ROM, range of motion.
Data from Schein AJ, Skalski MR, Patel DB, et al. Turf toe and sesamoiditis: what the radiologist needs to know. Clin Imaging 2015;39(3):380–9.

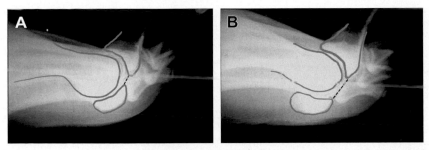

Fig. 6. Forced dorsiflexion lateral x-ray views with highlighted contour of the hallux sesamoid complex. (*A*) Normal. Note the normal distance between the sesamoid and 1st phalanx base (*dotted line*). (*B*) Abnormal. There is increased distance (lack of excursion) between the sesamoid and the 1st phalanx base indicative of SP ligament disruption (*dotted line*). (*Courtesy of* Thomas Clanton, MD, Vail, Colorado.)

accompanied by secondary hemorrhage into the underlying flexor hallucis brevis muscle belly. The finding can be visualized on sagittal and axial images (**Fig. 5C**). This proximal capsular injury is not as destabilizing as a SP ligament tear because of the overlying intact sesamoid attachments of the flexor hallucis brevis. As a result, there is no sesamoid retraction with this type of injury. A turf toe variation with valgus component to this injury can result in strain and tearing of the abductor hallucis tendon.

IS ligament rupture can result in widening of the interval between the medial and lateral sesamoids. IS ligament tear is best visualized on the coronal short axis images at the level of the sesamoids (**Fig. 4B**). Isolated IS ligament injury is a rare occurrence. IS ligament injury occurs with hallux dislocation and larger capsular rupture of the 1st MTP joint.

Severe valgus injury to the 1st MTP joint can result in tearing of the medial collateral ligament. This ligament typically tears proximally and is best appreciated on axial and coronal images (**Fig. 4C**). Associated traumatic hallux valgus deformity is important to report because such findings could favor surgical intervention.

Another variation of turf toe injury with combined valgus and dorsiflexion of the 1st MTP joint may involve the medial accessory collateral ligament with stripping of the capsuloligamentous complex from the medial border of the tibial sesamoid (**Figs. 4 and 7**). The presence of Sharpey fibers and their accompanying nerve endings at this capsuloligamentous peripheral sesamoid attachment render the site particularly sensitive and tender when injured.[19]

Turf toe injuries involving the lateral border of the 1st MTP joint are uncommon.

Varus forces may result in tearing of the adductor hallucis tendon and capsule from the lateral border of the fibular sesamoid or may also result in lateral collateral ligament tearing.

Forces contributing to turf toe may extend beyond the soft tissue of the plantar capsuloligamentous complex to involve the chondral surfaces and osseous structures of the joint (**Fig. 8**). The

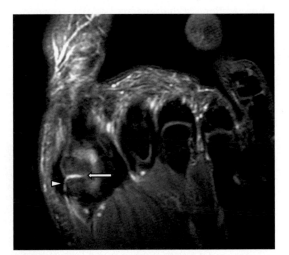

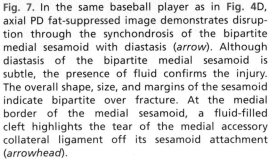

Fig. 7. In the same baseball player as in **Fig. 4D**, axial PD fat-suppressed image demonstrates disruption through the synchondrosis of the bipartite medial sesamoid with diastasis (*arrow*). Although diastasis of the bipartite medial sesamoid is subtle, the presence of fluid confirms the injury. The overall shape, size, and margins of the sesamoid indicate bipartite over fracture. At the medial border of the medial sesamoid, a fluid-filled cleft highlights the tear of the medial accessory collateral ligament off its sesamoid attachment (*arrowhead*).

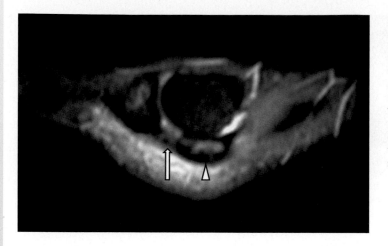

Fig. 8. Sagittal PD fat-suppressed image illustrates a mild turf toe injury characterized by a grade 1 medial SP ligament sprain (*arrow*) and medial sesamoid osseous contusion (*arrowhead*) in a gymnast. Medial SP ligament sprain is characterized by thickening, edema, and indistinct margin in this case. Subcutaneous edema is noted along the plantar surface of the 1st MTP joint from soft tissue contusion.

location and function of the sesamoids put them at a higher risk of injury relative to the 1st metatarsal and 1st proximal phalanx in the setting of turf toe.[19] The medial sesamoid is more frequently injured than the lateral sesamoid, likely secondary to its greater weight-bearing responsibility in the joint mechanics.[24] In a bipartite sesamoid, both parts are bridged by a synchondrosis. Similar to other locations in the musculoskeletal system, for example, at an accessory navicular, os trigonum, or os acromiale,[25] the synchondrosis can get disrupted. In turf toe, 2 distracted sesamoid fragments should always raise suspicion of disruption of the synchondrosis of a bipartite sesamoid with associated diastasis (see **Fig. 7**) versus a fractured sesamoid. Sesamoid diastasis and fractures are important in the discussion of turf toe because they represent indications for possible surgical intervention. Similarly, osteochondral injury, chondral surface disruption, and intra-articular loose body could alter therapy and warrant surgery. Severe turf toe is associated with joint instability. The untreated, chronically unstable turf toe leads to accelerated arthrosis, and ultimately to hallux rigidus. As elsewhere in the musculoskeletal system, early arthrosis in athletes, especially in young patients, suggests underlying trauma and secondary joint instability.[26] In cases of large

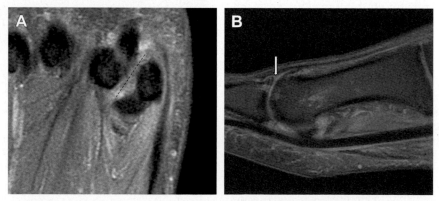

Fig. 9. PD fat-suppressed images. (*A*) Axial image offers a unique view of a large plantar capsular tear of the 1st MTP joint. The dotted line outlines the oblique course of the tear gap extending proximally from the torn lateral MT-S ligament, through the IS ligament defect, and to the torn medial SP ligament. (*B*) Sagittal image of the same case shows findings of untreated chronic turf toe characterized by the triad of arthrosis: dorsal cartilage loss to bone (*arrow*), joint space narrowing, and spurring. Hallux rigidus is a late manifestation of chronic turf toe.

Box 1
Diagnostic checklist for MR imaging turf toe
Structure
SP ligaments (medial and lateral)
MT-S ligaments (medial and lateral)
IS ligament
Collateral ligaments proper (medial and lateral)
Accessory collateral ligaments to the sesamoids (plantar medial and plantar lateral capsule)
Tendinous insertions and confluences with the plantar capsule (flexor hallucis brevis, abductor and adductor hallucis)
Sesamoids (medial and lateral)
Cartilage
Alignment

capsular tear, osteochondral injury and chondral wear occur classically along the dorsum of the joint in conjunction with dorsal impaction (**Fig. 9**).[5,14,27]

This review of turf toe anatomy and pathology should guide the MR interpretation of the 1st MTP joint (**Box 1, Table 3**).

Table 3	
What the clinician needs to know	
Grade of soft tissue injury	No, partial, or full-thickness tear
Extent of soft tissue injury	Structures involved
Location of tear (in case of surgical repair)	Structure torn from the sesamoid, phalanx vs metatarsal
Sesamoid retraction	Absence vs presence in case of SP ligament tear
Bone injury	Contusion, fracture, or diastasis of bipartite sesamoid
Chondral injury	Extent and grade of cartilage loss; acute vs chronic; presence of loose body
Alignment	Phalangeal subluxation or traumatic hallux valgus

SUMMARY

Forty years ago, turf toe was an esoteric diagnosis and MR imaging was in its infancy. Over time, both have progressed and crossed paths with their individual, impactful results in the world of sports and medicine. Turf toe is no longer a bucket diagnosis of a plantar plate injury in a football player on artificial turf. MR imaging has revealed what parts of the broader plantar capsuloligamentous complex are injured in a wide variety of athletes on multiple different surfaces. The additional details of subtle to severe turf toe injury and associated complications have increased MR imaging utilization. The resulting earlier, more accurate diagnosis has changed the course of conservative treatment and provided a road map for potential surgery. Giving athletes the opportunity for full recovery and decreasing the morbidity of this injury are the ultimate victories for all involved.

REFERENCES

1. Bowers KD, Martin RB. Turf toe: a shoe-surface related football injury. Med Sci Sports 1976;8(2):81–3.
2. Damadian RV, Goldsmith M, Minkoff L. NMR in cancer XVI. FONAR image of the live human body. Physiol Chem Phys 1977;9(1):97–100.
3. Wilson L, Dimeff R, Miniaci A, et al. Radiologic case study. First metatarsophalangeal plantar injury (turf toe). Orthopedics 2005;28(4):417–9.
4. Meyers MC, Barnhill BS. Incidence, causes, and severity of high school football injuries on FieldTurf versus natural grass: a 5-year prospective study. Am J Sports Med 2004;32(7):1626–38.
5. Clanton TO, Ford JJ. Turf toe injury. Clin Sports Med 1994;13:731–41.
6. Rodeo SA, O'Brien SJ, Warren RF, et al. Turf toe: an analysis of metatarsophalangeal joint sprains in professional football players. Am J Sports Med 1990;18(3):280–5.
7. McBride ID, Wys UP, Cooke TD, et al. First metatarsophalangeal joint reaction forces during high-heel gait. Foot Ankle 1991;11(5):202–8.
8. Clanton TO, Butler JE, Eggert A. Injuries to the metatarsophalangeal joints in athletes. Foot Ankle 1986;7(3):162–76.
9. Joseph J. Range of movement of the great toe in men. J Bone Joint Surg Br 1954;36:450–7.
10. Gregg J, Marks P, Silberstein M, et al. Histologic anatomy of the lesser metatarsophalangeal joint plantar plate. Surg Radiol Anat 2007;29(2):141–7.
11. Gregg JM, Siberstein M, Schneider T, et al. Sonography of plantar plates in cadaver: correlation with MRI and histology. Am J Roentgenol 2006;186(4):948–55.

12. Netter FH. Atlas of human anatomy. 6th edition. Philadelphia (PA): Saunders, Elsevier; 2014.

13. Schein AJ, Skalski MR, Patel DB, et al. Turf toe and sesamoiditis: what the radiologist needs to know. Clin Imaging 2015;39(3):380–9.

14. Watson TS, Anderson RB, Davis WH. Periarticular injuries to the hallux metatarsophalangeal joint in athlete. Foot Ankle Clin 2000;5(3):687–713.

15. Mason LW, Molloy AP. Turf toe and disorders of the sesamoid complex. Clin Sports Med 2015;34(4): 725–39.

16. McCormick JJ, Anderson R. Turf toe: anatomy, diagnosis and treatment. Sports Health 2010;2(6): 487–94.

17. Linklater JM. Imaging of sports injuries in the foot. Am J Roentgenol 2012;199:500–8.

18. Awh, M. 2012. Available at: www.radsource.us/clinic-turf-toe/. Accessed December 24, 2015.

19. Dedmond B, Cory J, McBryde A. The hallucal sesamoid complex. J Am Acad Orthop Surg 2006;14: 745–53.

20. Theumann NH, Pfirrmann CWA, Drapé JL, et al. MR imaging of the metacarpophalangeal joints of the fingers. Radiology 2002;222(2):437–45.

21. Jahss MH. Traumatic dislocations of the first metatarsophalangeal joint. Foot Ankle 1980;1(1):15–21.

22. Roedl JB, Gonzalez FM, Zoga AC, et al. Potential utility of a combined approach with US and MR arthrography to image medial elbow pain in baseball players. Radiology 2016. http://dx.doi.org/10.1148/radiol.2015151256.

23. Feuerstein CA, Weil L Jr, Weil LS Sr, et al. Static versus dynamic musculoskeletal ultrasound for detection of plantar plate pathology. Foot Ankle Spec 2014;7(4):259–65.

24. Oloff LM, Schuflhofer DS. Sesamoid complex disorders. Clin Podiatr Med Surg 1996;13(3):497–513.

25. Roedl JB, Morrison WB, Ciccotti MG, et al. Acromial apophysiolysis: superior shoulder pain and acromial nonfusion in the young throwing athlete. Radiology 2015;274(1):201–9.

26. Roedl JB, Nevalainen M, Gonzalez FM, et al. Frequency, imaging findings, risk factors, and long-term sequelae of distal clavicular osteolysis in young patients. Skeletal Radiol 2015;44(5): 659–66.

27. Kubitz ER. Athletic injuries of the first metatarsophalangeal joint. J Am Podiatr Med Assoc 2003;93:325–32.

The Role of Imaging in Determining Return to Play

Bethany U. Casagranda, DO*, Peter C. Thurlow, MD

KEYWORDS

- Return to play • MR imaging • Rotator cuff • Cartilage • Anterior cruciate ligament reconstruction
- Stress fractures • Concussion

KEY POINTS

- Return to play (RTP) means return to the preinjury level of athletic activity after sustaining an injury.
- The increasing level of competition among athletes and the pressure to return quickly after an injury makes RTP a particularly important subject for medical professionals involved in the treatment of musculoskeletal injuries.
- Balancing a quick return to maximal performance with the risk of reinjury or even the risk of worsening long-term injury is critical.
- The radiologist can help predict the appropriate RTP time for a specific subset of sports-related injuries.

INTRODUCTION

The increasing level of competition among younger and younger athletes, combined with the physical, emotional, and social stresses of athletes encumbered by injury, makes return to play (RTP) a particularly important subject for medical professionals involved in the treatment of musculoskeletal. From the first pitch of the Little League season to the last down in the Super Bowl, athletes are affected by injuries that may limit their participation or careers. Time is precious for a professional athlete, with a mean career length of 4.8 years for professional baseball pitchers and 3.5 years for a player in the National Football League (NFL).[1–3] Therefore, it is understandable that a fast RTP is desirable; but it has to be balanced with complete healing and recovery. The risk of reinjury or chronic injury has to be kept minimal to not jeopardize the athlete's health.

SHOULDER
Elite Overhead Throwers

Rotator cuff pathology is common in athletes performing repetitive overhead arm motions, such as baseball players, quarterbacks, tennis players, and swimmers.[1] Partial-thickness rotator cuff tears of less than 50% cross section of the tendon (**Fig. 1**) are often treated with arthroscopic debridement. Treatment of larger tears is heavily debated between debridement versus cuff repair. Although debridement of partial tears allows most players to return to some degree of play, only about half return to their previous level of competition.[1] RTP has been shown to be different based on the sport, with golf and football players halted for an average of 4 months and the tennis elite out of play approximately for 9 months. Although baseball pitchers return to some degree of play at 6 months, full throwing in baseball pitchers may take up to

Disclosure Statement: The authors have nothing to disclose.
Division of Musculoskeletal Radiology, Department of Radiology, Allegheny General Hospital, 320 East North Avenue, Pittsburgh, PA 15212, USA
* Corresponding author.
E-mail address: bcasagra@wpahs.org

Radiol Clin N Am 54 (2016) 979–988
http://dx.doi.org/10.1016/j.rcl.2016.05.003

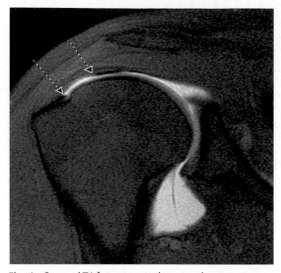

Fig. 1. Coronal T1 fat-saturated magnetic resonance arthrogram in a collegiate football player delineates the margins of a low-grade partial tear (*arrows*) involving the articular-sided fibers of supraspinatus. The torn fibers involve less than 50% cross section of the tendon.

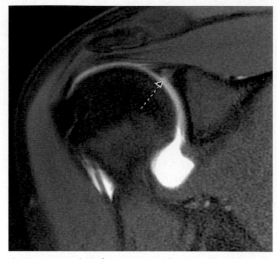

Fig. 2. Coronal T1 fat-suppressed magnetic resonance arthrogram shows contrast entering an isolated SLAP tear (*arrow*) of the superoposterior labrum in a high school football player.

1 year.[2] A recent study by the Jefferson group described a stress response across the immature acromial physis in adolescent baseball pitchers, which resulted in complete nonfusion and the development of an os acromiale in most affected patients later in life.[4] This occurred in young players throwing more than 100 pitches per month. Because of the high risk of nonfusion, the stress response across the immature physis was termed *acromial apophysiolysis*, similar to spondylosis at the pedicles of the lumbar spine (pars defects). It was shown that pitchers with acromial apophysiolysis were at high risk for rotator cuff tendon tears later in their mid 20s. Stress response and osteolysis at the distal clavicle is also seen in young overhead athletes but only in association with weight training, specifically bench pressing.[5]

Superior labrum anterior posterior (SLAP) lesions are part of the thrower's shoulder but are often seen in contact athletes as well.[3,6,7] The importance of separating the thrower from the contact athlete is illustrated by the different RTP times. A thrower's shoulder in the setting of an SLAP lesion often has several other concomitant injuries with a return-to-sport time of about 3 to 6 months but full throwing time of nearly 1 year.[3] However, the contact athlete with repair of an isolated SLAP lesion (**Fig. 2**) recovers quickly, with an average RTP time of 2.6 months.[7] Magnetic resonance (MR) arthrography is the imaging modality of choice for labral pathology and is also helpful for the evaluation of the postoperative shoulder.[3] Elbow injuries in overhead throwers, including

ulnar collateral ligament (UCL) tears, ulnar neuritis, posteromedial impingement, and myotendinous injuries are discussed elsewhere in this issue and have varying RTP times with full recovery after UCL reconstruction averaging around 1.5 years.[8]

KNEE
Anterior Cruciate Ligament Tears

A common injury affecting nearly all sports is the anterior cruciate ligament (ACL) tear. The ACL has 2 distinct bundles: the anteromedial bundle and the posterolateral bundle contributing to translational and rotational stability of the knee.[9] Operative and nonoperative treatments have been investigated in an attempt to expedite RTP. Nonoperative treatment has patients non–weight bearing for 6 weeks. Depending on the time of injury, this may allow the player to participate in part of the season. However, quick RTP has consequences, including recurrent knee buckling even while wearing a brace as well as progressive injury to the meniscus and cartilage.[10]

Operative treatment includes single, double, or selective bundle autograft or allograft reconstructions, with several factors affecting RTP. Elite athletes in the NFL return faster and perform better than earlier level athletes. This finding is thought be due to nonclinical factors helping the recovery, including physical conditioning, time, money, and rehabilitation resources. Interestingly, 2 factors strongly associated with RTP include the position of the professional football player and draft round. For example, wide receivers and quarterbacks have an RTP of 100% following ACL reconstruction, whereas offensive linemen fair at about 40%. First- and second-round draft picks RTP in 100% of cases with the sixth-round draft picks averaging 33% RTP.[2]

A recent literature review shows 40% of studies fail to provide any measure for RTP after surgery. Most studies (32%) determine RTP status after ACL reconstruction by using only postoperative time, with the common RTP time being 12 months. Only 13% of studies used at least one objective criterion, such as muscle strength and hop performance; but these common performance examinations have shown to be either not demanding enough or sensitive enough to identify differences between the postoperative and contralateral knee.[11,12] Bonfim and colleagues[13] reported altered knee kinematics up to 12 months, but sensory and motor deficits were appreciated as long as 30 months into the postoperative period. This finding is important because 12 months is likely too early for most athletes to RTP, and it has been shown that early RTP in reconstructed ACL knees is one reason for graft failure.[14] This finding is supported by a recent survey of patients at 12 months whereby two-thirds of patients had not returned to play. Of those that returned to play, only 33% attempted competitive sports. If a patient returned to play after 12 months, this did not predict how the patient would perform long-term. Despite the many advances in ACL reconstruction, less than 50% of athletes have returned to play when surveyed between 2 and 7 years following surgery.[14–16]

Other Common Knee Injuries

Other injuries, including closed degloving injuries (Moral-Lavallee lesions) and isolated lateral collateral ligament injuries of the knee, are managed nonoperatively with rapid RTP at the professional level (Fig. 3).[17,18] Although some cartilage injuries to the knee require surgical repair, studies show a high rate of RTP, often at the preinjury level.[19] Interestingly, a recent meta-analysis concluded that microfracture patients were least likely to RTP when compared with other operative approaches to cartilage repair.[20] Additionally, National Basketball Association (NBA) athletes have a higher reinjury rate and decreased athletic performance after undergoing microfracture when compared with NFL players and alpine skiers.[20] However, concomitant injuries and variable biomechanical stresses in different sports may confound these results. Younger age, shorter preoperative duration of symptoms, no prior history of surgical intervention, more rigorous rehabilitation protocols, and smaller cartilage defects (<2 cm^2) were all associated with better prognosis. Similar surgical cartilage repair techniques are used at the ankle and elbow. However, RTP outcome data are more limited at these locations. A recent retrospective study reported that 90% of professional athletes returned to the preinjury performance level at 12 months following autologous osteochondral transplantation.[21]

MR imaging diagnosis of the aforementioned knee injuries have been documented with high specificity and sensitivity.[22–24] At some institutions, standard MR sequences may be supplemented with a coronal oblique sequence (Fig. 4) for dedicated double-bundle ACL interrogation at the request of orthopedic surgeons who perform double-bundle and selective-bundle ACL reconstructions.[9]

LUMBAR SPINE

Back pain is a common ailment of athletes, with 9% to 15% of all athletic injuries involving the

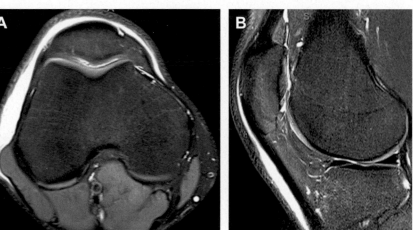

Fig. 3. Axial (A) and sagittal (B) T2 images illustrate fluid equivalent signal separating the subcutaneous fat from the underlying superficial fascia compatible with a closed degloving injury in a collegiate football player.

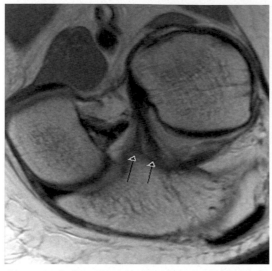

Fig. 4. A dedicated coronal oblique proton-density sequence separates the anteromedial and posterolateral bundles of the anterior cruciate ligament. *Arrows* point to the separated double bundle anatomy of the ACL.

spine, most treated conservatively. Common causes of athletic back pain include spondylosis, spondylolisthesis, and disc herniation.[25]

Spondylosis/Spondylolisthesis

Pars interarticularis fractures (**Fig. 5**) reveal themselves most commonly in sports with extension or extension/rotation forces on the lumber spine. Most patients do well with conservative treatment with RTP on average 9 to 12 months.

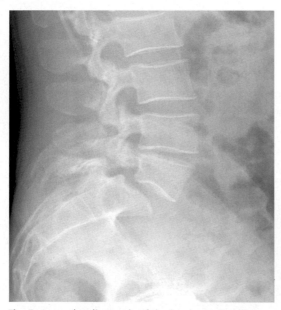

Fig. 5. Lateral radiograph of the lumbar spine demonstrating bilateral L5 pars interarticularis defects in 22-year-old male collegiate football player.

Conservative measures include rest and gradual rehabilitation. Conservative therapy success has been associated with early diagnosis, unilaterality, and absence of listhesis.

Surgery may be necessary in cases of nonunion with persistent pain, increase in listhesis, or development of neurologic deficits. Surgical options include pars repair or posterolateral fusion with or without decompression.[25] RTP averages 6 months. However, RTP to collision sports following spine fusion is highly controversial. This point is evident in the fact that 96% of professional team physicians surveyed downgrade the rating of players with known spondylolisthesis before the NFL draft.[26]

Lumbar Disc Herniation

Conservative treatment is attempted first for disc herniations, including antiinflammatories, rest, physical therapy, and therapeutic injection. Epidural steroid injections (**Fig. 6**) have proven to be an effective therapeutic option for disc herniation, with 89% successful RTP and less than one game missed following injection. Risk factors for failing injection therapy include disc sequestration and documented muscle weakness on physical examination.[27] If conservative treatment fails, surgical options include microdiscectomy or spinal fusion. One-level discectomy tends to have better RTP outcomes than multilevel cases.[28] RTP following microdiscectomy requires absence of pain and normal range of motion with 6 to 8 weeks recovery for noncollision sports and 3 months for collision sports.[29] Surgical fusion is used for more complicated cases with multilevel disc involvement or spinal instability. Ninety-one percent of surgeons allow for RTP to collision and noncollision sports within 1 year despite many critics questioning safety of return to collision sports following spinal fusion.[30]

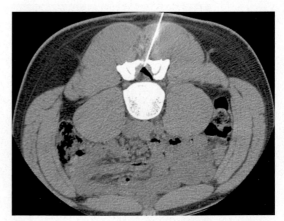

Fig. 6. Computed tomography–guided epidural steroid injection for treatment of lumbar herniated disc in a 19-year-old male collegiate football player.

One subset of elite athlete has been shown to greatly benefit from surgery for herniated disc: the NFL lineman. This particular athlete has an average body mass index of 40 with position requirements placing extraordinary demands on the lumbar spine during weight training and positional stance during play. Successful RTP numbers are approximately 81% following discectomy with or without laminectomy. Of the small subset that required revision, 86% were able to RTP.[31]

HAMSTRING

Almost any muscle or tendon can get injured during athletic activity, but the hamstrings warrant special attention because they are the most commonly injured group in athletes.[32] Why are the hamstrings so prone to sports-related injury? The tendons cross 2 joints and are subject to significant force from eccentric contraction during gait or running motion.[33] The clinical difficulty in hamstring injuries is balancing RTP with the risk of recurrence. There are no agreed-on criteria for safe RTP that eliminates the recurrence risk while allowing maximal performance.[32] Clinical predictors associated with RTP include time to walk pain free (<24 hours), history of prior hamstring injury, and the specific tendons injured.[34] Historically, semimembranosus injuries do well as opposed to lateral injures involving the biceps femoris, which carry a worse prognosis.[32,33]

Reviewing proximal hamstring anatomy, the 3 tendons originate from the ischial tuberosity as 2 discrete structures: the conjoined tendon formed by semitendinosus and biceps femoris as well as the more lateral origin of the semimembranosus tendon. Hamstring strains most commonly involve the myotendinous junction.[33]

The role of the radiologist is very specific in the setting of hamstring injury. Complete tears (Fig. 7), including proximal hamstring avulsions, must be recognized and treated operatively without delay. Partial tearing (Fig. 8) must be systematically described, including the specific tendons torn, the distance from the ischial tuberosity, and the length of the tear and the percent of tendon/muscle torn in cross section. Additionally, a clear distinction between disruption of the central tendon or injury to the adjacent musculature is critical in determining RTP. Comin and colleagues reported the mean RTP of 72 days (range 42–109 days) with central tendon disruption compared with the mean RTP of 21 days (range 9–28 days) in cases of partial hamstring tear in which the central tendon remained intact (Comin AJSM 2013).[35] Axial sequences on MR imaging can be obtained as a pelvis if comparison with the asymptomatic side is deemed helpful. However, spatial resolution will decrease with the larger field of view when compared with a dedicated MR hip protocol.

Imaging has also been used in treating hamstring injuries. The efficacy of ultrasound-guided hematoma aspirations and corticosteroid injections in the setting of acute injury have been debated in the literature.[33,36] Ultrasound or computed tomography (CT)–guided injection of autologous growth factors, including platelet-rich plasma (PRP), has gained popularity (Fig. 9). Several studies have discussed the healing potential of growth factor injections; however, randomized controlled trials have yielded equivocal results when compared with aggressive physical therapy alone.[37–40]

ANKLE
High Ankle Sprain

Inversion ankle sprains involving the anterior talofibular ligament and/or the calcaneofibular ligament are the most common ankle injuries with proven RTP success when treated conservatively.[41]

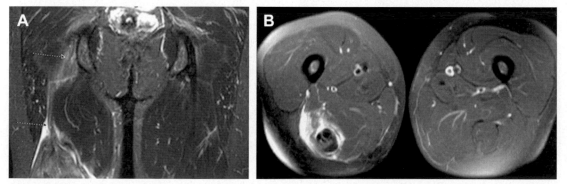

Fig. 7. T2 fat-suppressed images in the coronal (A) and axial (B) planes reveal a complete hamstring rupture from the right ischial tuberosity with approximately 13 cm retraction from the origin (arrows). No avulsion fracture was identified.

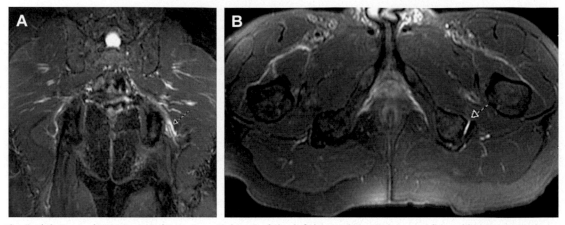

Fig. 8. (*A*) Coronal STIR image shows a partial tear of the left hamstring origin as evidenced by T2 hyperintense linear signal (*arrow*). (*B*) Axial T2 fat-suppressed images confirms a partial tear of the left hamstring (*arrow*).

However, the dreaded high ankle sprain involving the syndesmotic ligament complex is more common in collision sports and boot sports, such as skiing and hockey. High ankle sprains affect recreational and professional athletes alike with complications including delayed RTP, persistent pain, and long-term disability.[41,42]

The syndesmotic ligament complex is composed of 4 distinct structures: anterior inferior tibiofibular ligament (most commonly injured); posterior inferior tibiofibular ligament (PITFL); inferior transverse tibiofibular ligament, which is located inferior to the PITFL; and the most distal aspect of the interosseous membrane.[41]

Delay in diagnosis increases complication risks and delays recovery. Therefore, accurate imaging interpretation is critical. Imaging evaluation begins

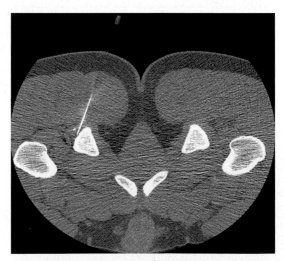

Fig. 9. A single axial image of a CT-guided autologous conditioned plasma injection for the treatment of a partial tear involving the left hamstring origin in an elite football player. (*Courtesy of* Dr Jeffrey Towers.)

with 3-view radiographs of the ankle (anteroposterior [AP], lateral, and oblique/mortise views) and at least 2 views of the tibia/fibula. Weight bearing is preferred but often not tolerated in the acute setting. The role of the radiologist is to identify fractures and evaluate the 3 classic parameters for syndesmotic injury, including tibiofibular clear space, medial clear space, and tibiofibular overlap. The tibiofibular clear space has been shown to be the most reliable when measured 1 cm proximal to the talar dome. Normal measurement is less than or equal to 5 mm on AP or mortise views. Normal medial clear space measurement is less than or equal to 4 mm. The tibiofibular overlap should always be present on all views. In severe cases, all measurements can be abnormal (**Fig. 10**A). Stress radiographs can be helpful when positive (**Fig. 10**B) but have a high false-negative rate.[41] MR imaging has yielded high interobserver agreement in evaluating for syndesmotic injury (**Fig. 11**) and sensitivities/specificities ranging from 93% to 100%. However, the association between MR imaging findings and clinical outcome or the need for surgical management has not been studied yet.[42]

Gerber and colleagues[43] described the West Point Ankle Grading system classifying syndesmotic injuries into 3 categories based on clinical stability. Their findings suggest syndesmotic injuries are more common than previously thought, and most patients with ankle injuries RTP prematurely. Persistent ankle dysfunction was seen in 40% of their patients 6 months after the initial injury. Grade 1 injuries are stable on examination with a good end point. Following 2 to 4 weeks of bracing, the patients can RTP once symptom free. Grade 2 injuries revealed mild laxity on examination and are treated with cast immobilization for 6 to 8 weeks or surgical consideration. Grade 3 injuries are frankly unstable

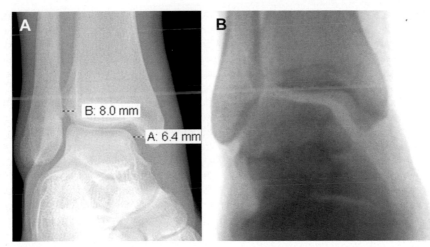

Fig. 10. (*A*) A mortise view of the right ankle reveals a severe syndesmotic injury with abnormal measurements of the tibiofibular distance and the medial clear space. There is very little overlap of the distal tibia and fibula, which normally is present on all 3 standard views of the ankle. (*B*) Stress view under fluoroscopy shows widening of the medial clear space with asymmetry to the mortise indicating instability.

and most often undergo surgical management with direct ligament repair or internal fixation.[41] At the authors' institution, direct ligamentous repair is rarely performed, and tightrope procedures or internal fixation are preferred. A recent randomized controlled

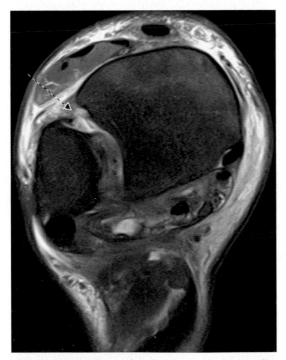

Fig. 11. MR imaging of the right ankle in an elite hockey player revealed various degrees of injury to all components of the syndesmotic ligament complex. This axial T2 fat-suppressed image shows a complete tear specifically of the anterior inferior tibiofibular ligament (*arrow*).

trial of ultrasound-guided PRP injection for grade 3 AITFL injury in elite athletes demonstrated shorter RTP, improved syndesmotic joint stability, and decreased long-term residual pain in the PRP group.[44]

Achilles Tendon Rupture

Achilles tendon rupture is specifically mentioned because it can be a career-altering injury as shown by an NFL documentation. Thirty-two percent of NFL players sustaining a complete Achilles rupture do not RTP. Of those who return, their power ratings were reduced by greater than 50%.[45,46] At the authors' institution, MR imaging is the most common modality used in evaluating the Achilles tendon with patients positioned in dorsiflexion.

HIGH-RISK STRESS FRACTURES

A common injury in athletes is the stress fracture. Certain bones are historically affected secondary to their location and forces placed on them during weight-bearing activity. The goal is to prevent complete fracture/bone failure with appropriate treatment based upon imaging findings and clinical evaluation. Stress fractures are defined as low risk or high risk based on the compression versus tension forces acting on the bone.[47] Kaeding and colleagues[48] proposed a management algorithm for stress fractures using these definitions.

Low-risk stress fractures can be managed based on symptoms. Many of these fractures will heal in 4 to 8 weeks if kept at a pain-free activity level. This limitation can be challenging in highly competitive athletes who want to RTP as soon as possible.[48]

High-risk stress fracture locations include the medial femoral neck, patella (**Fig. 12**), anterior tibial diaphysis, medial malleolus, talus, tarsal navicular, fifth metatarsal, and sesamoids. The risks and complications of these fractures include progression to complete fracture, nonunion, recurrence/refracture, and need for operative intervention. Therefore, imaging findings of a clear fracture line involving a high-risk bone often prompts operative management or at least immobilization with non–weight bearing.[48]

Radiologists can assist in the management of stress fractures by identifying low-risk versus high-risk bones and by identifying stress response before the development of stress fracture. Early diagnosis has shown early RTP[49]; when bone marrow edema is present without a fracture line, stress response is the likely diagnosis and should be communicated with the referring physician. When following up stress response/stress fracture cases, remember that imaging findings can continue to show abnormalities even when symptoms have improved.[49] Therefore, communication with the referring physician is critical in successful management of these patients.

CONCUSSION

Sports-related traumatic brain injury has become a popular media subject with a significant amount of recent research on the topic. Several sources agree that complete recovery is necessary before RTP. However, guiding safe RTP has been a clinical challenge. Traditional treatment and RTP decisions were based on clinical judgment and indirect

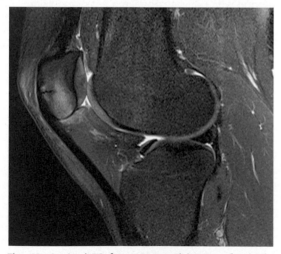

Fig. 12. Sagittal T2 fat-suppressed image of a high-risk stress fracture of the patella in a 22-year-old female collegiate basketball player.

measures, such as brief cognitive tests, loss of consciousness, headache, and amnesia.[50] The breadth of diagnostic modalities has increased with neuropsychological testing, balance testing, imaging, and physical examination with an emphasis on neurologic interrogation. The introduction of computerized testing to the comprehensive assessment of players who sustained a concussion has revealed devastating subclinical deficits, such as prolonged cognitive decline and strong correlation with depression/anxiety, substance abuse, and suicidal ideation.[50,51] Despite the disturbing information on the topic, athletes from all levels are returning to play prematurely. Athletic trainers admit to relying on symptoms over neurocognitive test scores in determining RTP; RTP guidelines are being ignored, with documented poor compliance found among high school athletes.[52,53]

Team approach to an athlete has never been more important than with concussion, as the consequence of early RTP can be fatal. Three major concerns with RTP include second impact syndrome (SIS), prolonged recovery from sequential concussions (postconcussion syndrome [PCS]), and chronic traumatic encephalopathy (CTE). SIS is devastating, with documented mortality of 50% and morbidity of nearly 100%. This syndrome is thought to come from incomplete recovery after the initial event. PCS describes prolonged symptoms after initial injury. If symptoms continue to persist, athletes may be out for the season or, in some circumstances, are advised to retire from the sport. CTE results from repetitive brain injury first described in boxers and recently recognized in the NFL. Symptoms include loss of intellect, memory, and balance as well as behavioral changes and symptoms resembling Parkinson disease.[54]

Imaging is leading the research in the concussion dilemma. Anatomic evaluation with head CT and MR imaging can evaluate for fracture, contusion, and hemorrhage. However, these studies are often normal when symptoms clearly reveal some degree of brain injury. Functional and metabolic imaging, such as MR spectroscopy, diffusion tensor imaging, functional MR imaging, PET, and single-photon emission CT, are currently being studied in hopes of improving the diagnosis and treatment of athletes with head trauma.[55,56]

REFERENCES

1. Reynolds SB, Dugas JR, Cain EL, et al. Debridement of small partial-thickness rotator cuff tears in elite overhead throwers. Clin Orthop Relat Res 2008; 466(3):614–21.

2. Shah VM, Andrews JR, Fleisig GS, et al. Return to play after anterior cruciate ligament reconstruction in National Football League athletes. Am J Sports Med 2010;38(11):2233–9.

3. Park HB, Lin SK, Yokota A, et al. Return to play for rotator cuff injuries and superior labrum anterior posterior (SLAP) lesions. Clin Sports Med 2004;23(3):321–34, vii.

4. Roedl JB, Morrison WB, Ciccotti MG, et al. Acromial apophysiolysis: superior shoulder pain and acromial nonfusion in the young throwing athlete. Radiology 2015;274(1):201–9.

5. Roedl JB, Nevalainen M, Gonzalez FM, et al. Frequency, imaging findings, risk factors, and long-term sequelae of distal clavicular osteolysis in young patients. Skeletal Radiol 2015;44(5):659–66.

6. Lyman S, Fleisig GS, Andrews JR, et al. Effect of pitch type, pitch count, and pitching mechanics on risk of elbow and shoulder pain in youth baseball pitchers. Am J Sports Med 2002;30(4):463–8.

7. Funk L, Snow M. S_AP tears of the glenoid labrum in contact athletes. Clin J Sport Med 2007;17(1):1–4.

8. Roedl JB, Gonzalez FM, Zoga AC, et al. Potential utility of a combined approach with US and MR arthrography to image medial elbow pain in baseball players. Radiology 2016;279(3):827–37.

9. Casagranda BU, Maxwell NJ, Kavanagh EC, et al. Normal appearance and complications of double-bundle and selective-bundle anterior cruciate ligament reconstructions using optimal MRI techniques. AJR Am J Roentgenol 2009;192(5):1407–15.

10. Shelton WR, Barrett GR, Dukes A. Early season anterior cruciate ligament tears. A treatment dilemma. Am J Sports Med 1997;25(5).656–8.

11. Barber-Westin SD, Noyes FR. Factors used to determine return to unrestricted sports activities after anterior cruciate ligament reconstruction. Arthroscopy 2011;27(12):1697–705.

12. Thomee R, Kaplan Y, Kvist J, et al. Muscle strength and hop performance criteria prior to return to sports after ACL reconstruction. Knee Surg Sports Traumatol Arthrosc 2011;19(11):1798–805.

13. Bonfim TR, Jansen Paccola CA, Barela JA. Proprioceptive and behavior impairments in individuals with anterior cruciate ligament reconstructed knees. Arch Phys Med Rehabil 2003;84(8):1217–23.

14. van Eck CF, Schkrohowsky JG, Working ZM, et al. Prospective analysis of failure rate and predictors of failure after anatomic anterior cruciate ligament reconstruction with allograft. Am J Sports Med 2012;40(4):800–7.

15. Ardern CL, Taylor NF, Feller JA, et al. Return-to-sport outcomes at 2 to 7 years after anterior cruciate ligament reconstruction surgery. Am J Sports Med 2012;40(1):41–8.

16. Ardern CL, Webster KE, Taylor NF, et al. Return to the preinjury level of competitive sport after anterior cruciate ligament reconstruction surgery: two-thirds of patients have not returned by 12 months after surgery. Am J Sports Med 2011;39(3):538–43.

17. Bushnell BD, Bitting SS, Crain JM, et al. Treatment of magnetic resonance imaging-documented isolated grade III lateral collateral ligament injuries in National Football League athletes. Am J Sports Med 2010;38(1):86–91.

18. Tejwani SG, Cohen SB, Bradley JP. Management of Morel-Lavallee lesion of the knee: twenty-seven cases in the National Football League. Am J Sports Med 2007;35(7):1162–7.

19. Mithoefer K, Hambly K, Della Villa S, et al. Return to sports participation after articular cartilage repair in the knee: scientific evidence. Am J Sports Med 2009;37(Suppl 1):167S–76S.

20. Campbell AB, Pineda M, Harris JD, et al. Return to sport after articular cartilage repair in athletes' knees: a systematic review. Arthroscopy 2016;32(4):651–68.e1.

21. Fraser EJ, Harris MC, Prado MP, et al. Autologous osteochondral transplantation for osteochondral lesions of the talus in an athletic population. Knee Surg Sports Traumatol Arthrosc 2016;24(4):1272–9.

22. De Smet AA, Blankenbaker DG, Kijowski R, et al. MR diagnosis of posterior root tears of the lateral meniscus using arthroscopy as the reference standard. AJR Am J Roentgenol 2009;192(2):480–6.

23. Halinen J, Koivikko M, Lindahl J, et al. The efficacy of magnetic resonance imaging in acute multiligament injuries. Int Orthop 2009;33(6):1733–8.

24. Laundre BJ, Collins MS, Bond JR, et al. MRI accuracy for tears of the posterior horn of the lateral meniscus in patients with acute anterior cruciate ligament injury and the clinical relevance of missed tears. AJR Am J Roentgenol 2009;193(2):515–23.

25. Alsobrook J, Clugston JR. Return to play after surgery of the lumbar spine. Curr Sports Med Rep 2008;7(1):45–8.

26. Shaffer B, Wiesel S, Lauerman W. Spondylolisthesis in the elite football player: an epidemiologic study in the NCAA and NFL. J Spinal Disord 1997;10(5):365–70.

27. Krych AJ, Richman D, Drakos M, et al. Epidural steroid injection for lumbar disc herniation in NFL athletes. Med Sci Sports Exerc 2012;44(2):193–8.

28. Wang JC, Shapiro MS, Hatch JD, et al. The outcome of lumbar discectomy in elite athletes. Spine (Phila Pa 1976) 1999;24(6):570–3.

29. Eck JC, Riley LH 3rd. Return to play after lumbar spine conditions and surgeries. Clin Sports Med 2004;23(3):367–79, viii.

30. Wright A, Ferree B, Tromanhauser S. Spinal fusion in the athlete. Clin Sports Med 1993;12(3):599–602.

31. Weistroffer JK, Hsu WK. Return-to-play rates in National Football League linemen after treatment for lumbar disk herniation. Am J Sports Med 2011;39(3):632–6.

32. Orchard J, Best TM, Verrall GM. Return to play following muscle strains. Clin J Sport Med 2005; 15(6):436–41.

33. Linklater JM, Hamilton B, Carmichael J, et al. Hamstring injuries: anatomy, imaging, and intervention. Semin Musculoskelet Radiol 2010;14(2): 131–61.

34. Warren P, Gabbe BJ, Schneider-Kolsky M, et al. Clinical predictors of time to return to competition and of recurrence following hamstring strain in elite Australian footballers. Br J Sports Med 2010;44(6):415–9.

35. Bowman KF Jr, Cohen SB, Bradley JP. Operative management of partial-thickness tears of the proximal hamstring muscles in athletes. Am J Sports Med 2013;41(6):1363–71.

36. Levine WN, Bergfeld JA, Tessendorf W, et al. Intramuscular corticosteroid injection for hamstring injuries. A 13-year experience in the National Football League. Am J Sports Med 2000;28(3): 297–300.

37. Lopez-Vidriero E, Goulding KA, Simon DA, et al. The use of platelet-rich plasma in arthroscopy and sports medicine: optimizing the healing environment. Arthroscopy 2010;26(2):269–78.

38. Mishra A, Pavelko T. Treatment of chronic elbow tendinosis with buffered platelet-rich plasma. Am J Sports Med 2006;34(11):1774–8.

39. MS AH, Mohamed Ali MR, Yusof A, et al. Platelet-rich plasma injections for the treatment of hamstring injuries: a randomized controlled trial. Am J Sports Med 2014;42(10):2410–8.

40. Hamilton B, Tol JL, Almusa E, et al. Platelet-rich plasma does not enhance return to play in hamstring injuries: a randomised controlled trial. Br J Sports Med 2015;49(14):943–50.

41. Press CM, Gupta A, Hutchinson MR. Management of ankle syndesmosis injuries in the athlete. Curr Sports Med Rep 2009;8(5):228–33.

42. Williams GN, Jones MH, Amendola A. Syndesmotic ankle sprains in athletes. Am J Sports Med 2007; 35(7):1197–207.

43. Gerber JP, Williams GN, Scoville CR, et al. Persistent disability associated with ankle sprains: a prospective examination of an athletic population. Foot Ankle Int 1998;19(10):653–60.

44. Laver L, Carmont MR, McConkey MO, et al. Plasma rich in growth factors (PRGF) as a treatment for high ankle sprain in elite athletes: a randomized control trial. Knee Surg Sports Traumatol Arthrosc 2015; 23(11):3383–92.

45. Parekh SG, Wray WH 3rd, Brimmo O, et al. Epidemiology and outcomes of Achilles tendon ruptures in the National Football League. Foot Ankle Spec 2009;2(6):283–6.

46. McCormick JJ, Anderson RB. Rehabilitation following turf toe injury and plantar plate repair. Clin Sports Med 2010;29(2):313–23, ix.

47. Boden BP, Osbahr DC, Jimenez C. Low-risk stress fractures. Am J Sports Med 2001;29(1):100–11.

48. Kaeding CC, Yu JR, Wright R, et al. Management and return to play of stress fractures. Clin J Sport Med 2005;15(6):442–7.

49. Webb BG, Hunker PJ, Rettig AC. Proximal femoral stress reaction in a professional football player. Orthopedics 2008;31(8):802.

50. Makdissi M, Darby D, Maruff P, et al. Natural history of concussion in sport: markers of severity and implications for management. Am J Sports Med 2010; 38(3):464–71.

51. Bailey CM, Samples HL, Broshek DK, et al. The relationship between psychological distress and baseline sports-related concussion testing. Clin J Sport Med 2010;20(4):272–7.

52. Covassin T, Elbin RJ 3rd, Stiller-Ostrowski JL, et al. Immediate post-concussion assessment and cognitive testing (ImPACT) practices of sports medicine professionals. J Athl Train 2009;44(6):639–44.

53. Yard EE, Comstock RD. Compliance with return to play guidelines following concussion in US high school athletes, 2005-2008. Brain Inj 2009;23(11): 888–98.

54. Doolan AW, Day DD, Maerlender AC, et al. A review of return to play issues and sports-related concussion. Ann Biomed Eng 2012;40(1):106–13.

55. Ellemberg D, Henry LC, Macciocchi SN, et al. Advances in sport concussion assessment: from behavioral to brain imaging measures. J Neurotrauma 2009; 26(12):2365–82.

56. Dimou S, Lagopoulos J. Toward objective markers of concussion in sport: a review of white matter and neurometabolic changes in the brain after sports-related concussion. J Neurotrauma 2014;31(5):413–24.

Index

Radiol Clin N Am 54 (2016) 989–996
http://dx.doi.org/10.1016/S0033-8389(16)30090-2
0033-8389/16/$ – see front matter